A profoundly human exploration of significant dimensions of experience touching many aspects of our being. It is a pleasure to wander and wonder with it through mysteries of human engagement.

Michael Eigen, author, *The Challenge of Being Human, Faith,* and *The Sensitive Self*

Psychoanalysis as a Spiritual Discipline

The great existential psychiatrist Ludwig Binswanger famously pointed out to Freud that therapeutic failure could "only be understood as the result of something which could be called a deficiency of spirit." Binswanger was surprised when Freud agreed, asserting, "Yes, spirit is everything." However, spirit and the spiritual realm have largely been dropped from mainstream psychoanalytic theory and practice.

This book seeks to help revitalize a culturally aging psychoanalysis that is in conceptual and clinical disarray in the marketplace of ideas and is viewed as a "theory in crisis" no longer regarded as the primary therapy for those who are suffering. The author argues that psychoanalysis and psychoanalytic psychotherapy can be reinvigorated as a discipline if it is animated by the powerfully evocative spiritual, moral, and ethical insights of two dialogical personalist religious philosophers—Martin Buber, a Jew, and Gabriel Marcel, a Catholic—who both initiated a "Copernican revolution" in human thought.

In chapters that focus on love, work, faith, suffering, and clinical practice, Paul Marcus shows how the spiritual optic of Buber and Marcel can help revive and refresh psychoanalysis, and bring it back into the light by communicating its inherent vitality, power, and relevance to the mental health community and to those who seek psychoanalytic treatment.

Paul Marcus is a training and supervisory analyst at the National Psychological Association for Psychoanalysis in New York City and co-chairperson of the discussion group Psychoanalysis and Spirituality at the American Psychoanalytic Association meetings. He is the author/editor of 21 books, including *Psychoanalysis, Classic Social Psychology and Moral Living: Let the Conversation Begin*.

Psychoanalysis as a Spiritual Discipline

In Dialogue with Martin Buber and Gabriel Marcel

Paul Marcus

Routledge
Taylor & Francis Group
LONDON AND NEW YORK

First published 2021
by Routledge
2 Park Square, Milton Park, Abingdon, Oxon OX14 4RN

and by Routledge
52 Vanderbilt Avenue, New York, NY 10017

Routledge is an imprint of the Taylor & Francis Group, an informa business

British Library Cataloguing-in-Publication Data
A catalogue record for this book is available from the British Library

Library of Congress Cataloging-in-Publication Data
Names: Marcus, Paul, 1953– author.
Title: Psychoanalysis as a spiritual discipline : in dialogue with
Martin Buber and Gabriel Marcel / Paul Marcus.
Description: Milton Park, Abingdon, Oxon ; New York, NY : Routledge, 2021. |
Includes bibliographical references and index.
Identifiers: LCCN 2020056648 (print) | LCCN 2020056649 (ebook) |
ISBN 9780367754006 (paperback) | ISBN 9780367754013 (hardback) |
ISBN 9781003162360 (ebook)
Subjects: LCSH: Psychoanalysis and religion. |
Buber, Martin, 1878–1965. | Marcel, Gabriel, 1889–1973.
Classification: LCC BF175.4.R44 M29 2021 (print) |
LCC BF175.4.R44 (ebook) | DDC 150.19/5–dc23
LC record available at https://lccn.loc.gov/2020056648
LC ebook record available at https://lccn.loc.gov/2020056649

ISBN: 978-0-367-75401-3 (hbk)
ISBN: 978-0-367-75400-6 (pbk)
ISBN: 978-1-003-16236-0 (ebk)

Typeset in Bembo
by Newgen Publishing UK

In memoriam
Distinguished Professor of Sociology,
William B. Helmreich, Ph.D.,
a brilliant, kind, and devoted friend,
who died of COVID-19 on March 28, 2020

Contents

Acknowledgements

I would like to thank my two thoughtful readers who critically commented on every chapter of my book, though I of course take full responsibility for its contents: my wife, Irene Wineman-Marcus, a child and adult psychoanalyst, and Distinguished Professor of Sociology, William B. Helmreich. Brendan Sweetman, Professor of Philosophy and the president of the Gabriel Marcel Society graciously read the first and last chapter. Without their helpful criticisms and suggestions, I doubt my book would be as good as it can be. I would like to also express my gratitude to my editor Jane Lerner and to Kate Hawes of Routledge for her continuing support of my work, as well as her superb staff who have brought this book to publication.

Chapter 1

Introduction

Psychoanalysis as a spiritual discipline

Contemporary "mainstream" psychoanalysis has been described by sympathetic scholars as in crisis.[1] As Marshall Edelson reflects, psychoanalysis is a "theory in crisis" characterized by "profound malaise" (1988, p. xiv), while Nathan G. Hale describes the psychoanalytic crisis as "a crisis of clashing theories, competing modes of therapy, and uncertainties of professional identity" (1995, p. 360). Twenty-three years after Hale's comment, the editors of the impressive anthology *Psychoanalytic Trends in Theory and Practice: The Second Century of the Talking Cure* (Etezady, Blon, & Davis, 2018) made a similar assertion: "Psychoanalysis has become a very diverse field with multiple schools of thought, each of which has its own theory and praxis (ibid., p. 476) ... [there is no] unified theory of psychoanalysis" (ibid., p. 478). The great W. R. Bion appears to have been aware **of** the aforementioned when he ironically quipped in 1990, "In the practice of psycho-analysis it is difficult to stick to the rules. For one thing, I do not know what the rules of psychoanalysis are" (1990, p. 139).[2]

Not only does psychoanalysis lack what Thomas Kuhn called a disciplinary matrix for its activities as a science, it "is too fragmented to be constituted as a unitary discipline" (Weinstein, 1990, p. 26),[3] but it has not been hospitable to heretical and dissident thinkers, thus "sucking the life" out of the psychoanalytic institute training experience (including some authoritarianism that has penetrated and blunted creativity (Kernberg, 1996)). As the great psychoanalytic theorizer of narcissism and borderline conditions, Otto Kernberg, recently noted in an interview, psychotherapy training in the United States is in serious decline (www.psychotherapy.net/interview/otto-kernberg, retrieved 5/12/19).[4] Psychoanalysis is hardly represented in the university training programs of psychiatrists and doctoral-level clinical psychology psychologists; it has instead been marginalized to institutes.[5] The average age of a trained American psychoanalyst is 66, which suggests cultural aging (four years ago it was 62), and the number of daily analytically oriented patients is 2.75 (i.e., at least three times a week) compared to 8 to 10 in the psychoanalytic glory days of the 1950s and 1960s (Leonard, 2015).

This book attempts to improve the dismal landscape of contemporary psychoanalysis by suggesting that a psychoanalysis that is animated by the powerfully evocative spiritual (and moral/ethical) insights of two great contemporary, deeply religious existential philosophers, Martin Buber and Gabriel Marcel,[6] can help reinvigorate a discipline and profession that is in a dire state, both in the "marketplace of ideas" and in terms of clinical practice. Indeed, Buber was a "believing" Jew (though not a religiously practicing one), and Marcel a "believing" Christian (a practicing one of a sort),[7] who were both trying to reach "believers" and "non-believers" in their writings. Their dialogical personalist philosophies provide a mighty intellectual and moral/ethical resource that can move psychoanalysis from its aspirational objectives to inspirational ones (Van Deurzen, 2012, p. 181). By claiming that human existence is fundamentally dialogue, I mean that it is "address and response, claim and counter-claim, pledge and promise." That is, the human person "is the only being who can address another, who can make promises, who is united with other men in bonds of covenant" (Pfuetze, 1967, p. 530).[8]

My book is a small contribution to the "revitalization" of psychoanalysis from its cultural aging, bringing it back into the light by communicating its vitality and power when viewed as a spiritual discipline. Buber and Marcel have a spiritual sensibility that is in many ways in sync with a psychoanalytic outlook: it can empower people to quest for truth actively, mindfully, and thoroughly through the challenging experience of critically reflecting on their own existential "situated-ness" in the world and the untapped, unrealized possibilities of their everyday lives (Van Deurzen, 2012, p. 181). Similar to philosophy, psychoanalytic theory and technique have not yet adequately assimilated the profundity of Buber and Marcel's insights into the ontological structure of human experience,[9] for example, the nature of relation/encounter and the act of distancing/detachment. Buber and Marcel's contribution to the I-Thou and I-It realms,[10] and to other central human experiences like love, hope, fidelity, and faith, has been regarded as so significant that it has been recently described as a "Copernican Revolution" in philosophy (Sweetman, 2008, p. 135).

Why use Buber and Marcel to enhance psychoanalysis?

As the philosopher/psychoanalyst (and member of a convent for 17 years in a previous life) Donna Orange, who highlights Buber in a short appreciative chapter, noted, "dialogic philosophy is a better resource than 'postmodernism' for our clinical practice" (2010, p. 12). Michael Eigen, a prolific analytic writer who approvingly cites Buber, also noted, "Clinically postmodernism hasn't added all that much for me" (1998, p. 184). Indeed, I wholeheartedly agree with Orange that Buber's (and even more so Marcel's) contribution "has gone largely unnoticed in the psychoanalytic world" (2010, p. 12).[11] This is especially noteworthy when we call to mind that Freud commented that the psychoanalyst can be described as a "secular pastoral worker" (Hoffman, 1998, p. 5).

Buber's notion of "healing through meeting" (Agassi, 1999 p. 17)[12] (aka, "dialogical psychotherapy" or some such variant, which has very low visibility as of late)[13] and related issues pertinent to clinical practice have been extensively written about, for example, by Leslie Farber (1956, 1966, 1967) and Maurice Friedman (1985, 1998),[14] and I have written the only book on Marcel that discusses psychoanalysis and the sacred (Marcus, 2013a; 2018). Yet no one has used these two religious existentialists in conversation with contemporary psychoanalysis or with each other, on such vitally important psychological themes to psychoanalysis as love, work, faith, and suffering, especially to the analyst/analysand interchange, as contained in this book. While there is much about which Buber and Marcel agree (there is a "spiritual convergence," says Marcel (1967, p. 41)), they differ too, as they are lodged in different intellectual traditions (unlike Marcel, Buber came from the Germanic intellectual atmosphere) and religions, and such a juxtaposition of outlooks makes for lively debate about summoning personal issues relevant to psychoanalysis.[15] These similarities and differences as they pertain to "the ontology of being human," as Buber called it (Mendes-Flohr, 2019, p. 50), or the "mystery of being" (the irreducible mystery of singularity, of the relation to the Thou), as Marcel called it, that is, the "interhuman" or "intersubjective" respectively, are common concerns of both of these path-breaking religious existentialists.[16] In addition, Buber and Marcel agreed on "the distinction between I-Thou and I-It relation, the inadequacy of conceptual knowledge to describe human experience in its fullness, and the identification of the transcendent dimension of human existence" (Sweetman, 2011, p. 132). Wood noted that "there is a remarkable parallelism" between Buber and Marcel on the "basic direction" of their thought, mainly because they were both "deeply religious thinkers" (1999, pp. 83, 94). Levinas concurs that "there is a remarkable commonality in the essential views of" Marcel and Buber (1994, p. 21), while most recently Treanor noted that "Buber remains philosophically close to Marcel" (2006, pp. 189–190).

For Buber, the "interhuman" is "the interactive region between persons in a genuine relationship [like the analyst/analysand], it is the spirit of 'the between,' through which a person can glimpse the unsayable ground, the 'eternal Thou,'" Buber's term for God (Kramer & Gawlick, 2003, p. 203). The "between" refers to "the immediate presence of unreserved, spontaneous mutuality common to each person yet beyond the sphere of either [as in the psychoanalytic interchange at its best]. Impossible to objectify, 'the between' is the most real reality of human existence, of being wholly and uniquely 'human' with humans" (ibid., p. 202). "Intersubjectivity" is defined by Marcel as "opening ourselves to others and the capacity to welcome them without being effaced by them" (Marcel, 1973, p. 39); as in a "loving heart," it is the starting point of his philosophy and my version of psychoanalysis (just as Freud advocated, Marcus, 2019). Intersubjectivity can be further described as "the infrastructure of spiritual life, an original human solidarity preceding the emergence of the ego and the conditions for its possibility" (Schmitz, 1984, p. 164). "We are not alone," says Marcel, and "that whatever we do we are responsible for what happens to others" (Marcel, 1973, p. 234). In fact, Marcel defined the human person as "homo viator," an "itinerant being" or "spritutal wanderer" on a "winding journey" in search for "something more," "something higher," and "something better" (Gallagher, 1962, p. 11). Marcel's preferred term for God was the "Absolute Thou."

In other words, for both Marcel and Buber, intersubjectivity and the interhuman, the bailiwick of all versions of psychoanalysis, are the opposite of self-centeredness and selfishness (i.e., inordinate narcissism and egocentricity, as analyst's would call such a way of being-in-the-world). Rather, they point to transcendence, to a "beyond," though not a literal supra-terrestrial, "not some other place, but an unknown and higher dimension of reality, attainable in and through human experience and existence" (Cain, 1979, p. 115). Transcendence is mainly a subjective sacred experience, where one apprehends what lies beyond creation and infinitely transcends it.[17] To "master otherness"—or at least become empathically attuned to animate and inanimate others, to the unseen and unevidenced God, and to the unconscious in oneself, "in a lived unity" as Buber noted (Mendes-Flohr, 2019, p. 188)—required fashioning a way of being-in-the-world that is other-directed, other-regarding, and other-serving, this being one of the key animating values in Marcel and Buber's oeuvres.[18] Indeed, Levinas thought that Marcel and Buber's "essential discovery" consisted of "affirming that human spirituality—or religiosity—lies in the fact of the proximity of persons, neither lost in the mass nor abandoned to their solitude" (1994, p. 21).

The fact that Buber and Marcel are deeply religious thinkers who are also steeped in secular philosophical thought is exactly why I chose them as my two intellectual touchstones to critically evaluate psychoanalysis, and ultimately to expand and enhance it as a spiritually animated discipline.[19] Both thinkers point to the possibility of transcendence, whether as a "believer" or a secularist, via critically reflecting on experience, rising above it and making it intelligible (Van Deurzen, 2012, p. 176). They do so by judiciously embracing a set of transformative valuative attachments and correlated actions that bring out the best in human relatedness. It should be noted that while Buber gave a set of lectures at the Washington School of Psychiatry and had a dialogue with Carl Rogers in 1957, he "was not a friend of psychoanalysis" (Friedman, 2013, p. 14). In fact, Friedman describes Buber as having a "distaste for Freudian theory," and claims that Buber confided to him that "most psychoanalysts, knowing me to be an 'adversary,' will deny having learned anything from me" (ibid., p. 88). Marcel respectfully mentioned Freud and psychoanalysis in passing (usually when talking about his own psychic pain as a child), but never in any depth or systematically as it pertains to his philosophical reflections.

By describing Buber and Marcel as religious, I do not mean I am advocating a return to formalized religion and the moralizing that is associated with the worst of institutionalized religion. Rather, by religiosity I mean to point to a form of faith, what Marcel calls "creative attestation," an act of creative witnessing to Beauty, Truth, and Goodness.[20] This mainly involves being ready, receptive, responsive, and responsible for and to the other, whether the other is a person, animal, thing, or the otherness of oneself (e.g., the other of internal dialogue, or the unconscious, the ground of being). Such faith is any act of putting oneself "at the disposal of something," "of giving oneself to, rallying to" (Marcel, 1964, p. 134) an act to which "I pledge myself fundamentally." That is, faith always has an "existential index," as it fully engrosses a person's power of being (Marcel, 2001, pp. 77–78). Faith thus involves a person's real-life, here-and-now promise to give oneself to and, says Marcel, "to follow" someone or something that one cherishes. Such opening up to, giving oneself, and following can be in the service of Beauty, as in the artist's courage to create; Truth, as in the whistleblower's courage to speak out against authority; Goodness, as in the soldier's courage to throw himself on a hand grenade to save his comrades; and in countless other less dramatically courageous everyday ways.

Put simply, the kind of religious faith or spirituality, as I prefer to call it, that Buber, Marcel, and I have in mind is a "bonding in and with being" (Buber's words) the archetypal religious action. And if one is a believer, this includes God's Presence refracted through the Presence of the other whom one encounters with the fullness of their whole being (Mendes-Flohr, 2019, p. 141). Marcel calls this "availability" *(disponibilité)*, "the self's participation in being or being-with" (Cain, 1995, p. 175), a dynamic, sensitive receptivity with a deeper and wider capacity for loving.

My book is about delineating the relevance of these and other central human experiences for the analytic dialogue and, more generally, for the art of living[21] a "flourishing" or "good life,"[22] for this is what I mean by maximizing psychoanalysis as a spiritual discipline. Such an approach includes, but goes beyond, the accepted claim that dialogical psychotherapy, in one form or another (e.g., relational and intersubjective approaches), is the main healing process in all versions of psychoanalysis and psychotherapy. That is, the five essential elements of psychotherapeutic support—presence, holding, caring, challenging, and confirming—are what matter most in terms of engaged interaction, what Buber and Marcel more aptly conceived as communion (Heery & Bugental, 2005, p. 287). As Freud noted, "What turns the scale is not intellectual insight, but the relationship to the doctor" (1916, p. 445), while Jung claimed, "Every psychotherapist not only has his own method—he himself is that method ... The great healing factor in psychotherapy is the doctor's personality ... theories are to be avoided, except as mere auxiliaries" (Jung, 1966, p. 88). Thus, the analyst's "personal psychology," his beliefs and values etcetera, is deeply implicated in all aspects of his clinical engagement (Renik, 1993, p. 553).

Buber and Marcel on spirituality

As I have noted, Buber and Marcel have a "remarkable parallelism" and "commonality" between "the basic direction" of their thought and its implications for fashioning a "flourishing" life. In particular, "both thinkers were interested in the question of wholeness, the wholeness of one's own being and one's relation to the wholeness of what is" (Wood, 1999, p. 83).[23] In Buber, this wholeness refers to the I-Thou relation, an entryway to the eternal Thou. For Marcel, the question of wholeness takes the form of centering on what he calls the "ontological mystery," an "ontological exigence," that is, an impulse or urge that is the "bedrock" of the human condition, an irrepressible need, even a "demand" for the presence of being, to say Thou (Marcus, 2013a, p. 66). For Buber and Marcel, wholeness thus suggests a relatively "seamless integration of body, mind and spirit" (Kramer & Gawlick, 2003, p. 99). Marcel clearly defines "thou" as "that which I can involve rather than that which I judge to be able to answer me" (Marcel, 2001, p. 48). *Thou* is a kind of invocation; it pleads "Be with me" (Gallagher, 1962, p. 25). For both Buber and Marcel, the term transcendence, at least in the full metaphysical sense, designates an otherness, even an absolute otherness.

Spirituality is a very difficult term to define, and there is no agreed-upon definition among scholars that I am aware of. In fact, most definitions of spirituality are only acceptable to their authors.[24] My working definition draws from Buber and Marcel, whose definitions are not exactly the same but point in a certain direction, or spiritual sensibility, that I will develop throughout the book, as I use this optic to critically evaluate and enhance contemporary psychoanalysis conceived as a spiritual discipline.

Briefly, for Buber, "spirit" relates to the wholeness of the person; it "is man's totality that has become consciousness, the totality which comprises and integrates all man's capacities, powers, qualities, and urges. Spiritual life is nothing but the existence of man, in so far as he possesses that true human conscious totality" (1948, p. 175). However, the mature Buber emphasizes that human wholeness is always merged with the real relationship to other living entities. In *I and Thou*, for example, Buber notes that spirit in its human expression is "a response of man to his *Thou*" (the Other) (1958, p. 39). Thus, wholeness and relation are inextricably connected for Buber (Friedman, 2002, p. 106). Spirit is thus "the word [the relationship to the world] … the Between binding man to the Other and opening out as a relation to Transcendence" (Wood, 1969, p. 74). "The man of spirit," says Buber, "is one whom the spirit invades and seizes, whom the spirit uses as its garment, not one who contains the spirt. Spirit is an event, something which happens to man. The storm of the spirit sweeps man where it will then storm on into the world" (Buber, 1957, p. 187).

While never formally defining spirituality, Marcel seems to mean a "spiritual attitude" (Anderson, 2006, p. 20), a way of being in the world that is passionately devoted to the intellectual and moral virtues, to Beauty, Truth, Goodness, and Justice, while at the same time being aware of the often conflicted, ambiguous, and ambivalent nature of such a way of being. As Marcel noted, "I wonder if we can define the whole spiritual life as the sum of activities by which we try to reduce in ourselves the part played by non-disposability [*indisponibilité*, roughly being emotionally unavailable and existentially disengaged]" (1965, p. 69). And again, "I think, that many enjoyments do not satisfy the whole of our being, that is to say our spiritual nature. They only satisfy us on condition that we have already put a great part of ourselves to sleep" (Marcel, 1952, p. 207). Finally, Marcel says that the spiritual attitude is "a spiritual dynamism of a completely different kind whose ground and main driving force is to be found in transcendence" (1964, p. 221).

Thus, Buber and Marcel believe that something like a "spiritual core" is the deepest center of the person (perhaps calling to mind Winnicott's "sacred core of the personality, the incommunicado self," Eigen's "living center" or "spiritual center" (Eigen, 1998, pp. 15, 58, 125) and Loewald's "ego core" (1962, p. 498)). It is in this domain that the person is open to the transcendental dimension; it is here that the person experiences ultimate reality. This includes the discovery of that core, the dynamics of its development, and its journey to the ultimate goal, however defined (the great religions and spiritualities of the world have magnificently detailed all of this). For a believer, it can focus on prayer and other inspiring rituals, but in whatever form this core takes, it pertains to spiritual direction (more this than a substance or endpoint), the various roadmaps of the spiritual journey, and the methods of progression in the spiritual ascent (Cousins, 1996, p. xii). For Buber and Marcel, all of this is encompassed in their dialectically and poetically expressed dialogical existentialism. They both shunned systematizing their philosophies, while they believed that the spiritual core or interior was the standard and criterion of reality and the external social world—what mattered most—was how this inner truth was enacted in real life, whether the other was honored and affirmed as a unique person (i.e., with openness, reverence and presence).

As I implied earlier, the central notion of the "transcendent" is much debated and hard to pin down. For example, Marcel was committed to what he called the "authentic, vertical transcendent," that is, "the transcendence, holiness, and sanctity of Christ and the martyrs" (Heffernan, 2017, p. 17). For Buber, it was "spiritual transcendence" with which we can genuinely reside in relationship, that is, there was a concealed power, spiritual in nature, which manifests itself in human life (Atterton et al., 2004, p. 9). Moreover, Judaism's "spiritual vocation" was less a legalistic project, as the ancient rabbis thought, than one mainly defined by a continuing quest to epitomize the ideal human community, that is, to be a "light unto the nations" (Mendes-Flohr, 2019, p. 115). The "nonbeliever" Albert Camus was committed to what has been called "horizontal transcendence" as manifested by charity, humanity, and solidarity (and these valuative attachments were of great concern to Marcel and most "believers"). Thus, for Marcel and Buber, transcendence is rooted in divinity, while for Camus it is rooted in history (Heffernan, 2017, pp. 20, 16). Transcendence and spirituality can thus be lodged in a religious or secular framework and sensibility, since for some individuals it is human society and the human being that are the ultimate transcending principle, the "ultimate concerns" (Van Deurzen,

2012, p. 172). The point is that one of the transformative goals of transcendence is to feel and act purposely in relation to what is judged as sacred and, thereby, meaningfully and soulfully rise above the triteness, sham, drudgery, and broken dreams of our everyday lives (ibid., p. 178).[25] As I shall point out throughout this book, transcendence is accessed through particular ethically animated valuative attachments in relation to the self, others, nature, life, and for that matter, anything one judges to "really matter" (Elkins et al., 1988, p. 10). The goal of psychoanalysis as I conceive it, at least in part, is to develop in the analysand the will and ability to transform his character so that he can transcend the worst of his outlook and behavior, his way of being-in-the-world, and be and do "better" as he construes it. Such an existential development is correlated with greater autonomy, integration, and humanity.[26]

While there are of course exceptions (Eigen, 2012), in general, psychoanalysis has given short shrift to the notion of spirituality per se, especially within the Judeo-Christian tradition (there has been more written on religion, admittedly in ambiguous if not conflated terms). However, Eastern religion/spirituality has been more frequently correlated and occasionally integrated into psychoanalysis, though this still takes in a small number of mainstream analysts who have a serious interest in spirituality (Vaidyanathan & Kripal, 2002, Hinduism; Molino, 2013, Buddhism). And while the Jungian analyst Lionel Corbett noted that "spirituality is no longer taboo among psychotherapists, and the importance of spiritual experience is increasingly discussed in psychoanlaytic writers such as Michael Eigen" (2018, p. 51), I believe it is a reasonable generalization that mainstream psychoanalysis has too frequently provided a superficial rendering of the homo viator and how his spiritual mode of comportment plays out in real life. For example, Stephen A. Mitchell (2002) notes in his book on love that "spirituality has certainly made something of comeback, in the broad spectrum of activities, from yoga to New Age crystals, from meditation to family genealogies," what he calls "popular spirituality" (p. 25). He does, however, note that these activities "point beyond everyday, mundane reality to something deeper, something transcendent," but that is all Mitchell has to say about the subject (p. 98). In two recent clinically focused introductory books on relational theory (Aron, Grand, & Slochower, 2018; Charles, 2018), there are no index entries on religion and spirituality, except the aforementioned two-page one on Jung (mainly about the numinous and mysticism) by Corbett in Charles's anthology. It should be mentioned that Buber seriously criticized Jung (and Freud) for his psychologism, using a strictly psychological frame and filter for making judgments and evaluations, including about the cosmic. Most importantly, psychologism left out the ontological dimension, the "superpsychic reality" (e.g., God), that "psychic statements … correspond" (Agassi, 1999, p. 69). Marcel, too, believed that the strictly psychological (and atheistic) observer has no special ability to judge the truthfulness of the theist's noumenal experiences, that is, he has no epistemic superiority over the other (Hernandez, 2011, p. 45). Moreover, both Buber (Zank, 2006, p. 64) and Marcel (Sweetman,

2008, p. 58) were critical of mysticism (or at least certain forms of mysticism) for a variety of reasons (as was Levinas).

Defining psychoanalysis as a spiritual discipline

It was Ludwig Binswanger who famously pointed out to Freud that a therapeutic failure they were conversing about could "only be understood as the result of something which could be called a deficiency of spirit" (1963, p. 1). Binswanger was surprised when Freud agreed, asserting, "Yes, spirit is everything" (ibid.). Freud further elaborated, "Man has always known he possessed spirit: I had to show him there is such a thing as instinct" (ibid.). Neville Symington, a member of the Middle Group of the British psychoanalysts and an ex-Catholic priest, noted that psychoanalysis was "a mature natural religion" (accessible to reason without drawing from revelation; Buber and Marcel would disagree)[27] and a "spiritual method relevant to the modern world" (1994, pp. 192, 137). Moreover, "psychoanalysis has a spiritual function," such that "purifying motivation" becomes "the organizing center of his activities." Finally, Symington notes that "moral development through the course of a person's life is only possible through the stewardship of a dedicated spirituality" (ibid., p. 47).[28] Following in the tradition of the great sages and religious leaders of the Axial period (Marcus, 2019; Symington, 2012), Symington believes that it is unbridled narcissism that is the main psychopathology animating all others. While one can certainly question the veracity of Symington's claims, he does put into sharp focus the fact that psychoanalysis can be reasonably conceptualized as a spiritual/moral venture, that is, it is concerned with "right" (e.g., "healthy," "adaptive," "normal") and "wrong" (e.g., "unhealthy," "maladaptive," and "abnormal") behavior and the "goodness" (e.g., other-directed, other-regarding, other-serving) and "badness" (e.g., inordinately, narcissism and selfishness) of character. Admittedly, these are intellectually, emotionally, and situationally lodged value judgments based on knowledge and critical discrimination made by the analyst and analysand. This being said, all analysts maintain that the psychoanalyst must be ever mindful of not becoming moralistic, that is, making reflexive judgments about an analysand's morality. Of course, reasonably distinguishing in a particular clinical context what constitutes psychoanalysis operating as a spiritual/moral venture versus a moralizing one, let alone distinguishing what instantiates these differences in the subtle registers of thinking, feeling, and acting, is a hugely difficult value judgment to make. While psychoanalysis shuns moralizing, Adam Phillips approvingly quotes Nina Coltart who said that it "may be defined as a moral activity," one in which symptoms are "disabling painful moral puzzles" (1994, pp. 138, 139). For example, in psychoanalytic theory, truth-telling is at best undertheorized and, at worst, has no means of effectively making a distinction between acts which are true and false to the self or sincere and insincere (especially if an analysand's "yes" can mean "no" and "no" can mean "yes," and "yes" may not mean this specific "yes" (Forester, 2000, p. 318)), even though psychoanalytic practice largely depends on the analyst being able to do so (Rycroft, 1995, p. 10). Thus, it is the analysand who ultimately determines what is true and sincere, just as it is the analysand who decides what kind of person to become (e.g., what constitutes a flourishing life).

In light of the aforementioned, psychoanalysis as I conceive it is a form of life, a meaning-giving, affect-integrating, and action-guiding resource for individuals who can appropriate the life- and identity-defining narrative of psychoanalysis when they seek to understand, endure, and possibly gain some mastery of the problems that affect, if not assault, the human experience of love, work, faith, and suffering (e.g., conflict, anxiety, despair, loss, and tragedy). As philosopher Pierre Hadot notes about ancient Greek philosophy, psychoanalysis can be understood as a "spiritual exercise," a tool for living life skillfully, more fully and wisely (1997, p. 83). The aim of a spiritual exercise is to foster a deep modification of an individual's way of "seeing and being," a decisive change in how one lives one's practical, everyday life. Michel Foucault (a student of Hadot's) also discussed spiritual exercises, calling them "technologies of the self": "an exercise of the self, by which one attempts to develop and transform oneself, and to attain a certain mode of being" (1989, p. 433). Most importantly, the objective of a spiritual exercise is "a total transformation of one's vision, lifestyle, and behavior" in the service of increased personal freedom and equipoise (Hadot, 1997, pp. 83, 103, 14) and, I would add, a less self-centric outlook and behavior. According to this view, as Levinas described "Jewish humanism" at its best, psychoanalysis is "a difficult wisdom concerned with truths that correlate to virtues" (1989, p. 275).

Psychoanalysis is a painful, deconstructive, demythologizing, and defamiliarizing process for acquiring greater self-awareness and self-understanding, especially of one's destructive unconscious emotional activity, one that transforms moral consciousness by expanding and deepening one's capacity to love. As Freud suggested, at least ideally, self-understanding leads to self-mastery, which leads to self-transcendence of one's impediments to being more other-directed, other-regarding, and other-serving (i.e., less crudely narcissistic and in other ways neurotically self-absorbed). In fact, Freud described psychoanalytic treatment as the "scientific cure by love" (McGuire, 1974, pp. 12–13). In this sense, psychoanalysis is animated by both the "love of wisdom" and the "wisdom of love," by Greek and Hebrew values (Levinas, 1981, p. 162), and is a powerful tool for the art of living a flourishing life as one construes and fashions it.

Structure of the book

Freud told Erikson that "love and work" were the central therapeutic goals of psychoanalysis (Erikson, 1959, p. 96), the two pillars for a sound mind and for living a flourishing life, and when Buber heard this, he "laughed and said that this was good, but not complete. He would say: work, love, faith and humor"

(Hodes, 1971, p. 134). I would add that the art of living requires the capacity for making suffering sufferable. Hence, this book has chapters on love, work, faith, and suffering (see Marcus, 2013b, 2019, for psychoanalytic studies of tragicomic humor and suffering, respectively), with each chapter providing psychoanalytic views of these central human experiences in a wide range of their permutations, followed by a Buberian and Marcelian critique and expansion/deepening, to be concluded with the implications for psychoanalytic treatment and the art of living a flourishing life. I have, where pertinent, drawn from research findings from personality/social psychology, organizational/industrial psychology, the empirical study of religion, and sociology to further illuminate and critically evaluate particular topics discussed by psychoanalysts and Buber and Marcel (my respectful attempt to be more "scientific").

In the last chapter, I attempt to integrate and expand the aforementioned into a version of psychoanalysis conceived as a spiritual discipline. I do this by answering three questions:

(1) What is the Buberian/Marcelian version of the world, their spiritualized conception of the human condition, and the central problematics that the individual struggles with within a larger social context?
(2) In light of this conception of the human condition, how is individual psychopathology (i.e., problems in living) understood?
(3) How does this conception of the human condition inform this type of clinical psychoanalysis as it attempts to alleviate individual psychopathology?

I very much want this book to be of lively interest to psychoanalysts and psychoanalytically oriented mental health clinicians, for it suggests a new direction that may be helpful to theoretically and practically re-enlivening psychoanalysis. By using a religiously inspired spiritual optic, one lodged in Buber and Marcel, two dialogical personalist giants—"the therapeutic community's conscience" (Orange, 2010, p. 10)[29]—my hope is that this book can be a small contribution towards reconceptualizing or at least significantly augmenting psychoanalytic theory and practice as a whole.

Notes

1 I am aware that what constitutes "mainstream" psychoanalysis is debatable, depending on one's perspective. There are a number of competing versions of psychoanalysis that have the loyalty of groups of analysts, for example, Freudian, Kleinian, Kohutian, Lacanian, Relational, Jungian, et cetera. This being said, I will focus on contemporary psychoanalytic theories and practices.

2 An example of what some may regard as conceptual disarray in psychoanalysis is the Oedipal complex. As Knafo and Moscovitz noted, "Today adherenance to the Oedipus complex, even by contemporary Freudians, is a hotly debated topic, with some insisting that it is central while others believing the concept needs to be revised or discarded" (2018, pp. 13–14).

3 How one defines psychoanalysis will differ greatly depending on the assumptions that one starts with and where one is culturally, geographically, and linquistically situated. In a word, "there are many Freuds" (Elliott, 2015 p. 180). Thus, I regard psychoanalysis as a "floating undefined signifier," a term that signifies that I read psychoanalysis, whatever it means, as historically contingent (Marcus & Rosenberg, in preparation).
4 The same can probably be said of much of the UK and the rest of Europe, though less so in South America.
5 Psychoanalysis has been marginalized by the biological revolution in psychiatry as well as the upsurge of cognitive behavioral therapy (including dialectical behavioral therapy) and related forms of efficacy-based psychotherapies (Harrington, 2019). The popularity of yoga, meditation, and other alternative therapies has also contributed to the downward spiraling of psychoanalysis as a "go-to" intervention.
6 Martin Buber (1878–1965) was a famous 20th-century philosopher, religious thinker, political activist, and educator. Austrian born, he lived most of his life in Germany and Israel, publishing in German and Hebrew. He is best known for his book *Ich und Du* (*I and Thou*), which differentiates between "I-Thou" and "I-It" modes of existence. Gabriel Marcel (1889–1973) was a prominent French philosopher, dramatist, and critic who was associated with the phenomenological and existentialist movements in 20th-century European philosophy and whose work and style are often described as Christian existentialism (Marcel preferred "neo-Socratic" because it suggested the dialogical, searching, and sometimes inchoate character of his reflections). His main book was the two-volume *Mystery of Being* (the Gifford lectures). Both philosophers had their heyday when they were alive, and have influenced many subsequent famous philosophers and others, such as Emmanuel Levinas and Paul Ricoeur. While Buber is better known, Marcel has recently been described as a "sorely neglected philosopher" (Treanor, 2006, p. 258).
7 Marcel did not sanction faith with pretensions to certitude, or faith that did not consider the limits of human reason. The limits of reason to generate the affirmation of being from the structure of thought preciesly manifests these limits (Treanor, 2006, p. 178). Buber had a similar outlook.
8 There are a number of different conceptions of dialogue and intersubjectivty in philosophy and psychology; Buber and Marcel thus represent one form lodged in this broadly defined tradition.
9 Buber and Marcel were in part reacting to Heidegger's philosophical reflections in their diverse writings, both praising his insights and criticizing some of his concepts. Both men regarded Heidegger's Nazi affiliations during World War II and his not repudiating his appalling behavior during the war as reprehensible.
10 Incidentally, as Marcel scholar Thomas Anderson noted, Marcel used the term "I-Thou" before Buber, but not before Kierkegaard (Marcus, 2013a, p. 159). In 1915 Marcel differentiated "between an I and a thou and an I and a he," eight years before Buber published *I and Thou* (Keen, 1967, p. 29).
11 As Oppenheim (2017) notes, in contemporary relational psychoanalysis there have been a few exceptions in terms of Buber. As far as I know, nothing has been written on Marcel and psychoanalysis except by me. In my last chapter I briefly discuss this underwhelming amount of Buberian/Marcelian scholarship as it relates to mainstream psychoanalysis.

12 This phrase emanates from the title Buber provided for a posthumous volume by the Swiss Jungian analyst Hans Trub, who integrated Jung and Buber.
13 Both Buber and Marcel maintained that a genuine dialogue must emanate from concrete experience and be addressed from such experience and not merely as an experience of thought, as is often the case with academic philosophers and sometimes analysts. Exactly what constitutes dialogue, let alone transformational dialogue in the therapeutic context, is still an open question which I touch upon in subsequent chapters (Cooper & Spinelli, 2012, p. 155).
14 Friedman, Buber's most important English-speaking translator/interpreter, makes brief mention of Buber and psychology in his last book (published in 2013); he died in 2012.
15 My book focuses more on the similarities of Buber and Marcel and much less on their differences. Specialists might find this approach plausible, but a trifle troubling. However, Marcel noted that his differences with Buber are more about details than about general orientation (Treanor, 2008, p. 111). Both philosophers can be described as "moral perfectionists" (Putnam, 2008, p. 59) in the sense that they tended to describe what is "best" about human being-in-the-world, both in terms of conscience/demands and "real life" behavior. They also, however, grappled with the "dark" side of human experience.
16 Buber also spoke about mystery, such as "primal mystery," in *I and Thou* (1958, p. 101), and Eigen (1998) alleges that "mystery is the core of consciousness, while we know around and through it" (p. 19).
17 Marion Milner (d. 1998), an analyst, noted that there is an inherent "search for transcendence," one that emanates from the unconscious, but is only genuinely realized through a unification of conscious and unconscious forces. Creativity is thus a "'religious' pursuit" (Raab, 2000, pp. 192, 187). This being said, Buber critically noted,

> The false prophets make their subconscious a god, whereas for the true prophets their subconscious is subdued by the God of truth, Who absolutely transcends everything discoverable in the psychic domain, and Who is recognized in this very transcendence as a vanguisher.
>
> (1949, p. 179)

18 Levinas can of course be included as one of the important philosophers of dialogue, and I will be drawing from him throughout this book. Levinas indicated that he was influenced by Buber and Marcel (he admiringly, though critically, wrote about both of them, calling Marcel's *Metaphysical Journal* a "sublime work"), and acknowledged their original contributions to philosophical anthropology (Atterton, Calarco, & Friedman, 2004; Levinas, 1994; Marcus, 2008, 2010). It is noteworthy that Buber, Marcel, and Levinas arrive at a very similar place in terms of praxis; they all concretely "lead us to the same generous, hospitable, and responsible conduct toward our fellows" (Treanor, 2008, p. 148). Treanor was comparing Marcel with Levinas, but Buber can reasonably be included.
19 Buber and Marcel were cognizant of the fact that no one perspective or system of thought will provide the answers to everything.
20 These terms are capitalized merely to point towards what I regard (as do Buber and Marcel) as desireable and praiseworthy valuative attachments; they are not meant to connote Platonic or Platonic-like ideals. For Marcel and Buber, Justice could also be included in witnessing.

21 The "art of living" is a phrase that deserves some clarification. Foucault aptly defines the phrase as "those intentional and voluntary actions by which men not only set themselves rules of conduct but also seek to transform themselves … and to make their life into an *oeuvre* that carries aesthetic values and meets certain stylistic criteria" (1990, pp. 10–11).

22 Following positive psychology, by "flourishing" I mean living "within an optimal range of human functioning, one that connotes goodness, generativity, growth and resilience" (Fredrickson & Losada, 2005, p. 678). Following Freud, by "good life" I mean a life characterized by deep and wide love, to work creatively and productively, a life that is also guided by reason and ethics and is aesthetically pleasing (henceforth, I will use the term *flourishing* as shorthand for these two related notions). I am aware, as the reader should be, that the aforementioned are suffused with moral beliefs, values, and ethical judgments, and are therefore perspectival and open to critical evaluation and challenge.

23 "Wholeness" has a long and complex history in psychoanalysis (as well as psychology and philosophy); it is one of those terms that is used differently by different authors. Self-psychologists have given a lot of attention to wholeness and related terms; for example, Strozier and colleagues (2020) noted that "the aim of successful treatment is the restoraton of the cohesion, integration and wholeness of the self rather than the unfolding of the transference neurosis" (p. 554) as in Freudian theory. In fact, these authors make the declarative statement that the "natural state of the self is one of wholeness, cohesion and integration," with "cohesion" being "ontological" (ibid.). Jung, too, made wholeness a key psychic achievement.

24 For example, Michel Foucault defines spirituality in a manner that is rooted in his study of ancient Greco-Roman philosophy: "As the subject's own transformation of his mode of being"; """The set of these researches, practices, and experiences, which may be purifications, ascetic exercises, renunciations, conversion of looking, modifications of existicence, etc., which are, not for knoweldge but for the subject, for the subject's very being, the price to be paid for access to the truth" (2001, pp. 178, 15).

25 As I have said, for Marcel and Buber, it is our behavior that affirms our commitment towards the transcendent, as opposed to our confessions to such a commitment. In this view, an atheist can act and thus be more like Christ than particular churchgoers. Moreover, as Richard Kearney noted, a person can disrespect others not merely by discounting their transcendence, but also by disrgarding their "flesh-and-blood thereness" (Treanor, 2008, pp. 284–285, 234–235).

26 I am aware that these terms, especially "humanity," are value-laden and depend on who is making the judgment. Indeed, one man's terrorist is another man's freedom fighter. This being said, both Buber and Marcel situate themselves in a broadly based humanistic tradition as they conceive it. They both were believing humanists, "the humanism of the 'life of dialogue'" (Friedman, 1967, p. 23).

27 Symington's notion of revelation appears to be rather limited and literal. For Buber and Marcel, revelation does come from "without" but not the way Symmington implies, as if man were a vessel that is filled or simply a mouthpiece of God. Rather, says Buber, "revelation seizes the human elements that are at hand and recasts them: it is the *pure shape of the meeting*" (Buber, 1967, p. 135). Likewise, for Marcel, revelation is only conceivable to the extent that it is addressed to a person who is

engaged (available) with the fullness of his whole being, who participates in the mystery of being.

28 In a letter to his friend and collaborator Wilhelm Fliess, Freud mentioned "in passing that psychoanalysis was akin to the ancient mystery rites" (Eigen, 1998, p. 13).

29 Orange was referring to Buber, but I believe that the less known Marcel can be aptly so characterized.

References

Agassi, J. B. (Ed.). (1999). *Martin Buber on psychology and psychotherapy. Essays, letters, and dialogues*. Syracuse, NY: Syracuse University Press.

Anderson, T. C. (2006). *A commentary on Gabriel Marcel's mystery of being*. Milwaukee, WI: Marquette University Press.

Aron, L., Grand, S., & Slochower, J. (Eds.). (2018). *De-idealizing relational theory. A critique from within*. London: Routledge.

Atterton, P., Calarco, M., & Friedman, M. (2004). Introduction. In P. Atterton, M. Calarco, & M. Friedman (Eds.), *Levinas & Buber: Dialogue & difference* (pp. 1–25). Pittsburgh, PA: Duquesne University Press.

Binswanger, L. (1963). (Trans. J. Needleman). *Being in the world*. New York: Basic Books.

Bion, W. (1990). *Brazilian lectures*. London: Karnac.

Buber, M. (1948). *The power of the spirit: Israel and the world: Essays in a time of crisis*. New York: Schocken.

Buber, M. (1949). *The prophetic faith*. New York: Harper & Row.

Buber, M. (1957). (Trans. M. Friedman). *Pointing the way. Collected essays*. Atlantic Highlands, NJ: Humanities Press.

Buber, M. (1958). (Trans. R. G. Smith). *I and Thou* (2nd ed.). New York: Charles Scribner's Sons.

Buber, M. (1967). *A believing humanism: My testament, 1902–1965*, New York: Simon & Schuster.

Cain, S. (1979). *Gabriel Marcel*. South Bend, IN: Regnery/Gateway.

Cain, S. (1995). *Gabriel Marcel's theory of religious experience*. New York: Peter Lang.

Charles, M. (2018). (Ed.), *Introduction to contemporary psychoanalysis*. London: Routledge.

Cooper, M., & Spinelli, E. (2012). A dialogue on dialogue. In L. Barnett & G. Madison (Eds.), *Existential therapy: Legacy, vibrancy and dialogue* (pp. 141–157). London: Routledge.

Corbett, L. (2018). Jungian approaches to psychotherapy. In M. Charles (Ed.), *Introduction to contemporary psychoanalysis* (pp. 33–52). London: Routledge.

Cousins, E. (1996). Preface. In P. H. Van Ness (Ed.), *Spirituality and the secular quest* (vol. 2, p. xiii). New York: Crossroad Publishing.

Edelson, M. (1988). *Psychoanalysis: A theory in crisis*. Chicago: University of Chicago Press.

Eigen, M. (1998). *The psychoanalytic mystic*. London: Free Association Books.

Eigen, M. (2012). *Kabbalah and psychoanalysis*. London: Routledge.

Elkins, D. N., Hedstorm, L. J., Hughes, L. L., Leaf, J. A., & Saunders, C. (1988). Toward a humanistic-phenomenological spirituality. *Journal of Humanistic Psychology, 28*(4), 5–18.

Elliott, A. (2015). *Psychoanalytic theory* (3rd ed.). London : Palgrave Macmillan.

Erikson, E. H. (1959). *Identity and the life cycle: Selected papers* (*Psychological Issues*, Vol. 1, No. 1, Monograph 1). New York: International Universities Press.
Etezady, M. H., Blon, I., & Davis, M. (Eds.). (2018). *Psychoanalytic trends in theory and practice: The second century of the talking cure*. New York: Lexington Books.
Farber, L. H. (1956). Martin Buber and psychiatry. *Psychiatry*, *19*(2), 109–120.
Farber, L. H. (1966). *The way of the will: Essays toward a psychology and psychopathology*. New York: Basic Books.
Farber, L. H. (1967). Martin Buber and psychotherapy. In P. A. Schilpp & M. S. Friedman (Eds.), *The philosophy of Martin Buber* (The Library of Living Philosophers Series, pp. 577–602). La Salle, IL: Open Court.
Forester, J. (2000). What kind of truth. In P. Brooks & A. Woloch (Eds.), *Whose Freud? The place of psychoanalysis in contemporary culture* (pp. 311–323). New Haven, CT: Yale University Press.
Foucault, M. (1989). The ethics of the concern for self as a practice of freedom. In S. Lotringer (Ed.), *Foucault live: Collected interviews, 1961–1984* (pp. 432–449). New York: Semiotexte.
Foucault, M. (1990). *The use of pleasure*. New York: Vintage Books.
Foucault, M. (2001). *The hermeneutics of the subject. Lectures at the College De France, 1981–82*. F. Gros (Ed.), (Trans. G. Burchell). New York: Picador.
Fredrickson, B. L., & Losada, M. F. (2005). Positive affect and complex dynamics of human flourishing. *American Psychologist*, *60*, 678–686.
Freud, S. (1916). *Introductory lectures on psycho-analysis*. In J. Strachey (Ed. & Trans.), *Standard edition of the complete psychological works of Sigmund Freud* (vol. 16, pp. 243–483). London: Hogarth.
Friedman, M. (1967). Martin Buber's credo. In M. Buber (Trans. M. Friedman), *A believing humanism—My testament, 1902–1965* (pp. 21–30). New York: Simon & Schuster.
Friedman, M. (1985). *The healing dialogue in psychotherapy*. Northvale, NJ: Jason Aronson.
Friedman, M. (1998). Buber's philosophy as the basis for dialogical psychotherapy and contextual therapy. *Journal of Humanistic Psychology*, *38*, 25–40.
Friedman, M. (2002). *Martin Buber: The life of dialogue* (4th ed.). London: Routledge.
Friedman, M. (2013). *My friendship with Martin Buber*. Syracuse, NY: Syracuse University Press.
Gallagher, K. T. (1962). *The philosophy of Gabriel Marcel*. New York: Fordham University Press.
Hadot, P. (1997). *Philosophy as a way of life*. Oxford: Blackwell.
Hale, N. G. (1995). *The rise and crisis of psychoanalysis in the United States*. New York: Oxford University Press.
Harrington, A. (2019). *Mind fixers: Psychiatry's troubled search for the biology of mental illness*. New York: Norton.
Heery, M., & Bugental, J. F. T. (2005). Meaning and transformation. In E. V. Deurzen & C. Arnold-Baker (Eds.), *Existential perspectives on human issues* (pp. 253–264). Houndsville: Palgrave Macmillan.
Heffernan, G. (2017). The meaningless life is not worth living: Critical reflections on Marcel's critique of Camus. *Marcel Studies*, *2*, 1–22.
Hernandez, J. G. (2011). *Gabriel Marcel's ethics of hope: Evil, god and virtue*. London: Bloomsbury.
Hodes, A. (1971). *Martin Buber: An intimate portrait*. New York: Viking.

Hoffman, I. Z. (1998). *Ritual and spontaneity in the psychoanalytic process: A dialectical-constructivist view*. Hillsdale, NJ: Analytic Press.
Jung, C. G. (1966). *Practice of psychotherapy: Vol. xvi, The collected works of C. G. Jung* (G. Adler & R. F. C. Hull, Eds. & Trans.), Princeton, NJ: Princeton University Press.
Keen, S. (1967). *Gabriel Marcel*. Richmond, VA: John Knox Press.
Kernberg, O. (1996). Thirty methods to destroy the creativity of psychoanalytic candidates. *International Journal of Psychoanalysis*, 77(5), 1031–1040.
Kernberg, O. (2019). Interview. Retrieved 5/12/19 from www.psychotherapy.net/interview/otto-kernberg
Knafo, D., & Moscovitz, S. (2018). Contemporary Freudian approaches. In M. Charles (Ed.), *Introduction to contemporary psychoanalysis* (pp. 13–14). London: Routledge.
Kramer, K. P., & Gawlick, M. (2003). *Martin Buber's I and Thou: Practicing living dialogue*. New York: Paulist Press.
Leonard, T. (2015). Retrieved 7/24/19 from www.spectator.co.uk › Features
Levinas, E. (1981). (Trans. A. Lingis). *Otherwise than being or beyond essence*. The Hague: Martin Nijoff.
Levinas, E. (1989). (Ed. Sean Hand). *Difficult freedom: Essays on Judaism*. Baltimore, MD: Johns Hopkins University Press.
Levinas, E. (1994). (Trans. M. B. Smith). Martin Buber, Gabriel Marcel and philosophy. *Outside the subject*. Stanford, CA: Stanford University Press.
Loewald, H. W. (1962). Internalization, separation, mourning, and the super-ego. *Psychoanalytic Quarterly*, *31*(4), 483–504.
Marcel, G. (1952). (Trans. B. Wall). *Metaphysical journal*. Chicago: Henry Regnery.
Marcel, G. (1964). (Trans. R. Rosthal). *Creative fidelity*. New York: Farrar, Straus and Giroux.
Marcel, G. (1965). (Trans. K. Farrer). *Being and having: An existentialist diary*. New York: Harper & Row.
Marcel, G. (1967). I and Thou. In P. A. Schilpp & M. S. Friedman (Eds.), *The philosophy of Martin Buber* (The Library of Living Philosophers Series, pp. 41–48). La Salle, IL: Open Court.
Marcel, G. (1973). *Tragic wisdom and beyond*. Evanston, IL: Northwestern University Press.
Marcel, G. (2001). *The mystery of being. Volume II: Faith and reality*. South Bend, IN: St. Augustine's Press.
Marcus, P. (2008). *Being for the other: Emmanuel Levinas, ethical living and psychoanalysis*. Milwaukee, WI: Marquette University Press.
Marcus, P. (2010). *In search of the good life: Emmanuel Levinas, psychoanalysis and the art of living*. London: Routledge.
Marcus, P. (2013a). *In search of the spiritual: Gabriel Marcel, psychoanalysis, and the sacred*. London: Karnac.
Marcus, P. (2013b). *How to laugh your way through life*. London: Karnac.
Marcus, P. (2018). Some reflections on how Marcelian thought can enhance psychoanalytic theory and practice. *Marcel Studies*, *3*, 1–16.
Marcus, P. (2019). *The psychoanalysis of overcoming suffering: Flourishing despite pain*. London: Routledge.
Marcus, P., & Rosenberg, A. (in preparation). *Psychoanalysis as a philosophical way of life*.
McGuire, W. (Ed.). (1974). *The Freud/Jung letters*. Princeton, NJ: Princeton University Press.

Mendes-Flohr, P. (2019). *Martin Buber: A life of faith and dissent*. New Haven, CT: Yale University Press.

Mitchell, S. A. (2002). *Can love last? The fate of romance over time*. New York: Norton.

Molino, A. (Ed.) (2013). (Eds. R. Carnevali, A. Giannandrea, & D. Yang). *Crossroads in psychoanalysis, Buddhism, and mindfulness: The word and breath*. Lanham, MD: Jason Aronson.

Oppenheim, M. (2017). *Contemporary psychoanalysis and modern Jewish philosophy. Two languages of love*. London: Routledge.

Orange, D. M. (2010). *Thinking for clinicians: Philosophical resources for contemporary psychoanalysis and the humanistic psychotherapies*. London: Routledge.

Pfuetze, P. E. (1967). Martin Buber and American pragmatism. In P. A. Schilpp & M. S. Friedman (Eds.), *The philosophy of Martin Buber* (The Library of Living Philosophers Series, pp. 511–542). La Salle, IL: Open Court.

Phillips, A. (1994). *On flirtation*. Cambridge, MA: Harvard University Press.

Putnam, H. (2008). *Jewish philosophy as a guide to life: Rosenzweig, Buber, Levinas, Wittgenstein*. Bloomington, IN: Indiana University Press.

Raab, K. A. (2000). Creativity and transcendence in the work of Marion Milner. *American Imago*, 57(2), 185–214.

Renik, O. (1993). Analytic interaction: Conceptualizing technique in light of the analyst's irreducible subjectivity. *Psychoanalytic Quarterly*, *62*(4), 553–571.

Rycroft, C. (1995). *A critical dictionary of psychoanalysis*. London: Penguin.

Schmitz, A. O. (1984). Marcel's dialectical method. In P. A. Schilpp & M. S. Friedman (Eds.), *The philosophy of Martin Buber* (The Library of Living Philosophers Series, pp. 159–176). La Salle, IL: Open Court.

Strozier, C. B., Strug, D., Pinteris, K., Kelley, K., & Mart, D. (2020). Termination in self psychology: Heinz Kohut's contribution. *Psychoanalytic Review*, *10*(6), 537–558.

Sweetman, B. (2008). *The vision of Gabriel Marcel: Epistemology, human person, the transcendent*. Amsterdam: Rodopi.

Sweetman, B. (Ed.). (2011). *A Gabriel Marcel reader*. South Bend, IN: St. Augustine's Press.

Symington, N. (1994). *Emotion and spirit: Questioning the claims of psychoanalysis and religion*. New York: St Martin's Press.

Symington, N. (2012). The essence of psycho-analysis as opposed to what is secondary. *Psychoanalytic Dialogues*, *22*, 395–409.

Treanor, B. (2006). *Aspects of alterity: Levinas, Marcel, and the contemporary debate*. New York: Fordham University Press.

Vaidyanathan, J. G., & Kripal, J. (Eds.). (2002). *Vishnu on Freud's desk. A reader in psychoanalysis and Hinduism*. Oxford: Oxford University Press.

Van Deurzen, E. (2012). Reasons for living: Existential therapy and spirituality. In L. Barnett & G. Madison (Eds.), *Existential therapy: Legacy, vibrancy and dialogue* (pp. 170–182). London: Routledge.

Weinstein, F. (1990). *History and theory after the fall*. Chicago: University of Chicago Press.

Wood, R. E. (1969). *Martin Buber's ontology: An analysis of* I and Thou. Evanston, IL: Northwestern University Press.

Wood, R. E. (1999). The dialogical principle and the mystery of being: The enduring relevance of Martin Buber and Gabriel Marcel. *International Journal for Philosophy of Religion*, *45*(2), 83–97.

Zank, M. (2006). Buber and *Religionswissenschaft*: The case of his studies on biblical faith. In M. Zank (Ed.), *New perspectives on Martin Buber* (pp. 61–82). Tubingen: Mohr Siebeck.

Chapter 2

The spirit of love

While Freud, Buber, and Marcel wrote robustly about the permutations of love, including how to expand and deepen this capacity, they all were fairly gloomy in their characterization of what they took to be the human condition and what was reasonably possible. Freud, for example, wrote, "The unworthiness of human beings, including the analyst, always impressed me deeply, but why should analyzed men and women in fact be better. Analysis makes for integration but does not itself make for goodness" (Hale, 1971, p. 188). Buber, sounding like Freud who described most people as "trash," "riff-raff," and "good-for-nothings" in his correspondences (Roazen, 2001, pp. 26, 27),[1] wrote in his "Autobiographical fragments," that most people were "tousle-heads and good-for-nothings," though he still loved them (Buber, 1967a, p. 38). Finally, Marcel described "the essence of our ["broken"][2] world is perhaps betrayal ... we live in a world where betrayal is possible *at every moment, in every degree*, and in every form" (Marcel, 1965a, p. 97).[3] Indeed, my three intellectual touchstones understood that there were powerful "dark" forces circulating in most individuals and in society that worked against the human capacity to love deeply and widely. And yet, Freud, Buber, and Marcel vigorously affirmed that it was precisely the capacity to give and receive love—especially giving for the latter two, which works against our narcissistic proclivity to be self-serving and selfish, however differently they conceptualized it—that centrally constituted a "flourishing" life. As Freud famously told Erik H. Erikson, "to love and work" were the central therapeutic goals of psychoanalysis, these being the twin pillars of a sound mind and artful living (Erikson, 1959, p. 96).[4]

In this chapter, I will first describe Freud's views on adult-to-adult love (often called "romantic love" or partnered monogamous relationships), followed by some of the post-Freudian formulations, including the analyst's so-called love of the analysand. By adult-to-adult love, I mean "evolved" love that often begins like the flash of kindling wood as passion, and morphs into the steady glow of the burning log, something kinder, profounder and more caring.[5] Next, I suggest in what ways the spiritual insights of Buber and Marcel can further illuminate, expand, and deepen how psychoanalysis conceptualizes the psychology of adult-to-adult love.[6] This includes mentioning some of the pertinent positive psychology research findings that both support and challenge certain psychoanalytic and Buberian/Marcelian claims. I will conclude by suggesting how Buber and Marcel's contributions, especially when they are supported by research findings, can be integrated into the clinical context and beyond.

Psychoanalytic reflections on adult-to-adult love

For Freud, as for all subsequent psychoanalysts, love has been approached mainly from the point of view of describing and understanding that which interferes and corrupts the capacity to love.

This can include, for example, issues related to "fantasy and actuality, sameness and otherness, bodies and emotions, love and hate, the controlled and the uncontrollable, pathos and guilt, safety and risk" and so forth (Mitchell, 2002, p. 29). Indeed, there is no body of knowledge that better depicts what St. Augustine called "disordered love," a lack of psychological fit between various human needs and wishes and the objects that can gratify them (Marcus, 2003, pp. 142–145). While psychoanalysis has in general been unsurpassable in explicating that which subverts evolved love, it has been much weaker in depicting what constitutes and sustains it. This trend is not unique to psychoanalysis, as empirical positive psychology researchers have noted, "Considering that love is so important to emotional well-being, it is surprising that comparatively little research has been devoted exclusively to it" (Compton & Hoffman, 2020, p. 141). What follows are some of the most interesting contributions of psychoanalysis to understanding what constitutes so-called "healthy/mature" love relations. My review of these contributions is meant to be illustrative, not complete, and it must be stated from the onset that the term "love" in psychoanalytic writings is as ambiguous and "up-for-grabs" as in philosophy and other disciplines. As Rycroft has noted, "Psychoanalysts have as much difficulty defining such a protean concept as do others" (Rycroft, 1995, p. 96). As a placeholder for this chapter, a serviceable psychoanalytic definition of love is: "A complex affective state and experience associated with primarily libidinal investment of objects. The feeling state is characterized usually by elation and euphoria, sometimes ecstasy, and on occasion pain" (Moore & Fine, 1990, p.113). "Mature love," says Kernberg, unifies the passionate nature of three interdependent, interrelated and interactive components: "the sexual relationship, the object relationship, and the superego [roughly the conscience] investment of the couple" (Kernberg, 1995, pp. 32–53).

Before presenting my illustrative review, however, it should be emphasized that each psychoanalytic account of love (and, for that matter, the chapters on work, faith and suffering) is largely controlled by its assumptions of what constitutes "the human condition" (or "human nature," as it is often called)[7] and, therefore, how it conceptualizes psychopathology or problems in living or with mental distress and treatment. Such "master narratives" (or perhaps more aptly, "morality plays") become the frame and filter for how love is seen to flourish and atrophy. For example, analysts have very different narratives about the self: the self that is fashioned by its defenses against instincts (Freud); the self formed by its inner objects (Klein); the self shaped by its internalized relationships (Kohut) (Jones, 1991, p. 135); and "the self as a narcissistic misrecognition, represented through the symbolic order of language" (Lacan) (Elliott, 2015, p. 123). Moreover, depending on which master narrative one is lodged in, the goals of psychoanalytic treatment tend to be conceptualized differently: We have "the taming of the beast within" through reason and love (Freud); the "mad person within raging about" who becomes transformed through compensatory reparative activities (Klein); the "discovery of the self within" and the development of compensatory self-structures (Kohut); and "to speak what [had] heretofore been unspeakable," to reclaim the voice of one's desires (Lacan) (Roth, 1998, p. 327).

Given that psychoanalysis does not have one notion of the human condition or human nature, but rather many—"Psychoanalytic models rest upon … irreconcilable claims concerning the human condition" (Greenberg & Mitchell, 1983, p. 404)—it is not surprising that it has been accused of being "too fragmented to be constituted as a unitary [scientific] discipline" (Weinstein, 1990, p. 26).

Sigmund Freud

For Freud, all love relations are "the finding of an object" that "is in fact a refinding of it" (Freud, 1953, p. 222), roughly analogous to the emotional experience of symbiotic togetherness with the mother or caregiver (Moore & Fine, 1990 p. 113). Moreover, the quest for the Oedipal object is an enduring embedded quality of all love relationships. While the frequently used term "object" in analytic writings is replete with a "myriad" of "ambiguities and confusions" (Akhtar, 2009, p. 192), and has an alienating if not dehumanizing "feel" to it, it can be serviceably defined as "that towards which action or desire is directed; that which the subject [the person] requires in order to achieve instinctual satisfaction; that to which the subject relates himself," most often a person, parts of a person or a symbolic equivalence of one or the other (Rycroft, 1995, p. 113). What this "finding/refinding" notion means in terms of establishing love relations is that to some extent the choice of our significant other repeats or calls to mind aspects of our childhood caregivers. Love, says Freud, "consists of new editions of old traits and it repeats infantile reactions," this being "the essential character of every state of being in love" (Freud, 1958, p. 168). That is, all love is based on infantile templates, is fundamentally a fixation on the parents, what Freud calls transference love. According to Reuben Fine, transference love and ordinary love only differ in terms of degree (Fine, 1979, p. 48).[8] The problem with this, of course, is that if we refind that which is "bad" from our childhood experiences, it usually leads to impoverished and/or destructive intimate relationships. The "trick" then is to refind in the significant other that which is consciously and unconsciously "good" from our childhood caregivers, so that we have a better chance of being relatively happy in our love relation. Most often, this "refinding" involves a subtle "refining" of earlier caregiver experiences, suggesting that the significant other is apprehended as a corrective emotional experience of a sort. For example, a man who refinds his "good" mother in a woman who has the best maternal qualities but is also capable of being a focus of passionate desire on the sexual level, has engaged in a refinding and refining (e.g., the fantasy that happily blends the "mother and whore" in the significant other). To attempt to refind the "impossible" significant other who will recreate the imagined perfection associated with the parent/child symbiosis is a doomed effort from the onset (Bergmann, 1987).

Freud's view of love is driven, if not limited, by his guiding assumption that man is fundamentally egotistical and pleasure-seeking. For Freud, all forms of love are seen as derivatives of instinct, and their function is to give instinctual gratification. In a sense, all love is love of a need-satisfying object.[9] Mature object love, in contrast to infantile, dependent, need-satisfying love, is love that recognizes the reality of the other, his otherness, and that he is a separate person with needs and wishes requiring and deserving gratification. Perhaps most importantly for Freud, the capacity for mature love requires object constancy, the capability to maintain an enduring relationship with a specific, single, separate other. This, in turn, presupposes the development of both a stable, structurally sound, coherent self and secure internalized object relations. "Normal" love, says Freud, thus results from the blending of caring, affectionate, and sexual feelings toward a person of the opposite sex. Its accomplishment is characterized by genital primacy in sexuality and by object love in relationships with others (Freud's heterosexual bias is exemplified. The term "significant other" could be used as a replacement for "opposite sex").

Thus, for Freud, love relations are conceptualized essentially as hedonistic and utilitarian, with the other viewed as a need-satisfying object: how can the other pleasure me, what can the other do for me? Freud's view of love tended to embrace such an outlook. In an improved variation on this conceptualization, in the "relational" psychoanalytic work of say Benjamin (1995, p. 29), Rubin (1996, p. 49) and Mitchell (2002), love relations are viewed largely in terms of a mutual instrumental calculus of two equal subjects who appreciate the uniqueness of each other, and give each other satisfaction. This surely goes further than the strict hedonistic-utilitarian view in that it acknowledges the other as unique in terms of desires, goals, values, and needs, and it makes satisfying those needs as important: "I am for you, you are for me," as Levinas put it (Robbins, 2001, p. 193). This is the love relation as symmetrically conceived. For Levinas (though less so and differently for Buber and Marcel), such a relational ethic is serviceable but does not go far enough, for it mistakenly treats entering the ethical realm (i.e., of moral principles) with becoming "good" (i.e., responsible for the other). The latter way of being-in-the-world, responsible subjectivity, points to transcendence. As Levinas pointed out, the love commandment ("Thou shalt love thy neighbour as thyself") "still assumes the prototype of love to be love of oneself," that is, "self-love is accepted as the very definition of a person." However, Levinas's conception of the ethical subject also asserts, "Be responsible for the other as you are responsible for yourself" (Levinas, 1987, p. 225).[10]

As Levinas further notes, while such a reciprocal approach moves in the direction of relating to the other as other, this view still subtly retains the wish to make the other the same, to totalize the other, and thus to open him or her to disrespect, disregard, de-individuation, and other forms of intersubjective violence. Such an ontologically based approach seeks to comprehend the otherness of the other by including him under a notion "that is thought within *me*, and thus is in some sense *the same* as me" (Atterton & Calarco, 2005, p. 10). To the extent that the other is construed in terms of his or her being and is comprehended and thematized on the basis of what he or she has in common with other beings, the other becomes conceptually the same as others, and therefore loses his uniqueness and individuality. According to Levinas, to comprehend the other in this way is roughly equivalent "to predicting, manipulating, controlling, even dominating the Other" (ibid., pp. 15, 16). Such a monological, non-I-Thou orientation can easily morph into something wretched and appalling: "I'll affirm you and allow you to exist if you become like me, think like me, do as I do, are my mental-spiritual clone" (Cain, 1996, p. 136). As we shall see, Buber and Marcel do not agree with Levinas's wholesale criticism of the mutuality/symmetrical approach, and I believe they are more plausible in terms of how "real-life" love relationships are enacted (e.g., via the testimonials of people in loving marriages or partnered monogamous relationships).[11] To love our significant other more than we love ourselves, to put their needs and desires before our own, especially in a sustained manner, seems like an impossible challenge for most people. In fact, the philosopher John D. Caputo, himself an admiring scholar of Levinas, claims that Levinas "weaves a fabulous, poetic story about absolute alterity" (otherness), which ultimately is not credible (Poole, 1998, p. 71). That is, Levinas's position is "inapplicable, unlivable, and utopian … there is a disconnect between his philosophy and our life" (Treanor, 2006, p. 123). Certainly, most of us can remember times when we acted altruistically, but such moments tend to be the exception rather than the rule. Still, Levinas's point, and I believe Buber and Marcel's, is that like the unreachable ideal of "free association," one should strive to be for the other before oneself, or as much as oneself, as much as possible, in part because this is the most promising basis for a love relationship that will endure and flourish.

For Freud, however, accomplishing hedonistic/utilitarian love is not simple; it requires resolving at a higher level of personality integration at least three aspects of love: "narcissistic versus object love, infantile versus mature love, and love versus hate" (Moore & Fine, 1990, p. 113). To the extent that love is dominated by inordinate, unhealthy, and pathological narcissism (e.g., self-centeredness and selfishness), infantile and dependent wishes and behavior (e.g., the other exists mainly to gratify our needs and wishes on demand) and hate (e.g., heightened ambivalence), one's love relation is doomed to failure, or at least much suffering. To the extent that it is animated by altruistic concerns (e.g., enhancing the other), is mature (e.g., recognizes that the separate other has needs and wishes worthy of gratifying), and is mainly affectionate (e.g., not corrupted by aggression), it is likely to succeed. For Freud, while all relationships are ambivalent, the ultimate pre-condition for maintaining a stable, healthy, mature love relation is that affectionate sentiments toward one's significant other be much stronger and more pervasive than the aggressive ones.

It is crucial to briefly contextualize Freud's views on love in terms of his broader version of the human condition and a flourishing life. As Wallwork (2005, p. 287) points out, for Freud the supreme moral criterion, what he took to be the "good" that reflected what humans strive for, was "happiness."

> [W]hat [do] men themselves show by their behavior to be the purpose and intention of their lives? What do they demand of life and wish to achieve in it? The answer to this can hardly be in doubt. They strive after happiness; they want to become happy and to remain so.
>
> (Freud, 1930, p. 76)

Wallwork further notes that for Freud, as was the case with Aristotle and other great humanist moral philosophers, happiness was in part conceptualized as "eudaimonia." However, eudaimonia is not simply a moment or experience of pleasure alone, but a "veritable form of life, a flourishing form of life capable of realizing the full range of possibilities for rational beings" (Robinson, 1997, p. 17).[12] As Wallwork succinctly puts it,

> Happiness for Freud is rather a matter of *functioning well* than feeling good. The mentally healthy person's happiness consists in the well-being that comes with certain forms of sublimation: loving and being loved, creative work, the pursuit of knowledge, freedom and aesthetic appreciation. These goods of life that make happiness possible are not instrumental to functioning well, but constituent aspects of happiness.
>
> (Wallwork, 2005, p. 287)

For Freud, love was perhaps the most important way of obtaining happiness—giving and receiving love. The "union of mental and bodily satisfaction in the enjoyment of love is one of its [life's] culminating peaks. Apart from a few queer fanatics, all the world knows this and conducts its life accordingly" (Freud, 1958, pp. 169–170). According to Freud, love is also crucial because it underpins other extremely important aspects of life and civilization. For instance, it libidinally binds and animates one's ties to family, friends, community and to the world at large. Without the force of Eros, Freud's poetic metaphor for the life-force and sexual instincts, civilization is doomed to be overwhelmed by the inherent aggressiveness and destructiveness that constitutes Thanatos, the Death Instinct.

Melanie Klein

For Freud, love relations, actually all human relations, largely reflect a utilitarian motive, that of using the other to gratify biologically endowed drives as a means to achieving one's end (i.e., a homeostatic drive-reduction paradigm). In contrast, Klein, drawing from psychoanalyst Karl Abraham, was attempting to comprehend the form of love "which *feels for* the object rather than the love" that Freud's classical model posed (Hinshelwood, 1991, p. 342). As Kleinian analyst Donald Meltzer points out, for Freud, love is like opening up a factory, of making a kind of capital investment bent on generating a profit. One does not invest one's libido unless one feels fairly sure that one will get back more than one gives. For Klein, love is conceptualized more in terms of bequeathing a charity (Meltzer, 1978, p. 84).[13] That is, says Alford, "Love gets from the very act of giving. It gets the opportunity to repair the self by repairing and restoring the world, or at least a little part of it" (Alford, 1998, p. 128). In the successful resolution of the depressive position (first experienced at about 6 months of age, according to Klein), an adult analysand is less prone to alternate so emotionally violently to hatred when their significant other's limitations become apparent; that is, there is a greater emotional stability. Such affect tolerance and a disinclination towards "emotional storms" contributes to a greater capacity for care and forgiveness (Hinshelwood, 1991, p. 344). For Klein then, love emanates from the infant's sense of gratitude toward the "good" mother, in Kleinian language, toward the satisfying "good breast." This feeling is the basis for the infant's and later the adult's "appreciation of all goodness in the self and in others" (Bergmann, 1987, p. 248).

Heinz Kohut

Kohut's psychoanalytic self-psychology claims that love is fundamentally establishing a "selfobject." A selfobject is someone who strengthens and sustains the sense of self, the self's cohesion, firmness, and harmony. The selfobject is psychically analogous to the oxygen we need to survive, and we are only mindful of it when we reflect on it, most often when there is a disruption in its psychic life-sustaining function (Kohut, 1971, 1977). As Wolf (1994) noted, selfobjects can be mainly mirroring (e.g., the subject feels validated), idealizable (e.g. the subject feels special), an alter-ego (the subject feels a twinship), and adversarial (e.g. the subject feels enlivening opposition and defiance). All of these selfobjects reinforce the vitality of the self. In infantile love, the significant other, the selfobject, mainly functions for my benefit and survival, a template rooted early in the childhood experience of the empathic, supportive, reassuring, and approving "good" mother or caregiver. In mature love, the self is better grounded, sustained, and strengthened and is thus capable of a more intense experience of receiving and giving love. In other words, for Kohut, in the love relationship one "refinds" the good mother or caregiver, the selfobject, the one who calls to mind, sustains, and strengthens structural self-coherence, energic vigor, aliveness, integration, and balance among the diverse elements of the self. For the love relationship to work, both people need to "refind" the self-selfobject relationships they had in their parent/caregiver-to-child relationships. For Kohut, the sense of comfort, healing, and happiness that characterize the best of love is precisely the byproduct of this mutual self-selfobject refinding.

Jacque Lacan

Lacan says it is "impossible to say anything meaningful" or intelligible about love (Evans, 1996, p. 103). For Lacan, love must be understood in terms of what he views as the larger ethical goal of psychoanalysis, namely, the discovery of the reality and truth of the Unconscious and its powerful interpretive grip over the subject (in Lacan's theory, the Unconscious is not instinctual, but rather linguistic, the impact on the subject of the trans-individual symbolic order) (Fryer, 2004, p. 190).[14] For Lacan, the self is always estranged from its own history, is shaped in and through otherness, and is embedded in a symbolic web, which is on the outside (Elliot, 2015, p. 108). Thus, as Evans points out, Lacan says love is situated as a "purely imaginary phenomenon" although it has an impact in the symbolic register (Evans, 1996, p. 103).[15] Love, for Lacan, "is autoerotic" and mainly has a "narcissistic structure" since "it's one's own ego that one loves in love, one's own ego made real on the imaginary level" (Lacan, 1991a, p. 142). As Lacan famously repeatedly said, "Loving is to give what one does not have" to someone who we don't know (Lacan, 2017, p. 194); in other words, the main thrust of loving is to embrace one's castration, one's lack, to deposit it into the other, and thus to imagine the other as capable of making this woundedness feel better or go away, a kind of illusory security-generating tactic.[16] Similar to Sartre, Lacan claims that love can never really be other than the demand to be loved, a claim based on a questionable assumption that, originally, I am for-myself rather than for-the-other, as Levinas vigorously affirms, and Buber and Marcel suggest, is the "highest" expression of love. Lacan further notes that "to love is, essentially, to wish to be loved" (Lacan, 1991b, p. 253).[17] For Lacan, love entails only "an imaginary reciprocity" and mutuality, the reciprocity between "loving" and "being loved," that, along with the "fantasy of fusion" with the loved other, mainly comprises the compelling illusion of love (Lacan, 1991b, p. 142). Lacan rejects Freud and other analysts who claim that love is a central clinical goal in psychoanalysis and, for that matter, a constituent aspect of living a flourishing life. Rather, he says that the aim of analysis is to reclaim the voice for one's desire by clarifying and making intelligible the familial experiences and knots, the governing signifiers, that have had such a powerful interpretive hold on one's way of being-in-the-world. As far as I can tell, this may or may not lead to a greater capacity and actualization of love in one's way of being-in-the-world. In fact, Mitchell notes that Lacan "seems never to have grasped the possibility of a genuine relatedness" (Mitchell, 2002, p. 50).

Very briefly, it is worth mentioning that Erik H. Erikson, the great ego psychologist, describes love as the key virtue, the ego strength that emerges after successful resolution of the intimacy versus isolation ego crisis, the sixth stage of human development of the life cycle. Erikson defines love as "mutuality of devotion forever subduing the antagonisms inherent in divided function" (Erikson, 1964, p. 129). Love thus involves a complementarity of identities: having both the ego strength to share identity for "mutual verification" of selected identity and drawing from the supportive and nurturing other "the strength to be 'self-ish'" (Monte, 1980, p. 256).

Also worth noting is that there has been an attempt to bring psychoanalysis in line with attachment theory, the view that the infant has a biologically driven need to have a secure, emotional bond with its mother or primary caregiver. Serious cognitive and emotional problems emerge if this maternal bond is not securely established. That is, if the infant does not develop a secure sense of the mother as a psychological parent who symbolizes nurturance and stability, psychic structure and object-relatedness can be damaged and truncated. For example, there is a correlation between flawed or failed childhood attachment, so-called insecure attachment, and problematic adult forms of relating. Anxious attachments often lead to dependent personalities, while avoidant attachments can lead to schizotypal, schizoid, narcissistic, and antisocial behavior. From the point of view of psychoanalytically glossed attachment theory, securely attached lovers establish a workable equilibrium between relatedness and self-dependency. As a consequence of this equilibrium, lovers have the will and ability to fashion sensible and mutually gratifying relationships, including engaging in joint novel activities and self-development. Pragmatically speaking, the securely attached lover honors their significant other's desire for alone and down time without resentment, while also demarcating time to engage with one another in pleasurable togetherness. Such an arrangement gives them both the chance for experiencing independence and interdependence.

Finally, psychoanalysts who have been influenced by "intersubjectivity" theory claim that psychic phenomena, such as between two lovers, should not be comprehended as separate from their interpersonal or relational matrix. That is, psychological events are not lodged "inside" a person, but are dialectally constructed experiences, unique to a specific interpersonal or relational context and setting, whether in real-life or therapy. Person (1988), for example, has described the experience of falling in love and how lovers generate an enlivened and enlivening two-person world, while also refashioning themselves in terms of self-development and self-enhancement. Mitchell (2002), coming from a relational perspective, discusses the impediments that comprise maintaining passion in love (e.g., being in love versus loving),[18] affirming the well-known observation that love involves a mixture of passion/romance and safety/security, depending on context and setting. Benjamin focuses on love as it relates to domination and the fact that it impedes the need for the dominated to acquire self-affirming recognition, through respectful (to-the-other's otherness) affective interplay and sharing (Benjamin, 1988, 1995).[19] As relational analyst Philip Bromberg noted, "Health is the ability to stand in the spaces between realities without losing any of them—the capacity to feel like oneself while being many" (Bromberg, 1993, p. 166).

Thus, one of the limitations in the theorizing on love in Freud, Klein, Kohut, Lacan, Erikson, and attachment/intersubjective theories, at least from the point of view of Buber and Marcel, is that all of these theorists, to some extent, treat the significant other reductively, mainly as a depersonalized love object, as a thing-like entity to be more-or-less crudely used for one's satisfaction. Even sophisticated relational theorists, like Benjamin, Rubin, and Mitchell, tend to view the other mainly as a source of reciprocal gratification of one's relational needs, which from a Buberian and Marcelian (and Levinasian) point of view frequently results in two people in a doomed arrangement of mutually instrumental use, unless perhaps, generously augmented by transcendence-pointing, other-directed, other-regarding, and other-serving considerations. As the lone voice of psychoanalyst Erich Fromm noted—similar to Levinas, Buber (whom he met) and Marcel—the active character of love can be described as "primarily giving, not receiving." Love is characterized by "care, responsibility, respect and knowledge." In essence, "to love means to commit oneself without guarantee, to give oneself completely in the hope that our love will produce love in the loved person. Love is an act of faith" (1956, pp. 22, 26, 128). That is, as Buber and Marcel have argued, while many philosophers, psychologists, and analysts claim that it's a fundamental fact of existence that one is an object for another, what is most important to understand is why that mode of comportment is never totally successful, how it ignores the interhuman, the mysterious realm of person-to-person contact (Wahl, 1967, p. 501).

The psychoanalyst's love of analysands

An illuminating way of understanding how love operates in the real world for the analyst is to briefly peek into the virtual world of the consultation room, and to consider the fact that many of the "most sophisticated psychoanalysts" claim, "usually to assure themselves, that they do, indeed, love their patients" and this has a therapeutic function (Friedman, 2005, p. 350). But what constitutes such love and how is it instantiated?[20]

First, it is important to mention that the analytic context is not one of two people coming together on a "level playing field," which greatly influences the power dynamics from the get-go. Such asymmetry is clearly to the advantage of the analyst; for example, the analyst is the "doctor" and the analysand is the "patient"; he is paid for his services and will typically end the treatment if not paid, and he takes the lead in scheduling the length,[21] frequency and time of sessions and vacations, the décor and structure of the waiting room and office (e.g., where the chairs are positioned) and its location (e.g., an alienating medical building versus a more comfortable home office). Such command and control over time/space and other contextual coordinates give alleged expressions of love from the analyst, and from the analysand to the analyst, a questionable basis for calling these expressions love, at least when love is conceptualized ideally as more or less symmetrical and reciprocal (the analyst is also more responsible for, and to, the analysand). While there is never complete equality or mutuality in a love relationship, or for that matter in any relationship, power relations are more easily reversible in other types of relationships. However, in the psychoanalytic relationship, the authoritative "doctoring" powers embedded in the situation often do not allow much if any room for the analysand to meaningfully interrogate, let alone seriously modify, the asymmetrical, non-reciprocal structure of the doctor-patient relationship. Of course, the analysand can leave his analysis, but this is easier said than done for a variety of reasons related to unconscious attachment and other issues. As Buber noted, similar to the teacher/student and pastor/parishioner relation, the therapist/client relation is constrained from the get-go in its mutuality potential by its social parameters, the "normative limitation of mutuality" (Buber, 1958, p. 132).[22] Put polemically, in some ways, an analyst who feels and or expresses love to an analysand may be roughly similar to a teacher with great affection for a student, a boss for an employee, or a cognitive-behavioral or other psychotherapist for his client or patient. That is, in all of these contexts, possibly in part because the power dynamics are asymmetrical from the start, the psychological conditions are fertile for the more powerful teacher, boss, therapist or analyst to feel and/or express so-called love (or, in extreme cases, enact it in real life, such as when an analyst, like Carl Jung, has an affair with his analysand or seeks her out after the analysis is over). As Freud allegedly told his colleague Max Eitingon, "The secret of therapy is to cure through love, and that with the greatest personal effort one could perhaps overcome more difficulties in treatment, but one would 'lose his skin by doing so'" (Grotjahn, 1967, p. 18).

Analysts have claimed that they provide the analysand with a "special kind of love" (Friedman, 2005, p. 349) that is central to their transformation and self-overcoming, their "cure" as a medicalizing analyst would say. This special kind of love has been described as a "*particular* kind of feeling" that the analyst typically has with "*all* of their patients" (Friedman, 2005, p. 349). What is important to grasp from the start is that for the analyst love is equated with a "feeling" that is "inside" the analyst, generated by his encounter with the analysand (a relational analyst would view this as a co-constructed moment, but still). This is in contrast to the Buberian claim that "feelings dwell in man, but man dwells in his love" (Buber, 1958, p. 14) and Marcel's claim that, "love moves on a ground which is neither that of the self nor of the other *qua* other; I call it the Thou" (i.e., the dynamic communion of mutual presence) (Marcel,

1965a, p. 167). These provocative and evocative Buberian and Marcelian claims will be elaborated in the next section.

Michael Balint (1949, p. 231) believed that the analyst's libidinalized relationship with the analysand, personified in the transference, is "exactly the same" as the analysand's toward the analyst, the difference being the analyst does not act on his desires and uses these erotic feelings to empathically assist him in the treatment of the analysand. In this formulation, love is equated with the erotic upsurge that the analyst feels and uses to helpfully animate his clinical interventions. While analysts are at times sexually attracted to their analysands (e.g., erotic countertransference), to claim that this is "exactly the same" as what the analysand who is in the middle of an erotically tinged transference feels, seems to be far-fetched in most cases. And if the analyst is contending with such high-octane erotic feelings, he is treading on very thin ice as an effective helper (e.g., he lacks disinterested interest, calmly and reasonably engaging the analysand).

Schaefer (1983) has emphasized that analysts typically demonstrate a concentrated attention, an intensely focused, empathic listening to the analysand, reflecting a deeply felt devotion or dedication that the analysand typically equates with an expression of love. As Paul Tillich noted, the "first task" of love is "to listen" (1954, p. 84). It is common knowledge that in a love relationship one has to be willing and able to empathically focus on the needs and desires of the other and not just one's own; and most significant others experience this as pleasurable and helpful.[23] However, how exactly this occurs is hard to formulate. Moreover, in Schaefer's view, this devotion and dedication has an ulterior motive, that is, it is the psychological staging-ground for the analyst convincing the analysand that one version of his "story," his narrative construction, is best for him because it is most likely to "work" in terms of the business of living. Whether such love is "really" love, or a skillful manipulation of some type, is open to debate, depending on whether you regard Schaefer's loosely aesthetic and pragmatic criteria as adequate in the therapeutic context (Kearney, 2002, p. 43).

It was Nacht (1962) who alleged that it is the analyst's "unconscious love that is basically responsible for cure," which sounds roughly like self-psychologies' emphasis on empathy and openness (Friedman, 2005, p. 354). The construct of "unconscious love" is admittedly hard to pin down. For example, if the love is unconscious, how does one know one feels or knows it? When is such unconscious love operative, what does it look like in specific relational contexts? Also, how does one know that the unconscious love is real or authentic and not a category mistake and/or a mainly self-serving imagining? Indeed, Nacht's formulation seems to boil down to a re-statement that the analyst loves the analysand in ways that he can't verbalize (e.g., unformulated or unthematized). However, it does not illuminate, let alone in a convincing manner, what this unconscious love is, how it is instantiated, and what situational forces are operative that evoke and/or support such a feeling. Nacht's view calls to mind Freud's advice to colleague Theodore Reik about choosing a career, by listening to "the deep inner needs of our nature," the unconscious, suggesting it is the wishes of the deepest part of one's personality that one has to somehow apperceive (Reik, 1983, p. 7). Indeed, researchers have shown that there are unconscious emotions, brain happenings that animate behavior and thought processes that are not conscious. Moreover, there are proven techniques that can strengthen or weaken the unconscious nerve signals lodged in the brain. These techniques "can transmute, enhance, weaken, or eliminate our hidden and not so hidden emotions," including love (Brogaard, 2015, p. 5); perhaps, this is what psychoanalysis, at its best, in part does.

Other theorists have described the "constant ['universally present'] love or love-like feeling that the analyst always has and always radiates" that enhance treatment (Friedman, 2005, p. 354). These include, for example, "contact feeling" (M. Gitelson); "a cathector of the patient" [investor of mental/emotional energy characterized by "love and respect for the individual and for individual development" (Loewald, 1960, p. 229]; "unconscious negotiations and 'winning' by the patient" that the analyst fosters within the transference/counter-transference context (L. Tower); the "mother of separation" (L. Stone), a view that calls to mind Winnicott's emphasis on the maternal function; and "a kind of love in which he [the analyst] is not personally concerned, although it *is* a deep feeling" that animates the analyst's effective interpreting function (H. Segal) (Friedman, 2005, pp. 353, 354, 356). And Aron noted, "Empathy, or analytic love, must be mutually given and mutually accepted" (1996, p. 136). For the most part, says Friedman, "After specific *feelings* are discussed, author after author concludes that love is embodied in the analyst's understanding, which in turn is in interpretations" (ibid., p. 356). Kohut and Loewald, for instance, suggest that the analyst's love is equated with the dedication to understanding the so-called objective truth of the analysand's individuality, with an eye to facilitating growth and development while appreciating the creative repository of the analysand's life trajectory. Efforts at empathic understanding tend to generate love or love-like feelings in analysts and others (ibid., pp. 357, 362).

In summary, while there are other analysts (Novick & Novick, 2000) who have contributed to answering the question, "What is unique about the psychoanalyst's love of his analysand," for the most part, it boils down to "affects" and an "elementary feeling" (Friedman, 2005, p. 373) that gets evoked when one is engaged with the analysand one is trying to deeply understand and help over a long period of time. No doubt, each of the aforementioned descriptions of the affects associated with this "special" (ibid., p. 349) kind of psychoanalytic love has some face validity, depending on the specific analysand/analyst context. Though it need not. For example, in my first two-year analysis as a young graduate student in New York, I experienced my interpersonal or relational analyst (as I would now call him) as a rather disengaged and uptight middle-aged man, although he could make some helpful suggestions to help me cope with my problems. My second analysis, this time with a Kleinian analyst during one of my years as a doctoral student in London, was like a "war zone," and I left the botched analysis more of a wreck because I experienced the analyst as mean and nasty. In my third analysis, two years with a well-known middle-aged female Freudian therapist while I was finishing my Ph.D., the treatment was like making love to and with a corpse, that is, it left me cold and lonely like a work of art, and was also unhelpful (actually, it made things worse). Finally, in my training analysis with an older Freudian male therapist which lasted a decade or longer, I experienced my analyst as kind and helpful, analogous to a loving parent, a wise teacher, a street-savvy, got-your-back "pal," and an unashamed pleasure-seeker who wanted me to develop the capacity to be likewise. From him I learned how to love more deeply and widely, and to be creative and productive in work; my faith was refound and refined, and my overall depressive comportment was transformed into one animated by tragi-comic attunement (Marcus, 2013b).

It also needs to be mentioned that much of what analysts claim they feel towards their analysands, their love or love-like feelings, bear a similarity to those in any of the helping professions who nurture individual growth and try, through understanding and the like, to resolve psychological and/or physical problems. Also worth noting is that like others in the helping professions, analysts can adequately give psychoanalytic love to their analysands while at the same time be deeply flawed in their willingness and ability to love outside the consultation room. As Freud wrote in a letter to his good friend James Jackson Putnam, "That psychoanalysis has not made the analysts themselves better, nobler, or of stronger character remains a disappointment to me. Perhaps, I was wrong to expect it" (Hale, 1971, pp. 163–164).

BUBER AND MARCEL ON LOVE

Buber

When putting forth Buber and Marcel's views on what constitutes love, we have to be willing and able to enter into a different "language game," one that is often poetic, metaphoric and at best suggestive, this being the preferred mode of communicating for these two God-infused, unsystematic dialogical personalist philosophers. Buber and Marcel's work thus has an ephemeral and hard to empirically verify quality to it, in part because they focus on how we personally experience, or rather participate (Buber and Marcel's preferred term), in the world (Sweetman, 2008, pp. 136, 138). Indeed, unless one has an "ear" for the "melody" of spiritual/religious language, one cannot adequately appreciate its powerful insightfulness regarding love. For ontological realities cannot be designated, as much as alluded to (Gallagher, 1962, p. 29). That being said, Buber and Marcel were not "Pollyanna-ish" men; they both suffered in their personal lives and did not shy away from engaging others who also suffered.[24] They also had long and happy marriages. Both Buber and Marcel were situationalists, that is, Marcel, for example, focused on embodied "situational involvement," such that "objects" of our experience have markedly divergent meanings to the person than the meanings presented in the mind's-eye of "clear and distinct" abstract ideas (Sweetman, 2008, p. 17). Such a willingness and ability to engage in understanding the phenomenology of "life in the raw" was Buber and Marcel's bailiwick, hence, they provide a way of thinking about love that is pertinent to mainstream "nuts and bolts" clinical psychoanalysis, including as it tries to reconstitute itself as a compelling spiritual discipline.

For Buber, to a large extent, what constitutes love is aptly evoked in a famous, though elliptical passage from *I and Thou*:

> Love ranges in its effect through the whole world. In the eyes of him who takes his stand in love, and gazes out of it, men are cut from their entanglement in bustling activity. Good people and evil, wise and foolish, beautiful and ugly, become successively real to him: that is set free, they step forth in their singleness, and confront him as *Thou*. In a wonderful way, from time to time, exclusiveness arises—and so he can be effective, helping, healing, educating, raising up, saving. Love is responsibility of an *I* for a *Thou*. In this lies the likeness—impossible in any feeling whatsoever—of all who love, from the smallest to the greatest and from the blessedly protected man, whose life is rounded in that of a loved being, to him who is all his life nailed to the cross of the world, and who ventures to bring himself to the dreadful point—to love all men.
>
> (1958, pp. 14–15)

In this evocative paragraph, we have many of the key notions that constitute what Buber means by love, including romantic love at its best.

Love involves taking a stand; this means that the person who is willing and able to love assumes a particular mode of comportment, a position, stance or bearing while in the presence of his dialogical partner (Kramer & Gawlick, 2003, p. 205). Such dialogical partners become "real" to him, they perceptually emerge as "free" in their "singleness," that is, their unique presence as a whole being, a *Thou*. Such a mode of comportment is when a person can be described as most wholly and uniquely "human" (ibid., p. 202). Love is "the revealing by two people of the *Thou* to one another" (Buber, 1958, p. 46). Buber suggests what this mode of comportment involves in terms of one's self-relation, by quoting a famous Hassidic story: Rabbi Zusya, who, on his death-bed, says: "In the world to come I shall not be asked: 'Why were you not Moses?' I shall be asked: 'Why were you not Zusya'" (Buber, 1995, p. 17). Exactly what it means to be a unique self is a complex matter raised by this story, just as it is to specify what it means to relate to another person in his unique presence, his "exclusiveness" as a whole being. For both Buber and Marcel, the "question of wholeness of one's own being and one's relation to that wholeness of what is" matters most, compared to solving piecemeal, abstract problems associated with philosophy as conceptual system (Wood, 1999, p. 83). Lacan, for example, claimed that psychoanalysis was not capable of making a broken person whole; in fact, he quips, "Have you ever encountered whole beings? I've never seen any. I'm not whole, neither are you" (Lacan, 1991b, p. 243). For Buber (and Marcel), any *I-Thou* relationship is spoken with the whole being, is mutual (this is a continuum notion), and the spirit does not reside in the I (hence, it is not a mere "experience"), rather, it is between the *I and Thou* (it is a "participation") (Buber, 1958, pp. 8, 10, 39). Also, every I-Thou relationship of existential contact eventually morphs back into an I-It relation, one of objective knowledge and abstract analysis (Marcel's "secondary reflection" presences the mystery of being and its personally engaged contemplation, that is, dwelling, not comprehending, versus "primary reflection," problem-solving cognition and detached analysis) (Sweetman, 2008, p. 140)—although the I-Thou is the superior, ontologically primary realm that emanates from the "inborn thou."[25] The "inborn thou" is the human tendency toward relationship in response to the parent or caregiver who effectively responds to the child's efforts to make a meaningful emotional connection (no doubt this notion has influenced the object relational and other psychoanalytic schools of thought). Indeed, relational analysts of different persuasions have exploited this theme that the self is, from the onset, constituted by and through its interactions with others (e.g., the relational, social, and linguistic influences), and that subjectivity is best understood in terms of intersubjectivity (Mitchell, 2000, p. 57).[26]

Most importantly, Buber says, "Love is responsibility of an *I* for a *Thou*," and without such a conviction, it is nearly impossible to engage in those actions that are correlated with love, "helping, healing, educating, raising up, saving."[27] Also worth noting again is that for Buber love is not a "feeling whatsoever," it is a way of being-in-the-world that can come easily to some whose circumstances tend to make it so (e.g., it is easy to love a healthy, attractive, successful, significant other, a child or grandchild or one's dog, as Freud described the most perfect love),[28] but for many of us, it involves engaging one's own and/or the other's suffering in circumstances that are very challenging (e.g., loving a significant other who has contracted a life-threatening illness or chronic disease that negatively impacts everyday living). Indeed, Buber makes it clear that love is not to be reduced to a feeling one has, usually experienced as a passing phenomenon by a lover, and mainly lodged in a sense of personal self-sufficiency. As Wood puts it, for Buber, "feeling is something that *occurs within* man as a psychological phenomenon," and there is no sure way of discerning authentic relation and fanaticism. That is, in both instances the self *feels* and judges itself as certain of its authenticity (Wood, 1969, p. 60). Buber comments on the category mistake of equating feelings and love:

> Feelings accompany the metaphysical and metapsychical fact of love, but they do not constitute it. The accompanying feelings can be of greatly differing kinds. The feeling of Jesus for the demoniac differs from his feeling

> for the beloved disciple; but the love is the one lone love. Feelings are "entertained"; love comes to pass. Feelings dwell in man; but man dwells in his love. That is no metaphor, but the actual truth. Love does not cling to the *I* in such a way as to have the *Thou* only for its "content," its object; but love is *between I* and *Thou*".
>
> (Buber, 1958, pp. 14–15)[29]

> Elsewhere, Buber says, "Living mutual relation includes feelings, but does not originate with them."
>
> (ibid., p. 45)

Thus, love for Buber is always "between *I* and *Thou*"; it is not something that one simply feels inside one's mind, or at least not only that, because love involves free, flowing, and unrestrained responsibility that one willingly embraces towards the one they call *Thou*. By "between," Buber means the impossible to objectify, "immediate presence of unreserved, spontaneous mutuality common to each person, yet beyond the sphere of either" (Kramer & Gawlick, 2003, p. 202), in which one assumes responsibility to and for the other. As Levinas notes, responsibility can be an expression of being-for-the-other before being-for-the-self, or at least as much as the self (Levinas, 1985). Such relationships, says Buber, are ultimately a result of will, of intention, of turning to the other in an open and welcoming manner, and "grace" that comes from the other. Grace is the spirit of "the between" that emanates from, motivates, and buttresses such genuine interhuman meetings (Kramer & Gawlick, 2003, p. 202). Relational grace points to the gift-giving character of genuine relation. Buber describes it is as a co-created irruption of divine immanence: "The creature waits for him. God waits for him. From him, from 'below,' the impulse toward redemption must proceed. Grace is God's answer" (Buber, 1960, pp. 122–123). Likewise, Marcel describes the "hidden impulse of grace" (Marcel, 1973, pp. 42–43), that is, to "a spiritual dynamism of a completely different kind from a mere psychological disposition whose ground and main driving force is to be found in transcendence" (Marcel, 1964, p. 221). What Buber and Marcel are suggesting is that we need to "open ourselves to those infiltrations of the invisible... the radiance of that eternal Light," that point to the spirit of Beauty, Truth and Goodness personified in love (Marcel, 2001b, pp. 187–188).

That Buber claims that "love is responsibility of an *I* for a *Thou*" helps explain his use of the previously mentioned crucifixion metaphor. That is, he means to suggest that to struggle to that "dreadful point" of loving—especially a hard-to-love other, or "all men" as Buber calls them—is an act of self-donation, of giving until it hurts, that calls a crucifixion to mind.[30] Such an act of self-donation "implies the constant risk of one's whole being in gift to one's fellows" (Moore, 1996, p. 118).[31] This is much more than mere feeling or affect, as usually conceptualized by analysts; it is an endangering, bold existential commitment of one's whole being in the present to one's dialogical partner, especially in terms of their vulnerability, weakness and neediness, in which one feels chosen and chooses, and which calls to mind a sacrifice. Such "sacrifice and risk" (Buber, 1958, p. 10) is a kind of suffering for the other's suffering, and it is this genuine relation, a real going to the other, a reaching to the other, that involves a significant personal cost on some level that points to Buberian love (Moore, 1996, p. 117). As the nineteenth-century Lithuanian rabbi Israel Salanter famously said, "The other's material needs are my spiritual needs" (Levinas, 1990, p. 99).

It was Maurice Friedman who pointed out that what Buber calls "experiencing the other side" can be viewed as "the essence of all genuine love" (Friedman, 2002, p. 102). "Experiencing the other side" bears a "family resemblance" to empathy, as analysts and others usually describe it, but it is also markedly different, and this difference is extremely important to Buber's conception of love. Indeed, accurate empathic immersion is a vital process for discerning what is perceived as the same in the self and the other, and thus it is necessary to create the sense of mutuality that is so important in love relationships. Empathy, a major concept in psychoanalytic theory and technique, has been defined in two major clinical texts as "the imagining of another's subjective experience through the use of one's own subjective experience" and "the ego's capacity to transiently identify with someone else in order to grasp his or her subjective experience" (Akhtar, 2009, p. 93; Person, Cooper, & Gabbard, 2005, p. 551). This being said, while empathy as psychoanalytically defined has its usefulness in terms of reinstating symmetry and mutuality between two lovers, it is a concept that Buber (as well as Marcel) has enlarged and deepened, which suggests why empathy as defined above may not be enough to "put things right" between conflicting lovers. Something "more," "higher," and "better" is required.

Let's use an evocative example of a man caressing a woman he is making love with and his singular goal being not to satiate his lustful sexual urge. This reflects a very different kind of meaning, in which the man makes giving the woman pleasure, satisfaction and comfort his priority, before seeking and concentrating on his own. In this context, the goal is to bring about the living presence of the one to the other, as a constant responsibility for the other's soul. Here, I am interested in mapping the subtle co-creative interplay of two subjectivities (Wyschogrod, 2000, p. 131), the sharing of worlds of subjective experience. Buber beautifully captures this form of caress:

> A man caresses a woman, who lets herself be caressed. Then let us assume that he feels the contact from two sides—with the palm of his hand still, and also with the woman's skin. The twofold nature of the gesture, as one that takes place between two persons, thrills through the depth of enjoyment in his heart and stirs it. If he does not deafen his heart he will have—not to renounce the enjoyment but—to love.
>
> (Buber, 1965a, p. 96)

Buber is making a crucial point here that psychoanalysis misses in its understanding of empathy, or at least underplays the ethically transformative potential of the erotic encounter: the need for a person to be able to "experience the other side" (ibid.). "Experiencing the other side," says Friedman, "means to feel an event from the side of the person one meets as well as from one's own side" (Friedman, 2002, p. 102). Most importantly, it involves what Buber calls "inclusiveness," which realizes the other person in the actuality and "presentness" of his being (Buber, 1965a, p. 97). "Confirmation," the affirmation, acceptance, and support of the other in his uniqueness, including challenging the other when required, is the main consequence of inclusion (Kramer & Gawlick, p. 202). For Buber, inclusiveness should not be confused with the psychoanalytic notion of "empathy," the defining means by which the data of psychoanalysis is collected according to self-psychologists. Empathy, say Buber and Friedman, implies the capacity to "transpose oneself over there and in there," into the dynamic structure of an object, to "the exclusion of one's own concreteness, the extinguishing of the actual situation of life, the absorption in pure aestheticism of the reality in which one participates" (Buber, 1965a, p. 97; Friedman, 2002, p. 102). Inclusion, says Buber, is the opposite of this: "It is the extension of one's own concreteness, the fulfillment of the actual situation in life, the complete presence of the reality in which one participates" (Buber, 1965a, p. 97). Put in more conventional psychological language, we can roughly say that such a recast notion of empathy involves both being able to put your self inside the other without losing your self and at the same time being able to put the other in your self without eradicating the other's difference and otherness. How a self's ego is supple enough to incorporate or, more aptly, embrace the other into its experience without having to project anything upon or into the other is not clear, nor is it agreed upon by most psychoanalytic and social psychological theoreticians on empathy (Todd, 2003).

In summary, Buberian love can be described as the full flourishing of the *Thou*-relation that is realized in meeting and thus transcends the phenomena, whether they are bodily or mental (i.e., it is not a mere feeling, though it includes it). Moreover, love involves embracing the totality of existential circumstances that constitute the whole person in his uniqueness, perceived as dialogical partner, in contrast to seeing the other as a mirror of one's self-serving needs and desires, a form of narcissistic monologue camouflaged as dialogue. Genuine dialogue, says Buber, means that "each of the participants really has in mind the other or others in their present and particular being and turns to them with the intention of establishing a living mutual relation between himself and them" (Buber, 1965b, p. 19). While this dialogical capacity involves the willingness and ability to "experience the other side," to openly give and receive what emanates from the other side, in some sense this is the phenomenological staging ground of Buberian love in its most evolved form. Genuine dialogue, admittedly a fleeting experience, says Buber, not only affirms the other as a whole person in his unique presence in the here-and-now, but involves the enactment in real life of responsibility to and for the other. As Wood puts it, "Love is the supreme articulation of the Between, Now, the Between in the Word [the domain of the Between, the primary relatedness binding a person to a person]: taking one's stand in the Word furnishes the basis for response to the Thou and it is only in terms of actual response that authentic responsibility occurs" (Wood, 1969, p. 60) Indeed, Shakespeare made a similar point when he succinctly said in *Two Gentleman of Verona* (Act I, Scene II), "They do not love [actually and completely] that do not show their love." Finally, for Buber, all love relations call to mind the eternal Thou, also called the "absolute Person," that is, God, conceived as the beginningless and endless Thou (the Person who can't be limited). "God is the Being that is directly, most nearly, and lastingly, over against us, that may properly only be addressed and not expressed" (addressed like a friend, parent or a child) (Buber, 1958, pp. 80–81). The eternal Thou can never morph into an It, it can never become an object of our experience, nor can it be exploited or used. That is, like Marcel's absolute Thou, Buber's eternal Thou is always veiled and obscure, and may stay completely nonreflective or intuitive (Anderson, 2006, p. 134). For Buber, the eternal Thou occurs via will and grace and can be glimpsed in every particular Thou in all genuine relationships: "Meet the world with the fullness of your being and you shall meet Him. That He Himself accepts from your hands what you have to give to the world is His mercy. If you wish to learn to believe, love!" (Buber, 1967b, pp. 212–213).[32]

Marcel

Love for Marcel is "the essential ontological datum," that is, it is intrinsic to the structure of human existence, of being-as-such, as he conceives it:

> Love, in so far as distinct from desire or as opposed to desire [i.e., pure passion, erotic attraction], love treated as the subordination of the self to a superior reality at my deepest level more truly me than I am myself, love as the breaking of the tension between the self and other, appears to be what we might call the essential ontological datum.
>
> (Marcel, 1965a, p. 167)

What Marcel means by love as "the essential ontological datum" is that it requires a commitment to, and a responsibility for, the other, one that can only be made when there is mindfulness "of the absolute value and eternity of the person loved" (Keen, 1967, p. 32). As Keen explains, love, also called "unconditional fidelity," affirms that the beloved is not spiritually destroyable: "To say that one loves a being … means … Thou, at least, thou shalt not die," as one of Marcel's characters says in a play (Marcel, 2001b, p. 61). What this means is that love is best understood as "a reality-relation, not an image or a memory of a shadow, but the 'still existing' of what 'no longer exists,' an *indefectible* [not affected by decay or failure] non-shadow, non-image" (Cain, 1995, p. 100). Any other assertion is a form of betrayal because to relinquish one's loved other when they die is to interpret "silence and indivisibility for annihilation" (ibid.). In the mind and heart of the lover, neither the passage of time or even actual death can ultimately destroy the trace of disclosed being of the beloved. While the lover knows that actual physical death is inevitable, in the most evolved form of love, the lover makes the astonishing demand for "everlastingness"; but most importantly, there is the heartfelt pledge that the co-created reality experienced within the relationship is inexhaustible and cannot be snuffed out by death (ibid.). It is, in part, for this reason that Marcel believed that love is the only way to effectively counter the dehumanizing objectification and problematization that so characterize contemporary relationships in our "broken world." The "broken world" refers to how we have been "leveled" as people according to our functionality (bureaucracy, technology, and social regimentation), and where betrayal and other forms of interpersonal treason are encouraged for practical purposes, such as getting ahead in a job or staying in a loveless marriage for self-serving financial reasons.

In his magnum opus, *The Mystery of Being*, Marcel states clearly what "genuine" love is, though he notes this is merely a "cut and dried answer" (because it suggests a dualist conception of the lover and the loved) that needs considerable elaboration:

> Under what conditions can love be known as genuine? At this stage of our investigation we may be satisfied with saying that my love is the more authentic according as I love less for my own sake, that for what I can hope to obtain from another, and more for the sake of the other.
>
> (Marcel, 2001b, p. 98)

Similar to Buber, and maybe before him, Marcel indicates that "it is possible to transcend the level of the self and the other; it is transcended both in love and in charity [i.e., self-donation, like love of God and neighbor]. Love moves on a ground which is neither that of the self, nor that of the other *qua* other; I call it the Thou" [what Marcel calls the domain of "mystery," Buber's "between," though Marcel also speaks about the "between" co-belonging"] (Marcel, 1965a, p. 167; Marcel, 1967, pp. 43, 46).[33]

In these two quotations, we begin to apprehend that all love involves a radical openness to the other, what Marcel calls "disposability" or "spiritual availability" (henceforth, "availability"). Availability is a certain kind of openness and receptivity to the other as exemplified in love, fidelity, faith (including grace), and hope. Such an existential preparedness involves being "permeable"; however, Marcel further refines his phenomenological analysis by using the evocative word "porosity," as easy to cross, infiltrate, and penetrate, to point to the inner state of readiness that makes the experience of love possible (Marcel, 1964, p. 87).[34] Marcel converges these notions in his discussion of love by describing love as equivalent to "communion." Communion can be roughly defined as the sharing of intimate thoughts and feelings, especially when the give-and-take is on a deeply psychological or spiritual level. While Marcel says communion emanates from love, in fact "communion is love" (Gallagher, 1962, p. 78). That is, while the other can be responded to as other (though not as an absolute or wholly other, which would make him or her inaccessible and un-addressable; Treanor, 2006),[35] there is the likelihood for communion between the self and other that acts like a modulating bridge between them as they engage in person-to-person participation. In other words, for Marcel, unlike perhaps Levinas, "the independent inner reality of the other person is not violated or diminished by his participation in an intersubjective relationship with the self, a relationship that takes place in a shared reality" (ibid., p. 100). Marcel does not hold that participation in shared reality, including a universal shared reality, inevitably means the loss or subversion of independent, individual realities or the other's otherness. In other words, universality is not to be confused with totality, as Levinas claims (ibid.).

In light of the aforementioned, the main aspects of Marcel's notion of love can be briefly summarized (Gallagher, 1962, pp. 78–79). First, love does not pertain to a hermetically sealed or monadic essence but, instead, opens up onto an infinity, a kind of presence which no kind of actuarial or calculative thinking can pin down or deplete. Second, the beloved is in a certain sense beyond anything except a superficial characterization—for example, she is sweet and funny—or judgment—for example, she acted mean and selfish—for this implies that the totality of what constitutes the beloved qua beloved can be objectified as if she were merely a finite thing or thing-like. And finally, love engages the being of the beloved and not simply one's notion, conception or idea of her. The beloved's presence is more than, and different than, what one can say in words, however well crafted (it is more presence than content, more testimonial than description).[36]

Thus, for Marcel, similar to Buber, love is the ultimate expression of intersubjective communion, an act of mutual, unique, non-objectifiable, and personal relationship in which two persons surrender themselves to each other's presence with the fullness of their whole being. For Marcel, love when experientially described "is a *union* of lover and loved, a participation of each in the reality of the other" (Anderson, 2006, p. 142), a co-created relationship in which paradoxically two people "become one while yet remaining two" ("each in being himself makes the other be") (Machado, 1961, pp. 55, 60).[37] Love thus reflects one aspect of the "mystery of being," an aspect of human experience that reassuringly points to an eternal, infinite, Divine reality which provides ultimate meaning, value and truth, what Marcel calls "ontological weight," to human existence (Marcel, 1965a, p. 103). "Real love," says Marcel, presupposes "the active recognition, in God and through God, of the bond which constitutes all real love" (Marcel, 2001b, p. 98). However, Marcelian love, conceived of as the "royal road" to access the "mystery of being," always includes fidelity and hope, which I want to briefly describe.

How can a partner astonishingly promise to love their significant other forever? For Marcel, fidelity, that free (and, most importantly, freely chosen), flowing, unrestrained self-donation, is an expression of one's intimate being, a self-giving that is grounded in the mystery of being, that "plenitude" that affirms our most profound exigence (irrepressible urge) as a person, our conviction that serving both the other and God (to the believer, or the transcendent for the non-believer) is the main purpose of our being in the world (for Marcel and Buber, it appears essence precedes existence, unlike the atheistic existentialists who believe existence precedes essence).[38] Put more straightforwardly, it is through the loving engagement with and belief in the finite empirical "thou's" goodness that one is able to assert, "I will love thee forever." A belief in the eternal goodness of the finite other is a form of bonding with and witness to the infinite, all-good God that is also supremely self-affirming to the believer. Fidelity, in part a volitional act of commitment and responsibility to and for the other, is rooted in a willingness to remain "available," "open," and responsive to the other's needs and wishes, often before one's own. Marcel calls this continuous, dynamic, transformative openness to participation and self-giving "permeability" (Marcel, 1964, p. 172). As Cain so aptly suggests, the type of promise-making that embodies the highest form of Marcelian fidelity "is an act of 'consecration' in response to the call or manifestation of transcendence ... a unity of personal decision and transcendent command is involved" (Cain, 1995, p. 124). In other words, "personal self-creation" as it applies to faithfulness in a relationship requires a receptivity "to transcendent, supra-personal reality" in which the person is ultimately satisfied. It requires "self-consecration and self-sacrifice to something beyond oneself—a 'creative fidelity' to being" (Cain, 1963, p. 81). According to Marcel then, fidelity to the empirical "thou," the loved other, calls to mind the "Absolute Thou," God, that transcendent reality of "infinite plentitude" (Marcel, 1964, p. 37), which is experienced as a cherished person intimately related to me (Anderson, 2006, p. 68). To reside in this dimension of the spirit characterized by fidelity to the thou/Absolute Thou is a manifestation of fidelity to being, to the peace of being. Being is an opaque fullness, fulfillment that quickens and refreshes as it points to the eternal/transcendent in one's existential circumstances (Gallagher, 1962). Anderson aptly summarizes why it is thus possible to promise unconditional fidelity to one's beloved (or good friend), why I feel compelled by the promise I made: Such a person experiences "albeit vaguely, both his being and his beloved's being participating in an eternal dimension of reality which can only be described as personal or supra-personal ['a supra-temporal depth of myself, my eternal being']—or, as he [Marcel] prefers to say, as an Absolute Thou. It is apparently in the veiled experience of such a Being, who is the absolute ground and guarantee of our fidelity, that we glimpse the promise that the complete fulfillment of our intersubjective union, and hence of ourselves, will take place in Eternity" (Anderson, 1985, pp. 280–281).

Thus, the person who lives his human and non-human relationships with "creative fidelity"—fidelity conceived of "as the hold the other has over us"—tends to experience his life at a "higher" level of autonomy and integration, at a "higher" register of being, certainly compared to someone who betrays the trust placed in me (Marcel, 1965a, p. 46). What is "creative" about "creative fidelity" is the lover's will and ability to engage in "constant reinvocation of the presence of the other," and not to be utterly reduced to two thing-like organisms emotionally blunted by everyday routine (Wood, 1999, p. 89). It is this theme of unfaithfulness—"betrayal as evil in itself," as Marcel describes it—that Marcel was deeply troubled about (Marcel, 1965a, p. 41). Betrayal for Marcel was a form of self-obsession or "self-worship," of "unavailability," of "closed-in-ness"; it is a way of staying riveted to the selfish self and indifferent to the other and the higher claims of intersubjectivity, an entitled way of being that claims through one's words and actions that "I am," rather than "we are." If, as Marcel says, "being," authentic selfhood "is the place of fidelity," then non-being, inauthentic selfhood is the place of betrayal.

And finally, Marcel claims that like fidelity, hope is always an aspect of love (in fact, fidelity/hope/love are deeply entwined).[39] Indeed, unlike desire, which is focused on what one wants for oneself (e.g., to possess a paramour), hope focuses on the we and the thou: "I hope in thee for us," an affirmation accentuating that to hope involves being other-directed, other-regarding and other-serving. While Marcel grasps that hope is a scale concept often enacted in trivial contexts (e.g. like hoping one's sports team wins), this is not the hope he is describing (Gallagher, 1962). "Hope," says Marcel,

> consists in asserting that there is at the heart of being, beyond all data, beyond all inventories and all calculations, a mysterious principle which is in connivance with me, which cannot but will that which I will, if what I will deserves to be willed and is, in fact, willed by the whole of my being.
> (Marcel, 1995, p. 28)

Hope is thus is an expression of that irrepressible human urge towards "something more," "something higher," and "something better," towards transcendence (that "unknown and higher dimension of reality attainable through human experience"; Cain, 1963, p. 115); it "is engaged in the weaving of experience now in process or, in other words, is an adventure now going forward" (Marcel, 1965b, p. 52).[40] Hope, says Marcel, is an "exigency," a fundamental impulse or striving of being, "a deep-rooted interior urge … an appeal" (Marcel, 2001b, p. 37) and thus is one of the fundamental ways in which freedom is affirmed. Hope, when it is joined with a robust imagination, generates the freedom to expand possibility: "I act freely if the motives of my act are in line with what I can legitimately regard as the structural features of my personality" (Marcel, 1973, p. 86). What needs to be emphasized here is that for Marcel hope is better conceived of as "hoping"; that is, the phenomenology of hope reveals that it is not simply a fixed idea that one possesses, but rather a processive, emergent and renewable psychological and behavioral activity that tends to upsurge in particularly challenging contexts,[41] in "extreme" situations of imprisonment. "Hope," says Marcel, "is a response to tragedy" (Pruyser, 1963, p. 92). While there is much more to Marcelian hope, perhaps the clearest summary of what Marcel is getting at, at least as it pertains to the love relationship, can be found in his masterpiece, *Homo Viator, Introduction to a Metaphysic of Hope*:

> We might say that hope is essentially the availability of a soul that has entered intimately enough into the experience of communion [the love relation] to accomplish in the teeth of will and knowledge the transcendental act [an act that is not restricted to what our desires are and what we reckon]—the act establishing the vital regeneration of which this experience affords both the pledge and the first-fruits [the love relation is an experience already ours, and also an inkling of what could possibly be].
>
> (Marcel, 1965b, p. 67)

Hope thus requires a willing receptivity and engagement with others; in fact, it is this aspect of hoping that Marcel claims is its foundation: "There can be no hope which does not constitute itself through a *we* and for a *we*" (Marcel, 1973, p. 143). Most importantly, in Marcel's ontology it is this characteristic of hope that points to God. For Marcel, it is one's relationship to others, most directly and profoundly one's loving relationships, those animated by Goodness, Truth, and Beauty, that are the "royal road" to the transcendent God. God, the Divine realm, can thus be conceptualized as "the 'Absolute Thou' who lurks in the truncated experience of presence felt as human communion" (Early & Gallagher, 2003, p. 134). Such a point of entry to the summoning God is not beyond everyday experience, but within it, what to the believer is embraced as moments of holiness (Marquez, 2017). "The way to heaven," Marcel warned, "is to dig down deep where you are" (Cain, 1963, p. 81). Marcel spoke of the "ontological exigence," an impulse or urge that was the bedrock of the human condition, an irrepressible need, even a "demand" for the presence of being. Marcel's "being is an 'Absolute Thou,' not the whole of reality, a particular being, not being in general," but rather his God is an impulse to which we are mysteriously tied, "immanent in yet transcending our experience, to which we have access by the act we are at liberty to realize or not" (Rosthal, 1964, p. xii). It is, as I have said, by way of communion broadly described, that one creatively pursues the Absolute Thou, a way of being that is also self-authenticating and the basis for one's self-presence (Pax, 1975, p. 20).[42] "Perpetual renewal," says Cain, "and continual self-intimacy" thus "go together" (Cain, 1995, p. 111). It is through the intimations of hoping and the cautious confidence regarding the future it implies that is the surest testimony of the Godly, mysterious realm (Cooper, 1998, p. 92). In a word, one becomes irrepressibly aware of the transcendent and bountiful nature of being, at its best. Love then for Marcel, like Buber, demands prior to anything else the free, flowing, and unrestrained availability enacted as the joyful welcoming of the other as Thou.

Implications for treatment

What then can a Buberian/Marcelian understanding of love offer to a psychoanalysis conceived of as a spiritual discipline? That is, while analysts tend to view love in terms of the individual's personal experience of it, a "spirituality of me," Buber and Marcel focus on the "spirituality of us," associated with the best of marriage or a partnered monogamous relationship (Mahoney, 2013, p. 365). In fact, in contrast to the *cogito ergo sum*, Marcel called his overall philosophy "a metaphysics of *we are*" (Marcel, 2001b, p. 10). Analysts, of course, have reaffirmed what Buber and Marcel and many love theorists before them have suggested, that the romantic love relation is a co-created, co-potentiating and co-occurring happening, that while fraught with possible impediments, as Freud claimed,[43] is perhaps the main port of entry to a modicum of experienced happiness. Indeed, as professor of family and consumer studies N.H. Wolfinger (2019, n.p.) noted in his recent analysis of survey marriage data, in general and in sync with prior research, married people [and by extension, I would add, those involved in a partnered monogamous relationship], both husbands and wives, are happier (and less unhappy) than their unmarried peers. "The story is straightforward: married respondents are much happier." Moreover, researchers have found that when a marriage is lodged in a relationship characterized by "mutual trust, good communication and healthy conflict management," it tends to be more satisfying for both partners regardless of the sexual orientation of the couple (Compton & Hoffman, 2020, p. 139). Indeed, while marriage was the accepted convention in the time in which they lived, Buber was happily married for 58 years ("marriage is the exemplary bond"; Buber, 1965b, p. 61), Marcel, for 28 years (his wife died before him), Levinas for 63 years, and Freud for 53. Here is what Freud's grieving widow Martha said about him in her 11/7/1939 letter to Ludwig Binswanger thanking him for his condolences:

> How good dear Dr., that you knew him when he was still in the prime of his life, for in the end he suffered terribly so that even those who would most liked to keep him forever had to wish for his release! And yet how terribly difficult it is to have to do without him. To continue to live without so much kindness and wisdom beside one! It is a small comfort for me to know in the fifty-three years of our married life not one angry word fell between us, and that I always ought as much as possible to remove from his path the misery of everyday life. Now my life has lost all content and meaning.
>
> (Grotjahn, 1967, p. 124)[44]

The aforementioned is noteworthy because it affirms the Buberian/Marcelian spiritual sensibility and valuative attachments pertinent to love: Freud's "kindness and wisdom," his lack of aggression towards Martha ("not one angry word"), the fact that he generated in Martha a wish to shield him from suffering, even to the point of her willingness to give him up rather than watch him suffer ("I suffer, therefore you are"), and the fact that he was the center of her universe are all tell-tale signs of an *I-Thou* relationship (as opposed to the *I* being the center of the universe in an *I-It* relationship). And finally, there is the fact that Martha's sense of "content and meaning" resides mainly in fidelity to the eternal memory of her loving service to Freud's best interests. As Mark Twain noted, "Love seems the swiftest, but it is the slowest of all growths. No man or woman really knows what perfect love is until they have been married [or in a partnered monogamous relationship] a quarter of a century" (Charles & Carstensen, 2002).

Buber and Marcel emphasize that spirituality involves the will and ability to restore the sacred into everyday life, what Marcel in affinity with Heidegger called affirming the "sacral dignity of being" (Marcel, 1973 p. 247). What this means is that the love relationship is to be regarded as reflecting the individual's quest for the sacred which Buber and Marcel (and Levinas) believe is the best of being human in the world. For all three philosophers, "holiness" in one's way of being-in-the-world is the ultimate ideal. Buber and Marcel describe holiness somewhat differently, but like Levinas, they all point in a certain direction, such that holiness includes, for example, hallowing the world, participating in a transcendent reality that evokes awe, love and fear, and being for the other before oneself. By sacred, Buber and Marcel are alluding to the perception of "something more," "something higher," and "something better," requiring cherishment and ethicality. For Buber and Marcel, both theistic believers in varying ways, the love relation is both an expression and affirmation of the human perception of a trace of the divine, transcendent reality, what they call God (e.g., the Eternal Thou or Absolute Thou), which summons the lover to being, first, other-directed, other-regarding, and other-serving (and if not first, then at least being-for-the-other as much as for oneself). This is the moment when *I-Thou*, even though by definition turns into I-It, nevertheless leaves a trace that ripples through one's whole being (one's feelings, thoughts, and actions), and becomes dispositional as opposed to a passing phenomenon (including relating to the It-world differently). Put simply, "Meeting with a Thou is thus not an aesthetic, but a *vocational* experience. It leads to a transformation of our lives," a more flourishing one (Wood, 1999, p. 88).

While Buber and Marcel stressed that the quest for the sacred/divine always travels through I-Thou relationships conceived of as one of mutuality and whole-subject-to-whole subject, Buber also believed that one could have an I-Thou relationship as he did, with say a tree, horse, cat, piece of mica, Doric pillar or a book; and Marcel implied that an I-Thou–like moment was possible when listening/playing music or watching/reading a great play. Researchers have noted that one of the factors that makes a flourishing marriage last (and I would assume, a partnered monogamous relationship) is that it is regarded by the parties as a "sacred institution" (or sacred bond, in secular language), a tangible sanctified result of a sacred gift from God (or its secular equivalent) (Lauer, Lauer, & Kerr, 1990). Feeling one is with one's "soulmate" can involve a God or God-like imagining, like "feeling blessed" or "relational grace," though a popular secular definition of "soulmate" points to a similar sentiment: "A soulmate is someone that just gets you. It's a connection of minds, a mutual respect, an unconditional love and a total understanding. It's about being yourself and knowing, not only that person is following and understanding your thoughts, but is right there with you, side by side" (www.refinery29.com>em-gb>soulmate-signs-definition retrieved 11/9/19).

While the previously mentioned "god talk" may trouble secular analysands and analysts, by God I mean the person's felt bond with the spirit of the sacred, understanding that people's conceptions and imaginings of God, whether "theistic or nontheistic, tangible or abstract, immanent or transcendent, personal or transpersonal," are diverse across persons, communities, and cultures (Mahoney, 2013, p. 369). In the positive psychology literature, defined as the search for personal strengths and virtues, there is a helpful distinction between two types of spirituality; both include a need and desire to relate to something greater than oneself that usually requires at least a modicum of self-transcendence. "There is no room for God in him who is full of himself," said Buber (2006, p. 102), and Marcel referred to "pride," the fantasy of self-sufficiency that manifests as "holding back" and "closed-in-ness," as lethal to a love relationship: "Where pride reigns there is no room for mercy [love]" (Marcel, 1973, p. 95). "Vertical transcendence" involves fostering a relationship with a spiritual being who is "higher" and "greater" than oneself, as in Buber's Jewish and Marcel's Christian view of God. When spirituality takes on a specifically religious expression, the quest for the sacred takes place in an institutional context like a church, synagogue, mosque or temple. "Horizontal transcendence" involves forming a relationship with a force that is more immanent in the world and is less often conceived of as a spiritual being. Taoism (a religion that Buber admiringly wrote about in 1910, early in his career)[45] views the *Tao* as the force that motivates and upholds the natural order of the universe (Compton & Hoffman, 2020, p. 395). As Buber said, "The atheist staring from his attic window is often nearer to God than the believer caught up in his own false image of God" (Margulies, 2017, p. 66). In psychoanalysis, the relational perspective has recently described the allegedly "universal … tragic and existential dimensions of the human condition" such as inner dividedness, hiddenness, self-deception, lack, loss and finitude (Slavin, 2016, p. 537), all themes that are profoundly discussed in the great ancient religious and spiritual wisdom traditions (Marcus, 2003). While these common existential themes are important to reckon with analytically (including regarding love), they are, in fact, interminable/unresolvable aspects of human existence, as we know it. However, such reflective activity that is linked to the otherness in oneself and others (a theme Buber and Marcel emphasized) was characterized by one relational analyst as "tragic in a deeply moving, ennobling, in what some might call a spiritual sense" (Slavin, 2016, p. 537).[46]

So, what specifically does the Buberian/Marcelian conception of love add to psychoanalysis conceived as a spiritual discipline? Briefly, Buber and Marcel have pointed to a spiritual sensibility, rooted in a transcendent domain of being-in-the-world that demands enacting a set of life-affirming and identity-defining valuative attachments which make loving behavior accessible in a sustained manner. Perhaps most importantly, responsibility for and to the other is the lynchpin of love in its most evolved form. As Oppenheim (2017, p. 130) noted, responsibility is an undertheorized notion in contemporary psychoanalysis, which has not entirely avoided the subject, but "usually appears in a limited form" (probably because it is associated with authoritarian moralizing). To further answer the earlier question, I will mention two important quotes from Buber and Marcel (the latter a paraphrase) which suggest, among other things, how a skillfully crafted, spiritual/religiously animated language can open up non-apprehended existential spaces in the analysand and analyst.

Buber noted that the "Dialogic is not to be identified with love. But love without dialogic, without real outgoing to the other, reaching to the other, the love remaining with itself—this is called Lucifer" (Buber, 1965b, p. 21). Marcel too claimed that he who rejects the absolute Thou (i.e., the loving Creator) and therefore centers himself solely on himself, closing himself in on himself, makes a decision that is "Demonic" (Marcel, 2001b, pp. 181, 194). As mentioned, for Buber and Marcel, this "reaching to the other" can in part be equated with embracing certain valuative attachments that are instantiated in the real-life, everyday love relations and called the "sacred emotions" that deepen and expand the spiritual connection between two lovers, for they personify "reaching to the other," if not being-for-the-other. As Aron notes, "Analysts must accept responsibility for the fact that it is their own personality, their own subjectivity, that underlies their values and beliefs, that infuses their theoretical convictions, and that forms the basis for their technical interventions and clinical judgments" (Aron, 1996, p. 259). A loving couple needs to be willing and able to sustain the difficulties that typically emerge in most love relationships (this is the bailiwick of psychoanalysis), what Sternberg in his triangular theory of love (1986; Sternberg & Hojjat, 1997) called assaults on "consummate love," the love that integrates passion (*eros*, erotic desire), intimacy (warmth, closeness, sharing), and commitment (deciding to sustain the relationship). But the kind of love relationship that Buber and Marcel were pointing to includes these critical factors, but strives for "something more," "something higher," and "something better." Paraphrasing Marcel, "You know you have loved someone when you have glimpsed in them that which is too beautiful, too true, and too good to die." Every love relation, infused with fidelity and hope, thus signifies a trace of eternity for Marcel. The way to access being-in-a-love-relationship is, in part, through the cultivation of, and attunement to, sacred emotions that point to "something more," "something higher," and "something better," such as gratitude, forgiveness, compassion, humility. A few brief comments on these sacred emotions are illustrative of how Buberian/Marcelian spirituality can be enacted in real life.

Gratitude, the willingness and ability to be thankful that evokes the wish to return kindness, has a central role in all ancient religious and spiritual wisdom traditions; it also has been regarded as important in contemporary secular contexts. For example, as early as the 1960s American psychologist Abraham Maslow emphasized that what he believed was the innate drive for self-actualization in part culminated in a person embracing a "count your blessings" outlook (Compton & Hoffman, 2020, p. 316). Likewise, Winnicott believed that the infant (and later the adult), if provided with the facilitating environment, has an "inherent potential to care about the (m)other," and that "goodness and morality and forward movement don't have to be taught, rather it is *there* waiting to be found and met" (Slochower, 2018, pp. 99, 100). Gratitude is an expression of this "goodness and morality," as Melanie Klein noted in her formulations of the infantile basis of gratitude: "A full gratification at the breast means that the infant feels that he has received from his love object a unique gift which he wants to keep. This is the basis of gratitude," an experience that is entwined with trust and generosity (Klein, 1957, p. 189).

Another way of thinking of gratitude plays off the ancient "count your blessings" notion that Maslow believed was part of self-actualization. For Buber and Marcel, such a saying is headed in the right direction when it comes to love but needs to be expanded by using a modern saying like: "When I count my blessings, I count you twice." The "you" denotes a person who acts as a blessing in someone's life, an acknowledgment that there is something miraculous-like that the person evokes by virtue of being in the person's life that deserves, if not demands cherishment, a manifestation of the "mystery of being," as Marcel calls it. The capacity to experience and express gratitude personified the spiritual sensibility that Marcel advocated, just as Maslow, Winnicott, and Klein believed that experiencing and expressing gratitude were important manifestations of a "mentally healthy" person. Indeed, empirical researchers have found that gratitude can function to sustain and improve romantic attachments and friendships (Algoe, Gable, & Maisel, 2010). Moreover, gratitude has been correlated with greater life satisfaction, optimism and more positive and less negative emotional experience (Emmons & Mishra, 2011). Such findings suggest the impressive role gratitude has in enhancing closeness and intimacy, along the lines of Buberian/Marcelian love (Compton & Hoffman, 2020, p. 317). Thus, what Buber and Marcel add to our understanding of gratitude is that when the significant other is viewed as "good," as deserving of our affirmation and cherishment, we are in fact allowing them to view themselves in the reflection of our high regard, which means that we assist them in becoming the best they are capable of being. This is an expression of the other-directed, other-regarding, and other-serving thrust of gratitude.

Forgiveness has been psychologically defined as

> a willingness to abandon one's right to resentment, negative judgment, and indifferent behavior toward someone who has unjustly injured us [from the point of view of the aggrieved party], while fostering undeserved [freely self-donated] qualities of compassion, generosity, and even love toward him or her.
>
> (Enright, Freedman, & Rique, 1998, pp. 46–47)

Indeed, as the well-known saying goes, there is no love without forgiveness and no forgiveness without love. Forgiveness expresses the renewal of hope, the summoning claim the other has on us, that is essential to any workable love relation. Indeed, in a love relation we all periodically feel unfairly treated, that is, narcissistically assaulted, or at least disrespected in terms of what we think we should be getting from our significant other—greater care, more accurate empathy, willingness to sacrifice and the like. Such narcissistic assaults tend to foster resentment, anger, revenge, and other forms of aggression that are common in intimate relationships in some form. However, the capacity to forgive, the compassionate reconfiguration of thought and feeling about the other that forgiveness requires, generates a new moral context for the interpretation of the other's hurtful behavior. When the aggrieved person chooses to give up *his* resentment, even hatred of the perpetrator for his misdeed, it signifies that he is, in effect, willing to deal with the pain that underlies the narcissistic rage evoked by his significant other's misdeed. Forgiveness increases one's range of alternatives just as it enhances one's freedom to grow and develop. It is the basis for the healing process that needs to occur to keep a love relation from disintegrating as a result of our all too human capacity to be destructive to our loved other. Both Buber and Marcel, lodged in the best of Hebrew and Christian Humanism, emphasize that forgiveness is not only one of the best ways to modulate distressing emotions like anger and resentment, which are ultimately self-destructive, but also strengthens our identification with the common humanity in the larger community and, therefore, deepens and expands our capacity for compassion, the lynchpin of spiritual valuative attachments that Buber and Marcel are committed to. In a word, forgiveness in a love relationship is aimed at "putting things right" between two lovers.

Compassion, often referred to as empathy in the analytic and psychological literature (not to be confused with Buber's "experiencing the other side"), involves the willingness and ability to engage another person's personal experience, in particular their suffering, that often leads to an upsurge to help make things better. Indeed, researchers have found a correlation between compassion and altruism that is decidedly operative in a love relation, such that one feels summoned to reduce one's partner's suffering through concrete ameliorative actions (Compton & Hoffman, 2020, p. 320). The Latin root for the word *compassion* means "suffering with" the beloved, calling to mind the great Biblical narratives in the Hebrew and Christian Bibles in which, for example, God had compassion on Israel and Christ God forgave you. Both Buber and Marcel would agree with Elie Wiesel, who described man's ethical outlook as it is instantiated in a love relationship, in which I choose to take on the burden of the other's suffering in compassion-infused fidelity and hope: "I suffer, therefore you are" (Berenbaum, 1994, p. 139).

Finally, we come to humility; a mode of comportment that empirical humility researcher J.P. Tangney said "is relatively rare" (2000, pp. 81–82). "True love," says Marcel, "is humble" (Marcel, 2001b, p. 83). By this, he means that in a love relationship the focus is on service to the honored other, without feeling that such sustained giving with the fullness of one's being is self-diminishing, or necessarily needs to be returned or even acknowledged. Humility for Marcel, like other Catholic thinkers, is conceived as a "moral virtue" by which a person freely embraces the profound and far-reaching idea that all of his "good—nature and grace, being and action—is a gift of God's creative and salvific love" (Gilleman, 2003, p. 205). For Marcel, the main thrust of humility is that it is "a mode of being" (Marcel, 2001b, p. 87) and not an isolated personality trait or character asset as it is usually conceived of in psychological and other circles. Rather, humility is best conceived of as an existential comportment that tends to animate a person's everyday way of thinking, feeling, and acting. Humility, continues Marcel, is "the act by which a human consciousness is led to acknowledge itself as tributary to something other than itself ... one from whom it holds its very being" (Marcel, 2001b, p. 88).[47] For Marcel, this "something other" is the absolute Thou, his term for God, and the apprehension of this divine being requires "creative receptivity" ["simultaneously throwing one's-self open and offering one's-self up," Marcel, 1965a, p. 188)], such that "the human creature turns humbly and freely towards Him from Whom it holds its very being" (Marcel, 2001b, pp. 88, 89). In other words, what Marcel is getting at is that to live humbly involves the mindfulness that the "I" is not the center of the universe. Marcel believes that "the ordering principle of the world is not in his own ego and in the powers of technology he controls" (1973, p. 211). In religious terms, this means to reject pride and the desire to replace God with oneself. The prideful being assumes an anthropocentric outlook; the humble person assumes a mainly theocentric one. In fact, Marcel decries what he calls "practical anthropocentrism," a derivative of the technological mindset in which "technical man" (Marcel, 2008, p. 55) conceives of himself as the only "giver and creator of meaning and value" (Keen, 1967, p. 11). Such a perspective, says Marcel, views the world strictly as neutral raw material to be transformed to satisfy self-serving desires. For the humble secularist, such a prideful mode of being means that rather than submit to the arbitrary and absolute determinism of reality, rather than modulating one's narcissism and egoism with a consciousness of being part of the universe that goes beyond the boundaries of one's individuality, what can be called a cosmic perspective, one denies the recognition of the smallness of one's existence compared to the eternally changing universe.

Final remark

Thus, while mainstream psychoanalysis has had "astonishingly little new thinking" about "sexual passion and enduring love" (Black, 2002, p. 12), and has mainly been involved in understanding "romance and its devaluation" (e.g., the lack of vitality and meaning) (Mitchell, 2002, p. 23),[48] Buber and Marcel made what Levinas called an "essential discovery" that has bearing on love in its most evolved expression (Levinas, 1994, p. 12). This "essential discovery" can have an antidote-like function, not only in suggesting a more profound understanding of love and its demise, but as Freud advocated, in making love central to the overarching goal of any successful analysis. That is, when it comes to love (as well as other matters of "ultimate concern" like work, faith, and suffering), the "essential discovery" is

> affirming that human spirituality—or religiosity—lies in the fact of the proximity [i.e., face-to-face meeting epitomized in love as responsibility for the other] neither lost in the mass nor abandoned to their solitude. This bespeaks both the religious significance of interhuman relations and, conversely, the original possibility and accomplishment of the relation-to-God (that relation to the Invisible, the Non-Given) in the approach of one person to another, addressed as *Thou*.
>
> (Levinas, 1994, pp. 21–22)

Thus, such spiritually animated love, one that has a "quasi-*aesthetic*" and "quasi-religious" dimension (Putnam, 2008, p. 61), can be the basis for the restoration, regeneration, and renewal of love. As Marcel would put it, "I belong to myself only as I do not belong to myself, as I give myself to otherness, and create myself, come into being and so belong to what I am" (Cain, 1995, p. 94). This is the moment when passion and enduring love exquisitely meet, when passion is hallowed and becomes spiritual connection and solidarity with one's *Thou*. At this moment, in the here-and-now of "whole fullness of mutual action," one feels, or rather "receives," an upsurge of an affect-integrating, action-guiding meaning that "has more certitude for you than the perceptions of your senses ... there is an inexpressible confirmation of meaning. Meaning is assured," and this has an eternal and infinite resonance to it, what points to the Divine or secular equivalent (Buber, 1958, p. 110). For example, the literal passionate "kiss" between lovers means something different than when it is simply a sexual urge hunting for lustful pleasure. Rather, the spiritual kiss can be viewed as a hugely subversive act of simultaneous, mutual, and intimate boundary crossing between two people. Such a life-affirming expression of transgressive and transfigurative Eros (Das, 2005, p. 179; O'Donohue, 1997, p. 32) involves both partners engaging with the fullness of their beings in an ardent interflow of other-directed, other-regarding, and other-serving feeling that "touches" the other's luminous inner divinity, and beyond. In this way, it is through the beckoning lips that the soul reveals itself as a sacred presence that summons the other to cherishment and service with both passion and a sense of urgency (O'Donohue, 2004, p.13). If the main purpose of the kiss is disclosure, that is, revelation, then the main content of such revelation is love (Putnam, 2008, p. 54). The spiritual kiss longs for the transcendent, to sense the heavenly presence in the earthly encounter with the loved other. Buber, Marcel, and Levinas all made the crucial point that when two people engage each other in love, whether love conceived as Buber's I and Thou, Marcel's unconditional creative fidelity, or Levinas's responsibility for the Other, it is in this love relation that an ultimately unthematizeable God comes to mind, that He is sensed as a living eternal Presence.[49] Buber noted, "He who loves a woman [any significant other], and brings her life to present realization in his, is able to see in the *Thou* of her eye a beam of the eternal *Thou*" (1958, p. 106). Indeed, the most porous exposure point on the literal face, where love and the trace of God are most manifested, is the lover's lips, the ultimate bodily signifier that points to the sacred presence of the Eternal. Playing off Marcel's aforementioned statement, "To love," and, I would add, to kiss, "is to say: thou, thou wilt never die." For Marcel then, but probably also for Buber, the spiritual kiss is the ultimate, intimate "eternal embrace" (O'Donohue, 2004, pp. 13, 41). It is nothing less than a "caesural" [a dislocating and liberating break or pause] (Fishbane, 2008, p. 33) and "fissure" (Putnam, 2008, p. 104), a threshold-crossing, category-breaking, grace moment when an encounter with the mysterious loved other reveals the glory of Divine tenderness.

Psychoanalysis would be well served to expand and deepen its understanding of love, both in terms of what is potentially life and identity-defining and affirming for the analysand post-analysis but, also, for the analyst as he relates to the analysand in a loving or love-like manner. That is, the art of living a flourishing life, one that correlates with a "difficult" happiness, entails the willingness and ability to deepen and expand one's capacity to fashion a subjectivity in which I-Thou becomes dispositional. In addition to insight and analysis, Buber and Marcel are pointing to the healing power of love, conceived as Being's lived participation in wholly and holy disclosure, truth and communion, when spirit miraculously becomes form.

Notes

1 For example, Freud wrote to Oskar Pfister, a Swiss Lutheran minister and lay psychoanalyst,

> I have found little that is 'good' about human beings on the whole. In my experience most of them are trash, no matter whether they publicly subscribe to this or that ethical doctrine or none at all. That is something that you cannot say aloud, or perhaps even think.
>
> (Freud, 1963, p. 61)

2 For Marcel, "We find ourselves in a broken world. We are dislocated. We are in exile," what calls to mind the Heideggerian "image of existential 'uprootedness'" (Lechner, 1984, p. 462). See for example Marcel (2008).

3 Marcel of course, recognized that betrayal can be refused or denied. Betrayal is manifested in at least two ways in psychoanalytic storytelling. As with all storytelling, the analysand targets his story to a listener, and in doing so he discloses the past, but also transforms it by converting it into something in the present act of speech which, inevitably, is somewhat different from what it actually was in the past. Such betrayal assumes, of course, that it is possible to have such accurate access to the actual past (Kearney, 2002, p. 165). Buber and Marcel imply that it is such betrayal that can be a source of existential guilt. Likewise, as Buber has noted, "The lie is the specific evil which man has introduced into nature .... In a lie the spirit practices reason against itself," and such self-betrayal, a kind of self-oblivion, can also lead to existential guilt as well as neurotic guilt as analysts describe it (Buber, 1953, p. 7).

4 Erich Fromm (1950) noted that "Analytic therapy is essentially an attempt to help the patient gain or regain his capacity for love" (p. 87). The main thrust of this claim has been reaffirmed by many analysts, especially those lodged in the relational perspective (Hoffman, 2011).

5 Love comes in many forms, none of them very clearly formulated, let alone with a consensus among philosophers, psychologists and psychoanalysts, of what love is and how it is instantiated. For example, Aristotle describes *eros* (erotic/romantic love), *agape* (selfless unconditional love), philia (brotherly or friendship love), and storge (familiar love). Buber and Marcel tend to focus on the last three forms of love, and less the bailiwick of psychoanalysis, erotic/romantic love. Similar to Levinas, Marcel (and less Buber) believed that erotic/romantic love was an especially ambiguous notion and prone to perversion and degradation (Treanor, 2006, p. 308). It is common knowledge that the love one feels for a significant other is different than towards say a stranger, a friend or the human community as a whole. Thus, love is best viewed as a "spectrum" notion, one that "comes in degrees" (Brogaard, 2015, pp. 165, 236).

6 For a very helpful exposition of Buber, Rosenzweig and Levinas's contribution to understanding relationships as it pertains to contemporary relational psychoanalysis, see Oppenheim (2017).

7 The term "the human condition" usually assumes that there is such a foundational entity; rather, what is taken to constitute "the human condition" depends on the theoretical and practical context that one is lodged in, including the particular episteme, or sociocultural reality. For example, "the human condition" of a religious

believer is a very different way of being-in-the-world and "language game" than the non-believer, though they probably agree on a number of points. From what I can tell, Buber and Marcel (and Levinas) may have an essentialist, or essentialist-like outlook; for example, there is a loving Creator or transcendent reality that one glimpses in a love relationship whether one knows it or not, or verbalizes it or not. That is, as Marcel believed, "Human existence by its very nature is endowed with value," especially when it is affirmed and confirmed in an *I-Thou* relationship (Sweetman, 2008, p. 61). Buber too, believed in "eternal values" and the "eternal norm" (Buber, 1965b, p. 116). Metcalfe & Game (2008), who draw from Buber, suggest that "by essence, we mean not identity but being-ness. The blanket usage of identity logic is apparent in the frequent equation of essence and identity" (p. 349).

8 Hans Loewald, trained as a traditional Freudian, has integrated other perspectives in a most original manner and has described the centrality of transference in comprehending the analysand qua person: "I shall try to develop the thesis that the concept of transference opened up the historical dimension of man's love life while at the same time disclosing the erotic dimension of his individuation and historicity, of his becoming what may properly called a self" (1978a, p. 32).

9 It was Erich Fromm, an enormously underappreciated post-Freudian psychoanalytic codifier and theoretician on love, who severely criticized Freud. In his gem, *The Art of Loving: An Enquiry into the Nature of Love,* he challenges Freud's physiological instinct-dominated view that human capabilities and inclinations for love and aggression are merely biological potentials. Rather, Fromm reconceptualizes all interpersonal relationships in terms of specific kinds of "being-with," modes of relatedness. In this context, love is one of the key characteristics of the "productive type." The productive person has achieved a high level of autonomy and personality integration: He is capable of being spontaneous, creative, positively related to others, transcendent, and grounded. He has a developed sense of personal identity and a stable though flexible frame of orientation toward living. Most importantly, following Freud, the productive person can love and work. "Mature love," says Fromm, "is union under the condition of preserving one's integrity; one's individuality." That is, "Love is an active power in man; a power which breaks through the walls which separate man from his fellow men, which unites him with others; loves makes him overcome the sense of isolation and separateness, yet it permits him to be himself, to retain his integrity" (1956, pp. 20–21). One can "hear" many Buberian/Marcelian themes in Fromm's formulations; he is a thinker who described himself as devoted to "nontheistic mysticism" and who as a child was raised as a religious Jew and, though he abandoned his Orthodoxy, maintained a strong interest in Biblical studies (Glen, 1962).

10 Buber has a similar point of view; "There is no self-love that is not self-deceit (since he who loves—and it is he who matters—loves only the other and essentially not himself), but that without being and remaining oneself there is no love" (1965b, 43).

11 For example, in contrast to Buber and Marcel's view of the I-Thou relationship, which is typically lodged in symmetrical (one possibility) and mutual subjectivities (there are gradations) that meet in the "between" (the I reaching towards the Thou), Levinas claims that it is the other person's radical alterity (i.e., his vulnerability and need to be tended to) that matters most, and that responsibility to the other does not seek symmetry, mutuality or reciprocity. Put differently, for Levinas, the person

has a fundamental obligation to be for the other, whereas for Buber and Marcel, what is fundamental is the relation, which includes cherishing and being for the other (Putnam, 2008, p. 75). In other words, while Buber/Marcel and Levinas have different ways of arriving at their relational ideal, they have similar conclusions in terms of what instantiates the I-Thou relation in "real life." As Putnam noted, it is wise to "see Buber as someone who identified a different 'I-Thou' relation than Levinas's, someone who identified a different sin qua non of the 'true life.'" Indeed, it is not a "competitive" matter, for "the ethical life has more than one sine qua non" (ibid., p. 99).

12 Aristotle's influence on Freud's view of happiness is considerable, and thus the former's view of happiness deserves a brief clarifying note. For Aristotle, says Robinson (1997, pp. 12–19), to achieve happiness one required excellence of character, that is, habits of virtue (the capacity of discerning and choosing the middle path between the extremes of excess and deficiency in one's behavior and emotions, including personal friendships and public life). The highest form of happiness for Aristotle was the contemplative life. Also worth noting is that for Aristotle happiness was the foundation for ethics, whereas for Freud ethics was based on the essential requirements of human cohabitation and survival.

13 I am paraphrasing from Alford (1998, p. 128).

14 What Lacan means by reality, truth and ethics is no simple matter; these important terms are hard to pin down in psychoanalytic writings, just as they are in philosophy and other disciplines. For example, are reality and truth discovered, as Lacan says, or socially constructed? Would Lacan agree with Buber who wrote, "The ultimate truth is one, but it is given to man only as it enters, reflected as in a prism, into the true life-relationships of the human persons" (1957, p. 79).

15 Briefly, according to Malcolm Bowie (1991, p. 92), the Imaginary is the realm "of mirror images, identifications and reciprocities." The Symbolic "is the realm of language, the unconscious and the otherness" that stays other.

16 I have drawn from Owen Hewitson—"What does Lacan say about … Love?"—who gives a good overview of Lacan's views on love. See Lacanonline.com.

17 Lacan's self-centric bias in his formulation of love, such as his claim that all desire is doomed to be a desire to consume the other, to make the other same, may reflect the fact that Lacan, a man "in constant need of admiration and power," as one author described him, seemed unable or unwilling to consider a more selfless for-the-other mode of being-in-the-world, as an authentic, non-neurotic human striving (Scarfone, 2005, p. 425).

18 In Barnes and Sternberg's (1997) two-factor theory of love, they called this "passionate" (erotically-based) and "companionate" (friendship-based) love, respectively. Likewise, Hendrick & Hendrick (1992) have described six love styles: *eros, storge, ludus, pragma, mania and agape*, all of which have some face validity and pertinence in real life, from what I can tell. Frederickson (2013) calls love "our supreme emotion," one that "springs up anytime any two people connect over a shared emotion" (p. 35). Gottman and Gottman (2018) have also done some interesting empirical work on marital stability and divorce. However, Buber and Marcel were pointing to a spiritual realm that is deeply personal and idiosyncratic, and therefore not easily empirically verifiable by positive psychology researchers.

19 Orange (2008) has raised some interesting questions about Benjamin's notion of mutual recognition.

20 I have organized this section by liberally drawing from Friedman's (2005) praiseworthy review of the psychoanalytic literature. Shaw (2003, p. 274), a relational analyst, also describes the alleged "therapeutic action of analytic love" beginning with Ferenczi's contribution to the present and mainly equating it with "mutual recognition," "empathic attunement" and "believing in him" [the analysand] with an attitude of "love and respect" for the analysand and his development, as Loewald described it. Finally, according to Vermonte, W.F. Bion claimed "the only link of a psychoanalyst with a patient should be the K-link (knowledge) and not Love or Hate" (Vermonte, 2019, p. 12).

21 It is worth noting that Lacan would on occasion abruptly shorten or end a session as a clinical tactic to destabilize the ego, the "enemy" structure in Lacan's theory (sometimes after a minute or a few seconds, although he also sometimes lengthened sessions), while Winnicott would often extend sessions during an analysand's regression as part of providing a better holding environment (this could include holding an analysand's head in his lap or touching her hand and having tea and cake after the session) (Luepnitz, 2018, pp. 122–123).

22 In a dialogue with Buber, Rogers claimed that full mutuality in the therapeutic context was possible; it can be "a meeting of two person on an equal basis, even though, in the world of *I-It* [viewing the other as an object or thing], it could be seen as a very unequal relationship" (Buber, 1965a, p. 173). Whether it is possible to have meaningful mutuality between analyst and analysand, at least in terms of some form of co-presence, give-and-take, or even reciprocal self-disclosure, when the relationship is decidedly asymmetrical in terms of power, is an open question to many analysts. Moreover, exactly what such terms symmetry/asymmetry, mutuality and reciprocity mean, let alone in the analytic context is hardly clear or agreed upon (Aron, 1996; Hoffman, 1998; Aron, Grand & Slochower, 2018).

23 It should be mentioned that empathy has its serious downside, both in terms of the self and the other, especially in terms of it being a basis for decisions, including in psychotherapy (Bloom, 2016). It has been suggested that empathy and emotional intelligence are "no contest for the hermitry that technology allows us to indulge in, or for the expectation of instantaneous responses from others" (Hong, 2019, p. 8). Stolorow et al. (1994) provided some cogent criticisms of how some self-psychologists use the term "empathic immersion."

24 As Buber's admiring biographer notes, like all human beings Buber had his personal deficiencies. He was "scarred by the wounds of his trouble childhood," such as the abandonment by his mother at age three. "He was at times narcissistic and self-absorbed," and he could be "inconsistent" in the eyes of some others "with his own demanding principles," thus reflecting "a failure to be truly dialogical" (Mendes-Flohr, 2020, pp. xvi, xvii). While there is much less written about Marcel, qua man, whose mother died when he was age four, he appears to have been a kind, hospitable and generous man, even adopting his only child, a son.

25 Putnam (2008, p. 62) claims that according to Buber, there can be a "demonic Thou" (1958, p. 68), that is, there can be an I-Thou relation say to a dictator, such as Napoleon who Buber cites. Putnam asserts that whether an I-Thou relationship is "good" depends on the appropriateness of the object chosen, though I am not sure that Putnam is reading Buber's passage the way it was intended.

26 As Mitchell noted, "An individual human mind is an oxymoron; subjectivity always develops in the context of intersubjectivity" (2000, p. 57), however, impersonal

situational forces (i.e., context and setting), such as those studies in the great "classic" social psychology experiments (Marcus, 2020), are also in play and profoundly impact decision-making and behavior.

27 Levinas made a similar claim in an interview: "The responsibility for the other is the grounding moment of love. It is not really a state of mind; it is not a sentiment, but rather an obligation" (Robbins, 2001, p. 133). He also approvingly notes in his discussion of Buber and Marcel that, "Love means, before all else, the welcoming of the other as Thou" (Levinas, 1976, pp. 5–6). Of course, specialists have noted that Buber and Levinas have some differences in their notions of love, though in most ways this appears to be philosophic hair-splitting compared to how such love is enacted in real life, my main concern in this book. In fact, in the latter part of his life, Levinas embraced Buber as an authentic ethical philosopher. See Atterton, Calarco, & Friedman (2004).

28 It is little known, let alone cited, that Freud wrote in a letter to Princess Maria Bonaparte in 1934,

> It really explains why we can love an animal … with such extraordinary intensity; affection without ambivalence, the simplicity of life from the almost unbearable conflict of civilization, the beauty of an existence complete in itself …. Often when stroking Jo-fi [his dog] I have caught myself humming a melody which, unmusical as I am, I can't help recognizing as the aria from *Don Giovanni*: 'a bond of friendship unites us both.'
>
> (Steadman, 1979, p. 108)

Also, it is easier to love a relatively healthy, cooperative, "high paying" analysand, compared to an unhealthy, oppositional, low fee one.

29 Marcel, too, notes that love is not merely a subjective feeling (though it is a feeling of full-bodied participation in the other), but rather the "active refusal to treat itself as subjective" (Anderson, 2006, p. 126). In other words, love is the belief that the beloved will not die because one has experienced something real in the beloved that contains eternal value, and it is precisely in love's refusal to treat itself as subjective that makes it a faith affirmation.

30 It is worth mentioning that Freud wrote in a letter to a colleague "the transference is indeed a cross" (1910, p. 39)

31 As Burston and Frie note, Buber (and Marcel) conceived of love as plentiful, substantial and perhaps above all, kind, "a voluntary process of witnessing, affirming, bestowing a sense of worth and recognition on other, analogous to gift-giving" (2006, p. 166).

32 Wood mentions that in Buber's refunctioning of Hassidic thought for the contemporary reader (i.e., in *Hassidism and Modern Man*), Buber claims that "in lovingly meeting with other persons or things, one releases from them the holy sparks that lie in their depths and which belong to the roots of one's own soul" (Wood, 1999, p. 86).

33 The "between" is quite likely the forerunner of "the third" in psychoanalytic theory. For Jung, "The confrontation of the two persons generates a tension charged with energy and creates a living third thing" (Jung, 1969, p. 90); for Lacan, the "the third" is viewed as that which sustains the relationship between the analyst and analysand from imploding; for Ogden, an object relational theorist, the intersubjective field refers to the co-created realm between the analyst and analysand in the service of

generating a novel shared reality of emotions, fantasies and thoughts. Benjamin also elaborates on the "interpersonal third" and the "moral third" (a moral component that animates the co-produced analytic encounter), which resembles what Buber (Oppenheim, 2017, pp. 57–58) and Marcel were describing, though the latter grounded the "between" in an absolutely trusting, dialogical relationship with God. It should be mentioned that the "analytic third" has been described as "a term difficult to define adequately and is used variously in the literature" (Hoffman, 2011, p. 128). Finally, Bolognini (2016) has written about the "interpsychic," an extended psychic realm (different from the intersubjective and interpersonal), referring to the joint functioning and reciprocal influences of two minds. While this transitional space is a form of relatedness and communication evident during therapeutic regression, Bolognini's fine distinctions strike me as rather torturous.

34 Winnicott describes a similar sense of aliveness when he prayed, "Oh God, May I be alive when I die" (Eigen, 1998, p. 15). This pithy statement calls to mind the words of Epictetus who after writing a death meditation, concluded "May death take me while I am thinking, writing and reading these phrases" (Foucault, 2005, p. 359).

35 Buber notes that "God is the 'wholly Other'; but He is also the wholly Same, the wholly Present … He is the *Mysterium Tremendum* that appears and overthrows; but He is also the mystery of the self-evident, nearer to me than my I" (Buber, 1958, p. 79). Marcel agrees with the main thrust of this observation (Treanor, 2006).

36 Both Buber and especially Marcel had a healthy distrust of language as being able to convey the irreducible presence of I-Thou as immediate co-presence and, for that matter, to meaningfully convey subjectivity in general. As Buber noted, "For in actuality speech does not abide in man, but man takes his stand in speech and talks from there; so with every word and every spirit" (1958, p. 39). Also, Buber and Marcel were well aware that language can be spoken with and through love (it's divine aspect), such as when the analyst speaks the truth, as he sees it, to the analysand in a loving manner (perhaps calling to mind the "magical-evocative aspects" of one's primary caregivers speech (Loewald, 1978b, p. 194); but it can also be spoken the in the opposite way, unethically, even violently. More generally, as Stanley Fish reflected on one of J.L. Austin's *How to Do Things With Words*, is there "a firm distinction between language that mirrors the world of fact and language that creates the facts to which it then refers[?]" (*The Week*, 11/8/19). And of course, all language reveals and conceals.

37 The great French idealist philosopher and Jesuit priest Pierre Teilhard de Chardin thought similarly: "Love alone is capable of uniting living beings in such a way as to complete and fulfill them, for it alone takes them and joins them by what is deepest in themselves" (Cousins, 1994, p. 180). For an interesting discussion of how the Christian narrative has impacted relational psychoanalysis, including its formulations of love between the analyst and analysand, and other Marcelian themes, see Hoffman (2011). Unfortunately, while Hoffman draws from the work of Paul Ricoeur, she does not mention Marcel who was an important philosophical influence on Ricoeur.

38 Eigen (1998) coming from a psychoanalytically-animated mystical perspective refers to "fidelity to this sacred something ["access eternity"], the very mystery of who we are" (1998, pp. 25, 24).

39 As R.G. Smith, Buber's translator, noted in *I and Thou*, both Jewish and Christian traditions are in play, including "having hope as one of its chief elements" (Smith,

1958, p. vi). It should be mentioned that in two important relational psychoanalytic books that centrally deal with hope, neither one mentions Marcel's pathbreaking work on hope in their index, a troubling omission in my view (Mitchell, 1995; Cooper, 2000). Hope has been undertheorized and hardly integrated into clinical analytic practice (Marcus, 2013a).

40 Vaclav Havel has defined hope in a manner than resonates with this aspect of Marcel's renderings, "It is not the conviction that something will turn out well, but the certainty that something makes sense, regardless of how it turns out" (Utne, 2020, p. A23).

41 Hope always has conscious, pre-conscious and unconscious aspects to it. As Erich Fromm points out, there are some individuals who feel consciously hopeful but may be unconsciously hopeless and others where it is the other way around (Fromm, 1968).

42 Marcel uses the term "Being" not only as a "God equivalent" but also to signify a certain kind of "fullness," "being-as-fullness," as well as "that in which we are always grounded, that in which we always stand." Busch further quotes Marcel as writing in *Being and Having* (p. 35), "We are involved in Being, and it is not within our power to leave it" (Busch, 1987, p. 15).

43 Such impediments include for example, believing that one is not lovable, undeserving of being loved, being unable to adequately give love, a fear of appropriating another's love, and the inability to sustain the preciousness of one's own love and the love of one's significant other, and for that matter, the love from others in general (Shaw, 2003). In one of his plays, Marcel describes people who love each other, "but not with the same kind of love, and never at any time finding themselves on the same plane of existence" (Lazaron, 1978, pp. 39–40).

44 It is worth mentioning that psychoanalyst W.F. Bion weighed in on the value of marriage. He told a single Michael Eigen who came to him for a consultation, "You know, you ought to get married .... Marriage isn't what you think it is. It's a relationship between two people speaking truth to each other, that mitigates the severity to yourself" (Eigen, 2014 p. 117).

45 Buber's early interest in Taoism influenced him in his later emphasis on personal oneness or completeness, the Tao as both transcendental and immanent, and the personal aspects of the divine. See Ebner (1994).

46 Aron, a relational analyst, noted that Buber's dialogic philosophy "most closely resonated with [a] relational psychoanalytic approach and its emphasis on mutuality" (1996, p. 154).

47 I am using Anderson's slightly modified translation of *Mystery of Being II* (2006, p. 140).

48 As Freud noted in *Civilization and Its Discontents*, written when he was 74, "The sexual life of civilized man is notwithstanding severely impaired; it sometimes gives the impression of being in process of involution [atrophy] as a function, just as our teeth and hair seem to be as organs" (1930, p. 105).

49 This is probably what Loewald (1978c, p. 69) was pointing to when he alleges that "intimations of eternity" are manifestations of the continuous presence of primary process cognition and the ego enhancement that is typical of primary narcissism, and are crucial to human growth as are the conscious executive ego functions and secondary process cognition

References

Akhtar, S. (2009). *Comprehensive dictionary of psychoanalysis*. London: Karnac.

Alford, C. F. (1998). Melanie Klein and the nature of good and evil. In P. Marcus & A. Rosenberg (Eds.), *Psychoanalytic versions of the human condition: Philosophies of life and their impact on practice* (pp. 118–139). New York: New York University Press.

Algoe, S. B., Gable, S. L., & Maisel, N. (2010). It's the little things: Everyday gratitude as a booster shot for romantic relationships. *Personal Relationships*, *17*, 217–233.

Anderson, T. C. (1985). The nature of the human self according to Gabriel Marcel. *Philosophy Today*, *29*(4), 273–283.

Anderson, T. C. (2006). *A commentary on Gabriel Marcel's* The mystery of being. Milwaukee, WI: Marquette University Press.

Aron, L. (1996). *A meeting of minds: Mutuality in psychoanalysis*. Hillsdale, NJ: Analytic Press.

Aron, L., Grand, S., & Slochower, J. (Eds.), (2018). *De-Idealizing relational theory. A critique from within*. London: Routledge.

Atterton, P., & Calarco, M. (2005). *On Levinas*. Belmont, CA: Wadsworth.

Atterton, P., Calarco, M., & Friedman, M. (Eds.). (2004). *Levinas and Buber. Dialog and difference*. Pittsburg, PA: Duquesne University Press.

Balint, M. (1949). Changing therapeutic aims and techniques in psychoanalysis. In *Primary love and psycho-analytic technique* (pp. 221–235). New York: Liveright, 1953.

Barnes, M. L., & Sternberg, R. J. (1997). A hierarchical model of love and its prediction of satisfaction in close relationships. In R. J. Sternberg & M. Hojjatt (Eds.), *Satisfaction in close relationships* (pp. 79–101). New York: Guilford.

Benjamin, J. (1988). *The bonds of love: Psychoanalysis, feminism and the problem of domination*. New York: Pantheon.

Benjamin, J. (1995). *Like subjects, love objects: Essays on recognition and sexual difference*. New Haven, CT: Yale University Press.

Berenbaum, M. (1994). *Elie Wiesel: God, the Holocaust and the children of Israel*. New York: Behrman.

Bergmann, M. S. (1987). *The anatomy of loving: The story of man's quest to know what love is*. New York: Fawcett Columbine.

Black, M. (2002). Foreword. In S. A. Mitchell, *Can love last? The fate of romance over time* (pp. 11–17). New York: Norton.

Bloom, P. (2016). *Against empathy. The case for relational passion*. New York: HarperCollins.

Bolognini, S. (2016). The interpsychic dimension in the psychoanalytic interpretation. *Psychoanalytic Inquiry*, 36(1): 102–111.

Bowie, M. (1991). *Lacan*. London: Fontana.

Brogaard, B. (2015). *On romantic love: Simple truths about a complex emotion*. Oxford: Oxford University Press.

Bromberg, P. (1993). Shadow and substance: A relational perspective on clinical process. *Psychoanalytic Psychology*, *10*(2), 147–168.

Buber, M. (1953). *Good and evil*. New York: Scribner.

Buber, M. (1957). *Pointing the way. Collected essays*. Atlantic Highlands, NJ: Humanities Press International.

Buber, M. (1958). *I and Thou* (R. G. Smith, Trans.). New York: Scribner.

Buber, M. (1960). *The origin and meaning of Hasidism* (M. Friedman, Trans.). New York: Horizon.

Buber, M. (1965a). *The knowledge of man: A philosophy of the interhuman* (M. Friedman, Ed.; M. Friedman & R. G. Smith, Trans.). New York: Harper & Row.
Buber, M. (1965b) *Between man and man* (R. G. Smith, Transl.). New York: Macmillan.
Buber, M. (1967a). Autobiographical fragments. In P. A. Schilpp & M. Friedman (Eds.), *The philosophy of Martin Buber* (The Library of Living Philosophers, vol. 12, pp. 3–39). La Salle, IL: Open Court.
Buber, M. (1967b). *On Judaism* (N.N. Glatzer, Ed.). New York: Schocken.
Buber, M. (1991). *Chinese tales*. San Jose, CA: Humanity Press.
Buber, M. (1995). *The way of man: According to the teachings of Hasidism*. New York: Citadel Press.
Buber, M. (2006). *The ten rungs & the way of man*. New York: Citadel.
Burston, D., & Frie, R. (2006). *Psychotherapy as a human science*. Pittsburgh: Duquense University Press.
Busch, T. W. (Ed.). (1987). *The participant perspective. A Gabriel Marcel reader*. Lanham, MD: University Press of America.
Cain, S. (1963). *Gabriel Marcel*. South Bend, IN: Regnery/Gateway.
Cain, S. (1995). *Gabriel Marcel's theory of religious experience*. New York: Peter Lang.
Cain, S. (1996). Dialogue and Difference. "I and Thou" or "We and They"? In M. Friedman (Ed.), *Martin Buber and the Human Sciences* (pp. 135–145). Albany: State University Press of New York.
Charles, S.T., & Carstensen, L. L. (2002). *Marriage in old age*. https://publishing.cdlib.org › ucpressebooks › view › brand=ucpress. Retrieved 12/6/19.
Compton, W. C., & Hoffman, E. (2020). *Positive psychology: the science of happiness and flourishing*. Los Angeles: Sage.
Cooper, D. (1998). Gabriel Marcel. In E. Craig (Ed.), *Routledge encyclopedia of philosophy* (vol. 6. p. 92). London: Routledge.
Cooper, S. H. (2000). *Objects of hope: Exploring possibility and limit in psychoanalysis*. Hillsdale, NJ: Analytic Press.
Cousins, E. (1994). *Christ of the 21st century*. London: Continuum.
Das, S. (2005). Kiss me, "Hardy": The dying kiss in the First World War trenches. In K. Harvey (Ed.), *The kiss in history* (p. 179). Manchester: Manchester University Press.
Early, T., & Gallagher, K. T. (2003). Marcel, Gabriel. In *The new Catholic encyclopedia* (vol. 9, p. 134). Detroit: Thomson/Gale.
Ebner, I. (1994). Martin Buber and Taoism. *Monumenta Serica*, *42*, 445–464.
Eigen, M. (1998). *The psychoanalytic mystic*. London: Free Association Book.
Eigen, M. (2014). *Faith*. London: Karnac.
Elliott, A. (2015). *Psychoanalytic theory* (3rd ed.). London: Palgrave Macmillan.
Emmons, R.A., & Mishra, A. (2011). Why gratitude enhances well-being. What we know, what we need to know. In K. M. Sheldon, T. B. Kashdan, & M. F. Stegar (Eds.), *Designing positive psychology: Taking stock and moving forward* (pp. 248–262). New York: Oxford University Press.
Enright, R. D., Freedman, S., & Rique, J. (1998). The psychology of interpersonal forgiveness. In R. D. Enright & J. North (Eds.), *Exploring forgiveness* (pp. 46–62). Madison: University of Wisconsin Press.
Erikson, E. H. (1959). *Identity and the life cycle. Selected papers*. New York: International Universities Press.
Erikson, E. H. (1964). *Insight and responsibility*. New York: Norton.
Evans, D. (1996). *An introductory dictionary of Lacanian psychoanalysis*. London: Routledge.

Fine, R. (1979). *History of psychoanalysis*. New York: Columbia University Press.
Fish, S. (2019). Best books chosen by Stanley Fish, *The Week*, 11/8/19, p. 24.
Fishbane, M. (2008). *Sacred attunement: A Jewish theology*. Chicago: University of Chicago Press.
Foucault, M. (2005). *The hermeneutics of the subject: Lectures at the Collège de France 1981–1982* (Michel Foucault Lectures at the Collège de France). F. Gros (Ed.), G. Burchell (Tr.). New York: Picador.
Fredrickson, B. J. (2013). *Love 2.0: Creating happiness and health in moments of connection*. New York: Plume.
Freud, S. (1910). Letter from Sigmund Freud to Oskar Pfister, June 5, 1910. *The International Psycho-Analytical Library*, 59, 38–40.
Freud, S. (1930 [1961]). Civilization and its discontents. In J. Strachey (Ed. & Trans.), *Standard edition of the complete psychological works of Sigmund Freud* (vol. 21, pp. 57–146). London: Hogarth.
Freud, S. (1953 [1949]). Three essays on the theory of sexuality. In J. Strachey (Ed. & Trans.), *Standard edition of the complete psychological works of Sigmund Freud* (vol. 7, pp. 130–243). London: Hogarth.
Freud, S. (1958 [1915[1914]). Observations on transference-love: Further recommendations on the technique of psycho-analysis III). In J. Strachey (Ed. & Trans.), *Standard edition of the complete psychological works of Sigmund Freud* (vol. 12, pp. 157–173). London: Hogarth.
Freud, S. (1963). *Psychoanalysis and faith. The letters of Sigmund Freud and Oskar Pfister* (H. Meng & E. L. Freud, Eds.; E. Mosbacher, Trans.). London: Hogarth (Original work published 1910).
Friedman, L. (2005). Is there a special form of psychoanalytic love? *Journal of the American Psychoanalytic Association*, 53, 349–375.
Friedman, M. S. (2002). *Martin Buber: The life of dialogue* (4th ed.). London: Routledge.
Fromm, E. (1950). *Psychoanalysis and religion*. New Haven: Yale University Press.
Fromm, E. (1956). *The art of loving: an enquiry into the nature of love*. New York: Harper Colophon.
Fromm, E. (1968). *The revolution of hope*. New York: Harper & Row.
Fryer, D. R. (2004). *The intervention of the other: ethical subjectivity in Levinas and Lacan*. New York: Other Press.
Gallagher, K. (1962). *The philosophy of Gabriel Marcel*. New York: Fordham University Press.
Gilleman, C. (2003). Humility. In B. L. Marthaler (Ed.), *The new Catholic encyclopedia* (vol. 7, p. 205). Detroit: Thomason/Gale and the Catholic University of America Press.
Glen, J. S. (1962). Erich Fromm: a Protestant critique. *Commentary*, *34*, 305–313.
Gottman, J., & Gottman, J. S. (2018). *The science of couples and family therapy: behind the scenes at the "Love Lab."* New York: Norton.
Greenberg, J. R., & Mitchell, S. A. (1983). *Object relations in psychoanalytic theory*. Cambridge, MA: Harvard University Press.
Grotjahn, M. (1967). Sigmund Freud and the art of letter writing. *Journal of the American Medical Association*, *200*(1), 119–124.
Hale, N. G. (1971). *James Jackson Putnam and psychoanalysis* (J. B. Heller, Trans.). Letter to Putnam, 6/17/1915. Cambridge, MA: Harvard University Press.

Hendrick, S. S., & Hendrick, C. (1992). *Romantic love*. Newbury Park, CA: Sage.
Hewitson, O. (2016). "What does Lacan say about ... love?" See lacanonline.com 6/27/16. Retrieved 9/10/19.
Hinshelwood, R. D. (1991). *A dictionary of Kleinian thought*. London: Free Association Books.
Hoffman, I. (1998). *Ritual and spontaneity in the psychoanalytic process: a dialectical-constructivist view* . Hillsdale, NJ: Analytic Press.
Hoffman, M.T. (2011). *Toward mutual recognition. Relational psychoanalysis and the Christian narrative*. London: Routledge.
Hong, E. (2019). Jorean's secret to happiness. *New York Times, Sunday Review*, 11/3/19, p. 8.
Jones, J. (1991). *Contemporary psychoanalysis: Religion, transference and transcendence*. New Haven, CT: Yale University Press.
Jung, C. (1969). *The structure and dynamics of the psyche*. In G. Adler & R. F. C. Hull (Eds. & Trans.), *The collected works of C.J. Jung* (vol. viii, pp. 3–553). Princeton, NJ: Princeton University Press.
Kearney, R. (2002). *On stories: Thinking in action*. London: Routledge.
Keen, S. (1967). *Gabriel Marcel*. Richmond, VA: John Knox Press.
Kernberg, O. (1995). Hatred as a core affect of aggression. In S. Akhtar, S. Kramer, & H. Parents (Eds.), *The birth of hatred: Clinical, developmental and technical aspects of intense aggression* (pp. 32–53), Northvale, NJ: Jason Aronson.
Klein, M. (1957). *Envy and gratitude and other works, 1946–1963*, New York: Free Press, 1975.
Kohut, H. (1971). *Analysis of the self*. New York: International Universities Press.
Kohut, H. (1977). *Restoration of the self*. New York: International Universities Press.
Kramer, K.P., & Gawlick, M. (2003). *Martin Buber's I and Thou: Practicing living dialogue*. New York: Paulist Press.
Lacan, J. (1991a). *The seminar of Jacques Lacan, book I: Freud's papers on technique, 1953–1954* (J. Forrester, Trans.). New York: Norton.
Lacan, J. (1991b). *The seminar of Jacques Lacan, book II. The ego in Freud's theory and in the technique of psychoanalysis: 1954–1955* (S. Tomaselli, Trans.). New York: Norton.
Lacan, J. (2017). *Formations of the unconscious: The seminar of Jacques Lacan, book V* (R. Grigg, Trans.). Cambridge: Polity Press.
Lauer, R. H., Lauer, J. C., & Kerr, S. T. (1990). The long-term marriage: Perceptions of stability and satisfaction. *International Journal of Aging and Human Development, 31*, 189–195.
Lazaron, H. (1978). *Gabriel Marcel the Dramatist*. Gerrards Cross: Colin Smythe.
Lechner, R. (1984). Marcel as radical empiricist. In P. A. Schilpp & L. E. Hahan (Eds.), *The philosophy of Gabriel Marcel* (The Library of Living Philosophers, vol. 17). La Salle, IL: Open Court.
Levinas, E. (1976). *Proper names* (M.B. Smith, Trans.). Stanford, CA: Stanford University Press.
Levinas, E. (1985). *Ethics and infinity: Conversations with Philippe Nemo* (R. Cohen, Trans.). Pittsburgh, PA: Duquesne University Press.
Levinas, E. (1987). *Time and the other (and additional essays)* (R. A. Cohen, Trans.). Pittsburgh, PA: Duquesne University Press.
Levinas, E. (1990). *Nine Talmudic readings* (A. Aronowicz, Trans.). Bloomington: Indiana University Press.

Levinas, E. (1994). *Martin Buber, Gabriel Marcel and philosophy: Outside the subject* (M. B. Smith, Trans.). Stanford, CA: Stanford University Press.

Loewald, H. (1960). On the therapeutic action of psychoanalysis. In *Papers on Psychoanalysis* (pp. 221–256). New Haven: Yale University Press.

Loewald, H. (1978a). *Psychoanalysis and the history of the individual: The Freud lectures at Yale*. New Haven, CT: Yale University Press.

Loewald, H. (1978b). Instinct theory, object relations, and psychic structure formation. In *Papers on Psychoanalysis* (pp. 207–218). New Haven: Yale University Press.

Loewald, H. (1978c). Comments on religious experience. In *Psychoanalysis and the history of the individual. The Freud Lectures at Yale.* (pp. 53–77). New Haven: Yale University Press.

Luepnitz, D. (2018). Toward a new middle group: Lacan and Winnicott for beginners. In M. Charles (Ed.), *Introduction to contemporary psychoanalysis. Defining terms and building bridges* (pp. 121–142). London: Routledge.

Machado, M. A. (1961). Existential encounter in Gabriel Marcel: Its value in psychotherapy. *Existential Psychology and Psychiatry*, *1*, 53–62.

Mahoney, A. (2013). The spirituality of us: Relational spirituality in the context of family relationships. In K. I. Pargament, J. J. Exline, & J. Jones (Eds.), *APA handbook of psychology, religion, and spirituality* (vol. 1, pp. 365–390). Washington, DC: American Psychological Association.

Marcel, G. (1964). *Creative fidelity* (R. Rosthal, Trans.). New York: Noonday Press.

Marcel, G. (1965a). *Being and having: An existentialist diary* (K. Farrer, Trans.). New York: Harper & Row.

Marcel, G. (1965b). *Homo viator. Introduction to a metaphysic of hope*. New York: Harper Torchbooks.

Marcel, G. (1967). I and Thou. In P. A. Schilpp & M. Friedman (Eds.), *The philosophy of Martin Buber* (Library of Living Philosophers, vol. 12, pp. 41–48). La Salle, IL: Open Court.

Marcel, G. (1973). *Tragic wisdom and beyond*. Evanston, IL: Northwestern University Press.

Marcel, G. (1995). *The philosophy of existentialism*. New York: Carol Publishing.

Marcel, G. (2001a [1951]). *Mystery of being. Volume I. Reflection and mystery*. South Bend, IN: St. Augustine's Press.

Marcel, G. (2001b [1951]). *Mystery of being. Volume II. Faith and reality*. South Bend, IN: St. Augustine's Press.

Marcel, G. (2008 [1952]). *Man against society*. South Bend, IN: St. Augustine's Press.

Marcus, P. (2003). *Ancient religious wisdom, spirituality, and psychoanalysis*. Westport, CT: Praeger.

Marcus, P. (2013a). *In search of the spiritual. Gabriel Marcel, psychoanalysis, and the sacred*. London: Karnac.

Marcus, P. (2013b). *How to laugh your way through life. A psychoanalyst's advice*. London: Karnac.

Marcus, P. (2020). *Psychoanalysis, classic social psychology, and moral living: Let the conversation begin*. London: Routledge.

Margulies, H. (2017). *Will and grace: Meditations on the dialogical philosophy of Martin Buber*. Rotterdam: Sense Publishers.

Marquez, G. G. (2017). Gabriel Marcel. *New World Encyclopedia*, n.p. www.newworldencylopdia.org/entry/Gabriel Marcel. Retrieved 11/10/19.

Meltzer, D. (1978). *The Kleinian development: Books I, II and III in one volume*. Perthshire, Scotland: Clunie Press.

Mendes-Flohr, P. (2020). *Martin Buber. A life of faith and dissent*. New Haven, CT: Yale University Press.

Metcalfe, A. & Game, A. (2008). Significance and dialogue in learning and teaching. *Educational Theory*, 58(3), 343–356.

Mitchell, S. A. (1995). *Hope and dread in psychoanalysis*. New York: Basic Books.

Mitchell, S. A. (2000). *Relationality: From attachment to intersubjectivity*. Hillsdale, NJ: Analytic Press.

Mitchell, S. A. (2002). *Can love last? The fate of romance over time*. New York: Norton.

Monte, C. F. (1980). *Beneath the mask: An introduction to theories of personality*, 2nd ed. New York: Holt, Rinehart and Winston.

Moore, B. E., & Fine, B. D. (Eds.). (1990). *Psychoanalytic terms and concepts*. New Haven, CT: American Psychoanalytic Association and Yale University Press.

Moore, D. J. (1996). *Martin Buber. Prophet of religious secularism*. New York: Fordham Univerity Press.

Nacht, S. (1962). Contribution to symposium on the curative factors in psycho-analysis. *International Journal of Psychoanalysis, 43*, 194–234.

Novick, J., & Novick, K. (2000). Love is a therapeutic alliance. *Journal of the American Psychoanalytic Association, 48*, 189–218.

O'Donohue, J. (1997). *Anam cara. A book of Celtic wisdom*. New York: HarperCollins.

O'Donohue, J. (2004). *Beauty: The invisible embrace. Rediscovering the true sources of compassion, serenity, and hope*. New York: HarperCollins.

Oppenheim, M. (2017). *Contemporary psychoanalysis and modern Jewish philosophy*. London: Routledge.

Orange, D. (2008). Recognition as: Intersubjective vulnerability in the psychoanalytic dialogue. *International Journal of Psychoanalytic Self Psychology*, 3, 178–194.

Pax, C. (1975). Marcel's way of creative fidelity, *Philosophy Today, 19*(1), 12–21.

Person, E. (1988). *Dreams of love and fateful encounters: The force of romantic passions*. New York: Norton.

Person, E. S., Cooper, A. M., & Gabbard, G. O. (Eds.). (2005). *Textbook of psychoanalysis*. Washington, DC: American Psychiatric Association.

Poole, R. (1998). The unknown Kierkegaard: Twentieth-century receptions. In A. Hannay & C. D. Marino (Eds.), *The Cambridge companion to Kierkegaard* (pp. 48–75). Cambridge: Cambridge University Press.

Pruyser, P. W. (1963). Phenomenology and dynamics of hoping. *Journal for the Scientific Study of Religion, 3*(1), 86–96.

Putnam, H. (2008). *Jewish philosophy as a guide to life: Rosenzweig, Buber, Levinas, Wittgenstein*. Bloomington: Indiana University Press.

Reik, T. (1983). *Listening with the third ear*. New York: Farrar, Straus and Giroux.

Roazen, P. (2001). *The historiography of psychoanalysis*. London: Routledge.

Robbins, J. (Ed.). (2001). *Is it righteous to be? Interviews with Emmanuel Levinas*. Stanford, CA: Stanford University Press.

Robinson, D. N. (1997). *The great ideas of philosophy, part 2* (course outline). Chantilly, VA: The Teaching Company.

Rosthal, R. (Trans.). (1964). *Introduction to G. Marcel's* Creative fidelity. New York: Noonday Press.

Roth, P. A. (1998). The cure of stories, self-deception, danger situations, and the clinical role of narratives in Roy Schaefer's psychoanalytic theory. In P. Marcus & A. Rosenberg (Eds.), *Psychoanalytic versions of the human condition: Philosophies of life and their impact on practice* (pp. 306–331). New York: New York University Press.

Rubin, J. B. (1996). *Psychotherapy and Buddhism: Toward an integration*. New York: Plenum.

Rycroft, C. (1995). *A critical dictionary of psychoanalysis*, 2nd ed. London: Penguin.

Scarfone, D. (2005). Psychoanalysis in the French community. In E. S. Person, A. M. Cooper, & G. O. Gabbard (Eds.), *Textbook of psychoanalysis* (pp. 423–433). Washington, DC: American Psychiatric Publishing.

Schaefer, R. (1983). *The analytic attitude*. New York: Basic Books.

Shaw, D. (2003). On the therapeutic action of analytic love. *Contemporary Psychoanalysis*, 39, 251–278.

Slavin, M. O. (2016). Relational psychoanalysis and the tragic-existential aspect of the human condition. *Psychoanalytic Dialogues*, *26*(5), 537–548.

Slochower, J. (2018). D.W. Winnicott: Holding, playing and moving toward mutuality. In M. Charles (Ed.), *Introduction to contemporary psychoanalysis: Defining terms and building bridges* (pp. 97–117). London: Routledge.

Smith, R. G. (Trans.). (1958). Preface. In M. Buber (1958), *I and Thou* (2nd ed., pp. v-xii). New York: Scribner.

Steadman, R. (1979). *Sigmund Freud*. New York: Paddington Press.

Sternberg, R. J. (1986). A triangular theory of love. *Psychological Review*, *93*, 119–135.

Sternberg, R. J., & Hojjat, M. (1997). *Satisfaction in close relationships*. New York: Guilford.

Stolorow, R., Atwood, G., & Bradchaft, B. (1994). (Eds.) *The Intersubjective Perspective*. Lanham: Jason Aronson.

Sweetman, B. (2008). *The vision of Gabriel Marcel: Epistemology, human person, the transcendent*. Amsterdam: Rodopi.

Tangney, J. P. (2000). Humility: Theoretical perspectives, empirical findings and direction for future research. *Journal of Social & Clinical Psychology*, *19*(1), 70–82.

Tillich, P. (1954). *Love, power and justice*. Oxford: Oxford University Press.

Todd, S. (2003). *Levinas, psychoanalysis, and ethical possibilities in education*. Albany, NY: SUNY Press.

Treanor, B. (2006). *Aspects of alterity. Levinas, Marcel, and the contemporary debate*. New York: Fordham University Press.

Utne, E. (2020). Feeling hopeless? Embrace it. *New York Times*, July 25, p. A. 23.

Vermonte, R. (2019). *Reading Bion*. London: Routledge.

Wahl, J. (1967). Martin Buber and the philosophies of existence. In P.A. Schilpp & M. Friedman (Eds.), *The philosophy of Martin Buber* (Library of Living Philosophers, vol. 12, pp. 475–510). La Salle, IL: Open Court.

Wallwork, E. (2005). Ethics in psychoanalysis. In E. S. Person, A. M. Cooper, & G. O. Gabbard (Eds.), *Textbook of psychoanalysis* (pp. 281–300). Washington DC: American Psychiatric Publishing.

Weinstein, B. (1990). *History and theory after the fall*. Chicago: University of Chicago Press.

Wolf, E. (1994). Selfobject experiences: Development, psychopathology, treatment. In S. Kramer & S. Akhtar (Eds.), *Mahler and Kohut: Perspectives on development, psychopathology, and technique* (pp. 65–96). Northvale, NJ: Jason Aronson.

Wolfinger, N. H. (2019). Are married people still happier? Institute for Family Studies. https://ifstudies.org>blog>are-married-people-still-happier. Retrieved 10/19/19.

Wood, R. E. (1969). *Martin Buber's ontology. An analysis of* I and Thou. Evanston, IL: Northwestern University Press.
Wood, R. E. (1999). The dialogical principle and the mystery of being. The enduring relevance of Martin Buber and Gabriel Marcel. *International Journal for Philosophy and Religion, 45*, 83–97.
Wyschogrod, E. (2000). *Emmanuel Levinas: The problem of ethical metaphysics* (2nd ed.). New York: Fordham University Press.

Chapter 3

The spirit of work

Psychoanalytic theory presupposes that a person's choice of career is lodged in conscious and, most importantly, unconscious processes, and this is one of the reasons that choosing an apt career and flourishing in it is so challenging. As Freud noted, "A man like me cannot live without a hobby-horse, without a consuming passion, without—in Schiller's words—a tyrant. I have found one ['working well, writing well']. In its service I know no limits" (1895 [1985], p. 129). Sounding similar to Freud who advocated choosing a career by listening to "the deep inner needs of our nature," the unconscious (Reik, 1983, p. 7), the great thirteenth-century Persian poet and Sufi mystic, Rumi, put it just right, "Everyone has been made for some particular work, and the desire for that work has been put in every heart. Let yourself be silently drawn by the stronger pull of what you really love" (https://resurrectionwaltz2013.wordpress.com/category/r-m.../page/24/, retrieved 10/29/19).

While Freud told Erik Erickson that "to love and work" were the central therapeutic goals of psychoanalysis, these being the twin pillars of a sound mind and for living the flourishing life (Erikson, 1959, p. 96), the fact is that in contemporary Western society, in say the last 25 years, many people have not experienced their work as particularly satisfying, let alone inspiring. From my experience as a psychoanalyst, analysands currently spend as much time speaking about their problems at work as they do about problems in their love relationships (and sometimes more). However, depending on which survey one peruses, a most recent one suggests that in the Trump era, job satisfaction has significantly increased (at least before the Covid-19 pandemic and upsurge of unemployment, and racial unrest). According to the highly respected non-partisan, non-profit think tank, The Conference Board, "Job Satisfaction in 2019," about 54 percent of American workers are satisfied with their employment (up three points from 2018, indicating one of the largest single-year increases in the survey's long history). Workers also report being considerably more relaxed about their job security. And millennials have reported an upsurge in confidence in relation to their wages. However, workers are most troubled by their current job's potential for future growth, with this being the most important indicator of job satisfaction. Moreover, over 60 percent reported feeling dissatisfied with their organization's recognition practices, performance evaluation process, and communication channels. Also, worth noting is that men generally feel better than women about manifold financial aspects of their work, such as wages and bonus plans (www.conference-board.org › press › pressdetail; retrieved 11/7/19).

Notwithstanding these encouraging statistics, this chapter is concerned with what psychological and contextual factors foster a person's love of their work as opposed to suffering through it. This is the problem of job satisfaction, as it is called in the psychology of work literature, a subject that should be of great concern to analysands (and their analysts), who are struggling to fashion a flourishing life, in part because of the massive amount of time the average person spends working during a typical week (Marcus, 2017). For example, a 2014 national Gallup poll put the average number of work hours at 47 hours per week, or 9.4 hours per day, with many respondents saying they work 50 hours per week. According to the Bureau of Labor Statistics, in 2018 the average 25–54-year-old (probably the bulk of analysands, patients, and clients) worked 40.5 hours a week. Indeed, the art of living a flourishing life requires the will and ability to navigate the workplace in a creative, skillful, and productive manner, and analysts can help potentiate this process (www.cnbc.com › 2017/05/03 › how-the-8-hour-workday-changed-h... retrieved 12/7/19).

While I will be summarizing some of the pertinent vocational and organizational research on job satisfaction, my main focus will be on what kind of "technology of the self" ("self-steering mechanisms" as Foucault called it (Rose, 1996, p. 29)) a person can implement that will likely help him to experience his everyday work as spiritually uplifting in the Buberian/Marcelian sense. That is, as "communion"—"being opened up and drawn in" (Buber, 1965, p. 91) or "opening-up and entering-in" ("availability" and "engagement" in Marcel's language) (Cain, 1963, p. 70)—that points to "something more," "something higher," and "something better" (i.e., it addresses the Eternal/Absolute Thou, the divine, or the transcendent). I will begin this discussion with Marcel's contribution on work as the created birthplace of the transcendent, followed by Buber's reflections on a specific type of work, what constitutes education, in particular, great teaching. "Education worthy of the name is essentially education of character," of the moral education of the "whole being of his pupil," said Buber (1965, pp. 104, 105), and this also is the main thrust of psychoanalysis at its best, at least as I conceive it.[1] I will conclude the chapter with some reflections on what Buberian/Marcelian spirituality can offer the analysand (and analyst) attempting to fashion a flourishing work life that goes beyond mere functionality, competence, even excellence, that has been aptly summarized in the many professional and lay publications on job satisfaction.

Job, career, calling

Before getting to the heart of this chapter, I want to briefly contextualize my subject in terms of the vocational and organizational psychology literatures. A very useful way of applying Freud's advice about choosing a career direction (let your unconscious decide, roughly the deepest part of your personality) involves distinguishing between a "job," a "career," and a "calling." As sociologists Bellah and colleagues (1986) first pointed out in their best-selling book, *Habits of the Heart: Individualism and Commitment in American Life*, a person with a "job" orientation to work is geared toward earning a living for himself and his family in order to prosper and to maximize their amount of leisure time. In other words, work is viewed strictly as a practical means to a financial end. Moreover, his sense of self is mainly defined by financial success, security "and all that money can buy" (p. 66). A "career" is a way to advance oneself in terms of accomplishment, status, and prestige. Such people mainly work in order to move up the hierarchical ladder, to be promoted, a competitive process they very much enjoy. The sense of self that is associated with a career is characterized by a broader kind of success than with a job, in that by attaining a degree of expanding power and competency, work itself becomes a way of sustaining self-esteem (ibid.). Individuals who have a "job" and "career" orientation toward work tend to have personal identities that do not significantly overlap with the actual work they do; to a large extent, they view what they do at work as distinct from the rest of their life (Berg, Grant, & Johnson, 2010, p. 974). They narrate their lives in terms of having a "work self" and a "non-work self," and rarely do they feel they are a "whole" or "complete self."

In contrast, a "calling" is a work orientation in which a person views their work as deeply satisfying and socially beneficial. That is, an individual chooses an occupation that he "feels drawn to pursue," often powerfully. He anticipates it to be "intrinsically enjoyable and meaningful," especially as a socially useful endeavor, and he views it "as a central part of his identity" (ibid., p. 973). As Bellah and colleagues (1986) noted, such work "constitutes a practical ideal of activity and character that makes a person's work morally inseparable from his or her life," and it links the person more intensely not only to his co-workers but to the larger community (ibid.). The highly regarded television special, *CNN Heroes: An All-Star Tribute*, hosted by anchorman Anderson Cooper, which honors everyday people who make remarkable contributions to humanitarian aid and a profoundly positive difference in their communities, is a wonderful example of the psychology of callings. In 2019, one hero brought transformative assistance to women and children by offering necessities, education, and job training to those in an economically deprived city; another offered restored RVs to displaced families after one of California's worst wildfires; a third offered psychological and practical tools and support to children grieving the loss of a parent or sibling, and a fourth gave a home to the pets of domestic violence victims so their owners could get their lives back on track (cnnpressroom.blogs. cnn.com › 2019/10/30 › top-10-cnn-heroes-of-2019; retrieved 12/12/19).

Perhaps surprisingly to some, research has demonstrated that about "one-third of workers, across a whole range of different occupations, view their job or career as a 'calling.'" For example, a public toilet cleaner or garbage collector is just as capable of experiencing their work as meaningful, if not as a calling, as, say, a doctor or member of the clergy. In other words, such a positive effect cuts across all socioeconomic levels (Hall & Chandler, 2005, p. 167; Stairs & Galpin, 2010, p. 161). From a Buberian/Marcelian perspective, the important point here in terms of the art of living a flourishing life, including its constituent realm of work, is that it is wiser to focus less on becoming a person of success ("the logos of things") and more a person of value (the "logos of the human") (Biswas, 1996, p. 228). That is, Buber and Marcel are emphasizing the importance of being able to justify one's existence not simply in terms of how others evaluate you in relation to surface material success, but in terms of self-judgment based on living a life of personal integrity and decency. This being said, it is rather troubling that one of the most prominent researchers on callings, Amy Wrzesniewski, in part defines the phenomenon as "an enactment of personally significant beliefs through work," and this is accepted without critical moral reflection (2012, p. 46). For such a definition would mean that an ISIS warrior engaged in violent *jihad* also views his work as a calling. Without acknowledging the moral values that are centrally contained in any definition of "calling," including how it is instantiated in "real" life, we are losing hold, at our peril, of the fact that every psychological construct is heavily value-laden and must be qualified and judged accordingly. Moreover, it is precisely a "lack of human values in depth," both professional and personal, that is often correlated with pathological behavior on the job, such as with narcissistic leaders who foster horrid relations throughout an organization. Such people are largely incapable of relating to others using reasonable ego-ideal criteria (a person's notion of ideal behavior developed from parental and social values) and super-ego standards, including "the inability to judge people in depth" (Kernberg, 1979, pp. 33, 35).

While the "job," "career," and "calling" work orientations represent distinct paradigmatic types, the fact is that for many people their work can be experienced at different times and in different contexts as being any one of these orientations or a combination of them. For example, a young, passionate congregational rabbi analysand of mine spoke in one session about his work as a way to make a good living so he could afford to send his five children to a first class *yeshiva* high school ("job"), about his wish to enlarge the membership and vitality of his small congregation as a way of showing his colleagues that he was made of the "right stuff" to be voted into a prestigious leadership position in a rabbinical association ("career"), and about his sacred duty and life commitment to significantly contribute to Jewish survival, continuity, and enhancement ("calling"). Indeed, research has shown that people who, for the most part, view their work as a calling fare better on the job and, for that matter, in the rest of life. Such people have higher levels of work, life, and health satisfaction as well as lower work absenteeism (and these findings remain constant when controlling for income, education, and type of occupation). They have higher levels of intrinsic work motivation, spend more time at work, even if they are not paid or in other ways compensated, report greater levels of passion for and pleasure in their work, feel stronger identification and engagement with their work, and perform at higher levels compared to their peers. Those with a "calling" orientation also are less inclined to suffer from stress, depression, and psychic conflict between the work and non-work realms of their lives (Wrzesniewski, 2012, p. 51).

In terms of flourishing on the job, what is most important about callings is "that *any* kind of work ['lofty to lowly'] can be a calling" (ibid., p. 47). That is, experiencing what one does as a calling largely depends on how one creatively conceives of the activity that one labels work. Put differently, when it comes to personal truth, it is a product of the imagination, that wonderful human capacity to form novel images and ideas in the mind:

> Three workers [were] breaking up rocks. When the first was asked what he was doing, he replied, "Making little ones out of big ones"; the second said, "Making a living"; and the third, "Building a cathedral."
>
> (Dik & Duffy, 2009, p. 424)

What this story highlights is the fact that what constitutes a calling depends on the individual's ability to project transcendent meaning, whether described in religious or secular language, into what he is doing. This involves a complicated deployment of matters connected to self-efficacy and agency in the psychic economy (Meissner, 1997, p. 37). As Heinrich Heine said, "The grandeur of the universe is commensurate with the soul that surveys it" (Gilbert, 1981, p. 131).[2]

Marcel on work as the creative affirmation of the transcendent

Drawing from Marcel's path-breaking formulations, I view creativity as having a central role in fashioning the flourishing life. By this, I refer to the individual's quest for what Marcel called "spiritual reality" and "spiritual illumination" (Marcel, 2001a, pp. 1, 13), a life that is characterized by "novelty, freshness, revelation," that intends the transcendent, and, perhaps most importantly, often leads to radical perspective-shifting, life-affirming self-transformation, and a "renewal of being" (Gallagher, 1962, pp. 84, 95). While a life that is narrated in terms of "spiritual reality" and "spiritually illumination" can be psychoanalytically viewed as merely a regressive manifestation of infantile wishes pertaining to mother/infant merging, or an indication of defensive idealization against aggressive wishes, I will instead mainly view such experiences as phenomenological, that is, as creative expressions that are authentically transcendent, certainly in the mind and heart of the person experiencing them (Akhtar, 2009, pp. 269–270). Most importantly, perhaps, it is the capacity for what Averill calls "emotional creativity," the psychological bedrock for a "renewal of being," that Marcel insinuates gives us access to the best of what is both "inside" and "outside" of ourselves, namely, the three virtues of Beauty, Truth, and Goodness,[3] which includes the workplace. Simply stated, emotional creativity refers to the capacity for "novel, effective and authentic" receptiveness, responsiveness, and responsibility, an openness, curiosity, and imagination that leads to a process of "spiritualization of the passions," to quote Nietzsche, that is, to "self-realization and expansion" and an increased "vitality, connectedness and meaningfulness" (Averill, 2009, p. 255). In short, I am talking about self-fashioning or self-creating, which, as Marcel sees it, always includes an other-directed, other-regarding, and other-serving thrust to it. Like Freud and Buber, for Marcel the fine arts are explicitly creative, but the creative impulse is also expressed in what can be broadly called the ethical sphere, in acts of hospitality, admiration, generosity, love, friendship, prayer, religion, contemplation, and metaphysics. Such ethically animated creative impulses can also be enacted in the workplace, whether by a volunteer doctor working with Ebola patients in West Africa, a policeman or fireman, or a graciously helpful clerk or doorman. In all such creative experiences of deep communion, of "being-with," of "self-donation to the thou, the spirit of encounter, co-presence, *engagement*" (italics in original; Miceli, 1965, p. 20) in Marcel's nomenclature, and more simply, the feeling of emotional and spiritual closeness, "*We do not belong to ourselves*: this is certainly the sum and substance, if not of wisdom, at least of any spirituality worthy of the name" (Marcel, "Foreword," in Gallagher, 1962, p. xiv).

In the vocational and organizational psychology literatures, the role of this kind of other-directed, other-regarding, and other-serving spirituality in the workplace has been conceptualized in terms of "the spiritualization of work," in which work is geared to "broader life fulfillment" rooted in promoting care and concern for family, colleagues, and the wider community. These include organizational strategies that demand ethical leadership, enhance employee well-being, facilitate sustainability, and are socially responsible, while they also uphold profits and revenue growth (Carroll, 2013, pp. 595, 597, 604). Prosocial practices, as they have been called (Dutton, Roberts, & Bednar, 2011, p. 159), are meant to shield and/or support the best interests of other people and provide a medium for employees to partake in routine helping and giving in the work context. Research has clearly shown that those employees who engage in regularly helping others and giving to a cause that transcends themselves are more likely to flourish in terms of job performance and job satisfaction. Moreover, engaging in prosocial practices in the work setting "often increases psychological and social functioning, as indicated by greater persistence, performance and citizenship behaviors on the job" (ibid.). Indeed, such a "for the other" comportment in the work setting also has its psychoanalytically conceived, exquisitely sublimatory, and self-reparative benefits, for it can stand for or replace a loved and loving internal object that enhances personality integration (Levine, 1997, p. 155). As English novelist George Eliot wrote in *Silas Marner*, "Everyman's work, pursued steadily, tends to become an end in itself, and so to bridge over the loveless chasms of his life" (1882, p. 121).

Delineating Marcelian creativity

Marcel notes in his magnum opus, *The Mystery of Being*, that there is an intimate connection between creativity and existence, a clarification that provides a helpful context for getting a better sense of how Marcel defines the notion of creativity, including as it applies to work behavior:

> A really alive person is not merely someone who has a taste for life, but somebody who spreads that taste, showering it, as it were, around him; and a person who is really alive in this way has, quite apart from any tangible achievements of his, something essentially creative about him; it is from this perspective that we can most easily grasp the nexus which, in principle at least, links creativity to existence, even though existence can always decay, can become sloth, glum repetition, killing routine. [Think of work "burnout" or bureaucratically induced alienation.]
>
> (Marcel, 2001a, p. 139)

To be a "really alive" person is to be someone who strongly feels, this being Marcel's main indicator of authentic participation in the mystery of being (roughly, being fully engaged in the experience of the here and now). A mystery "is something in which I am myself involved, and it can therefore only be thought of as a sphere where the distinction between what is in me and what is before me loses its meaning and its initial validity" (Marcel, 1965b). Authenticity, says Marcel, is the opposite of indifference—it is responsiveness, similar to how one watches a play, waiting for the story to unfold one sentence at a time (Marcel, 1973, p. 121). Such a person experiences his mind, body, and soul—his "self" in psychological language—deeply and joyfully, including those times when he feels threatened by the sham, drudgery, and broken dreams of his daily life. He exudes what Marcel calls "presence," that experience "of the immediate 'withness' of real being" (Cain, 1963, p. 28). Presence, says Marcel, is the

> sudden emergence, unforeseeable, salvific, of a form that is not simply traced, but wedded, that is to say, to and re-created from within and in which the entire experience, instead of being lost, instead of being scattered like sand and dust, concentrates itself, affirms itself, proclaims itself.
>
> (Marcel, 2005, p. 113)

Elsewhere, Marcel points out, presence "reveals itself immediately and unmistakably," for example, "in a look, a smile, an intonation or a handshake" (Marcel, 1995, p. 40). In addition to engaging in such novel, spontaneous self-creation, a "really alive" person is also willing and able to be self-consecrating and self-sacrificing (Cain, 1995, p. 104). He feels internally compelled to share this deep and joyful self-experience with others as a being among beings. The creative impulse, then, is best conceptualized as a relational moment, as being both self-affirming and other-directed, other-regarding, and other-serving: "The true artist" [in the broader sense, we can all be artists], says Marcel, "does not create for himself alone but for everyone; he is satisfied only if that condition is fulfilled" (Marcel, 1964, p. 47).

For Marcel, creativity is always a relational dynamic, whether conceived as "real," as in an act of love directed toward a significant other, or "imagined," as in an artistic vision that leads to the production of a work of art. In fact, any kind of work that has a reparative, healing, or in other ways uplifting ripple effect on others can be said to be creative, in part because it involves the persistent ethically animated deployment of thought, imagination, discernment, and decision making (Levine, 1997, p. 152). Thus, to create in whatever form is to refuse reducing the self and the other to the level of abstractions and objectifications (Marcel, 1964, p. 47). As Marcel says, such an alienating moment amounts to "the denial of the more than human by the less than human" (ibid., p. 10). Indeed, Primo Levi made a similar observation as it pertains to work: "I am persuaded that normal human beings are biologically built for an activity that is aimed toward a goal and that idleness, or aimless work (like Auschwitz *Arbeit*), gives rise to suffering and to atrophy" (1996, p. 179).

What are some of the key general characteristics of creativity, characteristics that Marcel suggests make the notion so summoning and enlivening, even when we simply hear the word "creativity"? Creativity is associated with "novelty, freshness, revelation," as Gallagher aptly summarized it (1962, pp. 84–85). Creativity is novel in the sense that it points to that which is unique, original, and different, always in a thrilling, self-renewing way. It is fresh in the sense that it calls to mind that which is eternal; that is, the creative experience is unaffected by the passage of time, like when creating or encountering a great piece of music or art. Finally, creation gives a person the feeling of being in a state of "beholding," looking at or hearing something amazing and exciting, and the sense that he has been given an irresistible, magical gift that makes him feel "anew and beyond beginnings" (ibid., p. 85). As Mother Teresa said about her work with the poor, "The miracle is not that we do this work, but that we are happy to do it" (www.catholicbible101.com/motherteresaquotes.htm; retrieved 12/23/19. Indeed, any act of kindness in the everyday workplace reflects a similarly praiseworthy sentiment.

In creation, whether one is the creator or the person who witnesses creation and its product, the experience is that one has engaged "the source, the beginning, which is also the end." As Gallagher further notes, "One who stands in the source transcends time"; however paradoxically, "We need time to stand in the source" (1962, p. 85). Put somewhat differently, in creativity, the creator surrenders himself to something other; he puts himself at the service of something, a source that transcends while at the same time depends on him (Cain, 1995, p. 104). Marcel notes, for example, that for the artist there is an encounter with "the original mystery, the 'dawning of reality' at its unfathomable source." Moreover, he says, "The artist [or any vocation that is experienced as a calling] seems to be nourished by the very thing he seeks to incarnate; hence the identification of receiving and giving is ultimately realized in him" (Marcel, 1964, p. 92).

In the act of creation, ironically, one does not feel as though one is giving up anything vital of the self, even as there is hard work and output that is required to create. Rather, the act of creation makes one feel as though one has become more bountiful, has a more plentiful supply of something that is judged by the creator as good and feels significantly healing. Calling to mind Klein's description of the depressive position and the reparative capacities that emanate from it, in Marcel's language we could say that such a creative person, conceived as a *homo viator*, a spiritual itinerant or wayfarer, has decisively moved further along his internal journey from "existential brokenness," from experiencing his life as having "lost its inner unity and its living center" (Marcel, 1963, p. 91) to a greater "ontological fullness" (Cain, 1995, p. 84). As the great Irish playwright George Bernard Shaw remarked, "I am of the opinion that my life belongs to the community, and as long as I live, it is my privilege to do for it what I can. I want to be thoroughly used when I die. For the harder I work the more I live. I rejoice in life for its own sake" (www.rebellesociety.com › troublemakers; retrieved 12/24/19).

As I suggested earlier, Marcel notes that the creative experience fundamentally changes the experience of time during the creative act and its witnessing. Creativity does not take place in time as conventionally conceived, as a dimension that enables two identical events occurring at the same point in space to be distinguished, measured by the interval between the events. Rather, time tends to feel without beginning or end, being bathed in the eternity of the creative activity and its result. Such an experience of immediate, present time is the opposite of the way time is experienced in ordinary life, especially in an overly routinized activity where one feels bored because the activity is predictable, monotonous, and unchanging. The point is that creation renews, replenishes, and enlivens, while routine atrophies, empties, and deadens.[4] As Gallagher aptly puts it, all creative activities—in the fine arts, in contemplation, in love, or in encountering a beautiful sunset—"are absolute beginnings which thrust me into the plenitude [a palpable sense of 'fullness' or completion] which is beyond beginnings … wherever there is joy, there is being: for wherever there is joy, there is creation" (Gallagher, 1962, p. 87).

In the workplace, this experience of time has been formulated by scholars in terms of "flow" (or being in the "zone"), that condition of heightened focus, concentration, and immersion that also takes place in play and art. As the originator of this notion Mihaly Csikszentmihalyi pointed out, it is precisely the total absorption with an activity and the situation one is in that is the basis for optimal performance, learning, and the experience of joy and other positive affects (Nakamura & Csikszentmihalyi, 2009). Marcel's observations about how time is experienced during creativity also resonates with the construct of a psychological state called "work engagement." This concept is roughly defined as "a psychological presence in a role," or "being there," and refers to the degree to which workers are "attentive, connected, integrated, and focused on their role performances." Greater work engagement is associated with better job performance and increased job satisfaction (Rothbard & Patil, 2012, pp. 56, 57). As Marcel's observations suggest, during the creative act and its witnessing, one is more of a "visionary" in time perspective, as it has been called in the psychology of work literature. That is, such a person resides in a different dimension of the spirit, in a deeper form of attunement, and thus is able to intuit things that have not yet come into being. This is different than the "realist," who is bound only to the present and who cautiously proceeds as required, or those individuals who mainly dwell in the past to animate their way of engaging the present (Marianetti & Passmore, 2010, p. 193).

Another important aspect of all creativity, as Marcel construes it, is that the division of giving and receiving is overcome. Marcel makes this point in reference to hospitality, providing a friendly welcome and kind, generous treatment offered to a guest or stranger, or for that matter, a co-worker, colleague, or boss:

> If we devote our attention to the act of hospitality, we will see at once that to receive is not to fill up a void with an alien presence but to make the other person participate in a certain plenitude. Thus the ambiguous term, "receptivity," has a wide range of meanings extending from suffering or undergoing to the gift of self; for hospitality is a gift of what is one's own, i.e., of oneself . To provide hospitality is truly to communicate something of oneself to the other.
>
> (Marcel, 1964, pp. 28, 90)

What Marcel is getting at in this excerpt is that to be hospitable, to "receive" someone, is to open oneself to the other, to let the other into one's inner reality, that is, to literally and symbolically let the other into one's "home," that place where one finds refuge and feels most safe and secure. To "receive" a visitor, I must unlock the door and allow him in, clutch his hand, and openly and responsively give myself to him (Cain, 1979, p. 27). Feelings of vitality and generosity spontaneously emerge. In other words, hospitality is both a moment of receiving and giving, of being receptive and responsive, but also of being responsible to, and for, the other. At this juncture, receiving and giving are impossible to tell apart. Marcel puts this point succinctly:

> I can only grasp myself as being—on condition that I feel; and it can also be conceded that to feel is to receive; but it must be pointed out at once that to receive in this context is to open myself to, hence to give myself, rather than undergo an external action.
>
> (Marcel, 1964, p. 91)

Thus, it is a psychological paradox that to give the best of oneself is the surest way one can receive. Research inspired by Frederickson's "broaden and build" theory has found that, in the workplace, institutionalized care-giving and supportive attachments and other prosocial behaviors that are rooted in heartfelt collective values which reflect "organizational virtuousness" generate upward emotion spirals, so compassion begets compassion among employees (Lilius, Kanov, Dutton, Warline, & Maitlis, 2012, pp. 276, 278).

Marcel further elaborates this crucial fusion between giving and receiving when he discusses the example par excellence of work, namely, the artistic process, that "mysterious gestation" that makes the creation of an artistic work possible (1965a, p. 25). According to Marcel,

> That which is essential in the creator is the act by which he places himself at the disposal of something which, no doubt, in one sense depends upon him for its existence, but which at the same time appears to him to be beyond what he is and what he judged himself capable of drawing directly and immediately from himself [i.e., from his personality].
>
> (ibid.)

Marcel notes that while the creative act involves what he calls "the personality" of the artist—his inner resources broadly described—at the same time, as all artists will tell you, "Creation depends in some way upon a superior order" (ibid.), a transcendent realm, perhaps God, as Michelangelo and Bach thought and felt, or the unconscious or collective unconscious, as Freud and Jung might have called it. According to Marcel,

> it will seem to the person that sometimes he invents the order ["giving"], sometimes he discovers it ["receiving"], and reflection will moreover show that there is always a continuity between invention and discovery [what "callings" researcher Wrzesniewski referred to as discovering and creating], and that no line of demarcation as definite as that ordinarily accepted by commonsense can be established between the one and the other.
>
> (ibid.)

The point is that in ultimate domains of being, such as creativity, the creator simultaneously and indistinguishably receives and gives as he fully engages the creative process, right up to the last brushstroke, note, word, or prosocical act in the workplace. Put somewhat differently, the creative "action is neither autonomous nor heteronomous" (Gallagher, 1962, p. 88). Artistic creation feels as if it is not simply one's own possession, "it testifies to a gift from transcendence, even though the reception of the inspiration is itself an act of the" artist (ibid.). The great German psychiatrist/philosopher Karl Jaspers made a similar observation when he wrote, "There where I am myself I am no longer only myself" (ibid., p. 91). Transcendence, in other words, particularly in the creative realm broadly described (including in the workplace), refers to "that which is not myself but which can never be external to myself" (ibid., p. 93). Extrapolating from this point, we could say, as Marcel wrote, that the most receptive and responsive person, the one who is able to engage life openly with the fullness of his whole being, is also the most creative (1965a, p. 264). It is within this context that the creator enters the realm of "creative testimony" or "creative attestation," that existential place "where the human person bears witness to the presence of being" (Cain, 1979, p. 75).

Finally, for Marcel, creativity, especially in the ethical realm, emanates from and is intimately involved in cultural beliefs and values. While an extensive discussion of the complex and murky subject of beliefs and values is well beyond the scope of this chapter, by cultural beliefs I simply mean any statement that attempts "to describe some aspect of collective reality," beliefs largely being the basis for our social construction of everyday reality, including its less common aspects, such as spirituality or cosmology (Johnson, 1995, p. 24). By cultural values I mean those "shared ideas about how something is ranked in terms of its relative social desirability, worth or goodness" (ibid., p. 309). Most importantly, for Marcel, values, which he closely links to being and creativity, can be psychologically viewed as the core components of a clustering of beliefs that direct behavior on a long-range basis toward a particular goal. A value, says sociologist Barry Barnes, is "a cluster of accepted modes of action" (1983, pp. 29–30), while Richard Rorty notes that beliefs are "successful rules for action" (1990, p. 65). For Marcel, the domain of being, of "fullness" and transcendence, of which creativity is one of its most exquisite points of entry and expression, is always embedded in and animated by values. In fact, for Marcel, values are the same as, or at least strongly point to, being and transcendent reality. "Being cannot be separated from the exigence of being ... the impossibility of severing being from value" (Marcel, 2001b, p. 61). And elsewhere he notes, "For what we call values are perhaps only a kind of refraction of reality, like the rainbow colors that emerge from a prism when white light is passed through it" (Marcel, 2008, p. 122). In other words, creativity, whether in the artistic or ethical realms—and this includes everyday life in the workplace—is always intimately connected to such concrete values as Beauty, Truth, and Goodness, those sacred values being the basis for living with a sense of transcendent meaning and purpose. For Marcel, the process of integrating these higher values into one's artistic endeavors and intersubjective relations, as Bach did in his music, Jesus did in his relationships, and Mother Teresa did in her tireless work with the poor, involves both actively inventing usable truths and discovering universal truths, a fundamentally active, dynamic, creative process that is both self- and other-affirming. Put differently, the self that is creatively attained, including in the workplace, is spiritual; this is a self that cannot be objectified, for it has become realized "in perpetutity by reinscribing oneself in the eternal" (Rodwick, 2013, p. 127).

Buber on some ethical elements in teaching

While Marcel, qua philosopher, envisioned himself to be less a teacher as conventionally defined and more an "awakener," he nonetheless implied that being a great teacher (in his case, of philosophy) also required being a "seeker," engaged in what he called a "vocation" (1973, p. 19).

Buber too viewed the teacher at his best as pursuing a calling, and it is in part for this reason that I want to summarize Buber's observations about what constituted this specific kind of work, the great teacher who was trying to awaken his students to the "growth of the spirit" (Buber, 1965, p. 89).[5]

Buber would quite likely agree with the late A. Bartlett Giamatti, a professor of English Renaissance literature and president of Yale University: "Teachers believe they have a gift for giving; it drives them with the same irrepressible drive that drives others to create a work of art or a market or a building" (Malikow, 2010, p. 42).[6] Indeed, for Buber, like pastors, psychotherapists, and parents, teachers have an asymmetrical relationship in terms of responsibility to their students; they ideally give without expecting or needing reciprocation from those in their charge. A teacher should lack Eros (self-serving desire) and the will to power in his way of relating to his students. While Buber's I-Thou relationship between, for example, lovers is rooted in mutuality, reciprocity, and equality, the "subspecies" of I-Thou relationships between teacher and student work a bit differently, though also reflecting the teacher's genuine responsibility. "Genuine responsibility," said Buber, "exists only where there is real responsibility. Responding to what? To what happens to one, to what is to be seen and heard and felt" (Buber, 1965, p. 16). In other words, the work of education, the teacher's calling, is the "growth of the spirit" via communion, "freedom in education [as opposed to coercion, brainwashing, or propaganda] is the possibility of communion" (ibid., pp. 89, 91). In this section, I want to briefly describe some of the qualities of mind and heart that a teacher has as he tries to morally educate his students, Buber's main focus suggests that the teacher is animated by the "instinct for communion" (ibid., p. 88), which points to "something more," "something higher," and "something better," to addressing the Eternal Thou, the divine, or the transcendent. This is when the teacher's comportment is inspired and inspiring, reflecting a relationship to the totality of circumstances that constitutes his work as a calling. Indeed, in his description of the teaching practice, Buber employs evocative language that he used in *I and Thou* to suggest a sense of revelation. Revelation is less about specific content than about a powerful Presence often sensed in contexts of great Beauty (e.g., the Sistine Chapel), Truth (e.g., the iconic video of the lone man resisting the tanks at Tiananmen Square), and Goodness (e.g., Mother Teresa selflessly tending to the poor and sick): "Wherever the action of nature as well as spirit is perceived as a gift, Revelation takes place" (Buber, 1973, p. 26). Revelation can be described as welcoming the wholly new with a dedicated openness to dialogue. Similar to the receiver of revelation, the student is transformed from the dialogical encounter with the teacher with a plenitude of trust and meaning. One can think of *Mr. Rogers' Neighborhood* as an everyday placeholder. Indeed, Fred Rogers was an icon for his commitment to the best interests of children, as manifested in his creativity, kindness, and spirituality (he graduated from Pittsburgh Theological Seminary and was ordained a minister of the United Presbyterian Church at age 35, always renewing his ordination via regular church attendance). Affectionately described as "America's favorite neighbor," he exploited his varied talents to inspire, nurture, and educate.

Following his assumption about what constitutes the human condition, his philosophical anthropology of personhood,[7] Buber believed that education was *not* mainly about the appropriation of knowledge and the received wisdom of the day, the enhancement of creativity, or even about changing the internal world of the student—all important aspects of the educational process—but rather, it was the transcendent goal of modifying the way students relate to others, such that they can enter into dialogical relationships. The teacher, conceived of as a change agent, is thus willing and able to use his own personhood, including his strongly felt, flexibly and creatively applied, transcendent-pointing moral beliefs and values, that are primarily other-directed, other-regarding, and other-serving, to create genuine mutuality between himself and his students, a relationship lodged in trust. Buber wrote that while a teacher does not typically choose his students—that is, they are the other to him as he is to them—the great educator views "each of these individuals as in a position to become a unique, single person, and thus the bearer of the special task of existence which can be fulfilled through him and through him alone" (Buber, 1965, p. 83). The teacher's task is to create the psychological and moral conditions of possibility for the aforementioned to be actualized in his students, and this centrally means acting as role model for confirmatory relations. Confirmation means the teacher takes a stand in the presence of the student, being to being, affirming, accepting, and supporting him in his uniqueness, and challenging him when it is required (Kramer &Gawlick, 2003, p. 202).

As already mentioned, trust is a key notion for Buber as it relates to the educational process. The teacher has to be perceived by the student as utterly devoted to his best interests, and this involves the student experiencing him as a stable, reliable potential presence. As Buber noted, "Trust, trust in the world [faith in the world in which one resides], because this human being exists—that is the most inward achievement in education" (1965, p. 98), for it gives a student a feeling of acceptance and self-confidence. This demands that the teacher be willing and able to "remain truly present" as a whole person to the student, as he has "gathered the child's presence into his own store as one of the bearers of his communion with the world, one of the focuses of his responsibilities for the world" (ibid.). Another way of putting this is that the teacher engages in "inclusion" (a concept described in depth in Chapter 2). Inclusion means "making present," the act of imagining what the person before you thinks, feels, and experiences (i.e., engaging his otherness), not as detached analysis or abstract content, but as living engagement without relinquishing one's own existential position (Kramer & Gawlick, 2003, p. 203). One could say inclusion has a "family resemblance" to empathy conventionally understood (but not exactly), "the act of putting oneself in the Other and that of putting the Other into oneself" in the service of enhancing the other (Todd, 2003, p. 153), though for Buber this is what the teacher does but not the student, reflecting the asymmetric responsibility of the relationship. In contrast to inclusion, empathy involves the endeavored participation in the inner experiences of the other, such that provisionally one person becomes identical with the other or, at the minimum, attempts to do so. As Friedman notes, through engaging the otherness of the student, the teacher realizes his own real and imagined limitations, but also "recognizes the forces of the world which the child needs to grow and he draws the forces into himself. Thus, through his concern with the child, the teacher educates himself" (Friedman, 2002, p. 208). Indeed, Levinas's observation, "The other is … the first rational teaching, the condition of all teaching," cuts both ways (Levinas, 1969, p. 203).

Thus, for Buber, education as conventionally conceived includes, for example, conveying knowledge, the so-called truths, values, and creative problem-solving skills necessary to function in a democratic society. He acknowledges a potentially useful role for these reality-based student acquisitions in educational settings and beyond. However, he believes that this educational approach alone situates the student too much in the It-world, characterized by subject-object separation, objectification, and monology. Rather than reaffirming a mode of education that is mainly geared to acquisitions and accomplishing ("achievement" and "success"), in education at its best, the teacher-student relation must be lodged in genuine dialogue. As Silberstein further noted, "Insofar as people actualize themselves by relating to the student as an I to a You [Thou], the teacher helps the student to actualize the inherent capacity [the 'inborn Thou'] to relate dialogically [i.e., immediately and mutually] to the world and to other people" (Silberstein, 1989, p. 190). It is the teacher's responsibility to generate the psychological and moral context for dialogue to take place between himself and his students in the service of character building. "The great character," says Friedman, "acts from the whole of his substance and reacts in accordance with the uniqueness of every situation"; each situation demands heartfelt presence and responsibility for himself and for the well-being of others (Friedman, 2002, p. 214). Moreover, educating the great character demands that a teacher be willing and able to discern appearance and reality, that which is true and false and right and wrong. Admittedly, these are judgments that one makes with great deliberation (including regarding normative considerations), criticality, and in "fear and trembling" (e.g., that one can have it all wrong). Detailing exactly how this is accomplished is beyond the scope of this section. However, Buber makes it clear that for the student to engage in genuine dialogue/relation, the teacher must, for example, act as an intermediary between the student and the external world, which includes offering critical and instructive interventions as he educates the student:

> The educator gathers in the constitutive forces of the world. He distinguishes, rejects and confirms in himself, in his self which is filled with the world. The constructive forces are eternally the same: they are the world bound up in community, turned to God. The educator educates himself to be their better vehicle.
>
> (Buber, 1965, p. 101)

Notwithstanding Buber's claim about "eternally the same" "constructive forces" "turned to God" and elsewhere, "God has one truth, the Truth, but He has no system" (Simon, 1967, p. 544),[8] a questionable assertion for most postmodernists; what Buber is emphasizing about the teacher's role has been aptly summarized by Hodes, who quotes Buber in their conversation:

> Everything depends on the teacher as a man, as a person. He educates from himself, from his virtues and his faults, through personal example and according to circumstances and conditions. His task is to realize the truth in his personality and to convey this realization to the pupil.
>
> (Hodes, 1971, p. 127)

Perhaps most importantly, all of the aforementioned requires exquisite emotional/intellectual attunement to the ethical potential of education, what has been called the "ethical turn" in educational theory and other disciplines. The "ethical turn" comprises critically reflecting on the ways in which we conceptualize otherness and how our encounters "with otherness leave intact or challenge the very differences that categorize the Other as other" (Todd, 2003, p. 2). While Todd has been greatly influenced by Levinas, much of what she describes is in sync with Buber's approach to education. For like Levinas, Buber recognized that affirming and respecting the otherness and difference of the student, an otherness and difference which reflects what Buber and Marcel called the "mystery" of existence (e.g., the other as never completely knowable, the transcendence of the other, including over me, as Levinas radically claimed), is the main thrust of the education of character. This is the difference between learning "about" a student, an I-It approach mainly geared to the teacher's mastery and control, and learning "from" a student, which, of course, is an intensely emotional engagement that includes Buberian inclusion, love, managing closeness/distance, guilt/reparation, humility, and the like. The latter especially requires respectful listening, being ready (vulnerable and open), responsive, and responsible to the other and maintaining otherness and difference; it is conceived as a non-coercive and non-violent option, while the teacher works toward the education of character (ibid.). In a sense, this involves reciprocity (e.g., being moved by the other), enlarged self-awareness, and the willingness and ability to risk and sacrifice, as in all Buberian-like dialogical participation (Ehrenberg, 1992, p. 48). For Buber, the education of character, what Todd calls "moral education," profoundly "becomes identified as the domain of educational knowledge that can aid students in the practice of living" a flourishing life (Todd, 2003, p. 5). Moreover, this educational knowledge, conceived as teacher-derived and inspired ethical "knowledge in practice" (ibid., p. 6), is intimately linked to actualizing genuine community and social justice. Silberstein, a Buberian scholar, called this "education for community," a "radical restructuring of modern society," along the lines of biblically inspired justice and love (Silberstein, 1989, p. 187).

While there is much more to what constitutes a great teacher, I have given the reader a sense of what Buber thought was important about the educational process. However, the question remains: What from a Buberian point of view motivates and instantiates a great teacher, one who experiences teaching as a calling that points to "something more," "something higher," and "something better," to addressing the Eternal Thou, the divine, or the transcendent?

Teaching as a calling is another way of describing the teaching process as a spiritual vocation in which the teacher strives to affirm the students' quest to connect to something larger than themselves—that is, to fashion an affect-integrating, meaning-giving, action-guiding way of being that allows them to engage in a flourishing life, in part, as Freud described it: a life characterized by deep and wide love, to work creatively and productively, one that is also guided by reason and ethics and is aesthetically pleasing. This means, in part, the teacher is a transmitter to the student of the best of his strongly felt, flexibly and creatively applied, transcendent-pointing moral beliefs and values that are primarily other-directed, other-regarding, and other-serving. "What we term education, conscious and willed, means *a selection by man of the effective world*" (Buber, 1965, p. 85). Indeed, Buber was fond of quoting the great nineteenth-century Polish Hassidic Rabbi Simcha Bunam as saying, "If someone is merely good, he is a beggar; if he is merely pious, he is a thief; and if he is merely prudent, he is an unbeliever" (Simon, 1967, p. 545). In other words, it is through having integrated these three qualities instantiated in everyday life (i.e., love of man) that a spiritual aspirant can best serve God (i.e., love of God). "The educational directive," said Buber, "is the way from 'below' to 'above'" (ibid.). The teacher never does this value-transmission, of which he is the living embodiment, in a heavy-handed manner (e.g., no ethics "right and wrong" teaching, sermonizing, "fire and brimstone," and the like), but rather always indirectly and gently, and within the context of the dialogical participation with the student who is discovering the values and his own unique relationships to truth, through his own experience with the teacher (whose job is to elicit it) and capacity to reason. It is through this dialogical process with his students (a kind of reciprocal interaction) that the teacher feels or senses the upsurge of joy that gives him a deep and abiding justification to his existence. As Fred Rogers said, this can be conceptualized as engaging in "love without an agenda": "Mutual caring relationships require kindness and patience, tolerance, optimism, joy in the other's achievements, confidence in oneself, and the ability to give without undue thought of gain." Moreover, and this is one of the take-home points for this section about work as a calling, again quoting a Buberian-sounding Mr. Rogers, "The connections we make in the course of a life—maybe that's what heaven is" (Zlotnick, https://twentytwowords.com › incredibly-inspiring-mr-rogers-quotes-that-wil...retrieved 12/18/19). In fact, Buber put this point just right by saying that the teacher's "real goal" (in terms of education of character), acting from the "whole of his substance," from his personhood, the goal in which in his "destiny lies the very meaning of his life's work," is that he helps the student "back to his own unity [roughly the integration of being, life, and action, an identity grounded in responsibility and love] … to put him again face to face with God" (Buber, 1965, pp. 113, 117). "The highest form of education is this: existential unity," a unity of actuality and potentiality, in which the teacher facilitates the student's "becoming" via his encounter with the student (Simon, 1967, p. 544). "Becoming" can be roughly thought of as the upsurge of autonomy, integration, and humanity, rooted in what Buber called "the presence of universal values and norms of absolute validity" (Buber, 1965, p. 108).[9] As Erich Fromm noted, when the teacher has faith in the child's potentialities, education in contrast to manipulation occurs, "Education is identical with helping the child realize his potentialities" (1947, p. 207). Needless to say, this includes moments of high conflict (which can be perspective-shifting, soul-deepening educational moments), in which the teacher and student fight for truth as they see it, but the teacher must always be generous in victory and loving in defeat, so that the student never closes down to further dialogue about moral conundrums.

It should be mentioned that Buber's reflections on education in *Between Man and Man* in many ways were a forerunner of the findings of those empirical researchers interested in religion and spirituality in educational settings (Rockenbach & Townsend, 2013). For example, in their path-breaking work, Love and Talbot (1999; Love, 2019) put forth a workable definition of spirituality (admittedly, an ambiguous and debated notion, especially when compared to religion) in terms of five important features: 1) an inner process of questing/fashioning a sense of personal authenticity, genuineness, and wholeness as a critical component of identity construction; 2) the process of persistently transcending one's self-centric outlook (i.e., inordinate narcissism, egocentricity); 3) the creation of enhanced connectedness to one's self and others via robust relationships and communal engagement; 4) the process of finding/creating meaning, purpose, and direction in one's existential odyssey; and 5) developing a greater receptivity to an unseeable, unevidenced pervasive power, essence, or center of value that transcends human existence and rational comprehension (this can be called God, the divine, transcendent, or something else by a non-believer).

Indeed, the aforementioned appears to correlate with many of the descriptions and formulations of Buber (and Marcel). In terms of the focus of this chapter, helping the analysand (or for that matter, the ordinary person) to experience work as a calling, what personifies the dialogical nature of education as Buber describes education of character is that the teacher, like his students, is a *homo viator*, a spiritual pilgrim. That is, the teacher's outlook and behavior, including his mode of self-comportment, the questions he raises, and the educational "headspace" he creates for his students, will convey that he too is a *homo viator* and that he and his students are dialogical partners in nurturing each other's inner lives—and most importantly, they are "faithfully, and open to the world and the spirit," where "living truth arises and endures" (Buber, 1965, p. 99). That is, what is life-affirming and identity-defining for the teacher and, in part, joyfully motivates him to press on educating his students year after year in challenging institutional circumstances is the realization that they have a common ground of sacred interconnectedness: connectedness to self, to the natural world, and to diverse others in a pluralistic community, connecting via service and social justice, and of course connecting to spiritual support networks, all in the service of creating a mode of being-in-the-world animated by the spirit (or Spirit) (Rockenbach & Townsend, 2013, p. 586). It is through such meetings that the teacher can both apprehend and fashion his everyday work as a calling.

Implications for treatment

What then can the analyst help to potentiate in the analysand so that he is willing and able to embrace without reserve an outlook and behavior that allows him to experience his work as a calling? As I have emphasized, work experienced as a job (or even a career) feels like being obligated to do something for a paycheck, while work experienced as a calling feels like being graced to do something that can make a positive difference (i.e., it reflects one's core beliefs and values). While this is a complex and challenging question that in part involves the murky issue of choosing the "right" career in the first place ("What do you want to be when you grow up?"), a subject I have dealt with elsewhere and is beyond the scope of this chapter (Marcus, 2017), I want to mention a few aspects of the aforementioned outlook and behavior that is correlated with experiencing work as a calling, a constituent aspect of a flourishing life. For if the analysand (with the analyst's help) can discern what it is in his mode of comportment to work that needs to be actualized (and impedes him), he has a better chance of potentiating in his everyday work its spiritually animated dialogical potential as conceived by Buber and Marcel.

According to researchers Hagmaier and Abele (2014), a person's job can be aptly described as a calling if it has three specific elements: 1) a sense of a perfect or near-perfect "fit" between the person's skills and interests and the demands of the job; 2) a sense of meaning/purpose and altruism (i.e., prosocial behavior) in the work; and 3) the sense of a life- and identity-affirming transcendent animating/shepherding force (e.g., suggesting Marcel's previously mentioned "spiritual reality" and "illumination" and Buber's "eternal values"). The researchers reported (based on respondents' self-reporting) that people with a calling described having a greater sense of engagement with their work, in addition to a higher sense of self-congruence, that is, the perception that their "real" self is in accordance with their view of their "ideal" self. The respondents also reported more life satisfaction or happiness. Other vocational psychologists have similarly noted that those who view their work as a calling had three critical elements: 1) an "action orientation," that is, a more assertive-like "doing" mode versus a more passive-like "being" one; 2) "a sense of clarity of purpose, direction, meaning, and personal mission"; and 3) a "personal intention," or what calls to mind the notion of agency, a wish to fashion the world into an improved place (Compton & Hoffman, 2020, p. 250).

Following Marcel (and in many ways Buber), I have suggested that creativity, conceived as "creative testimony" especially but not only in the ethical realm, is the dimension of the spirit from which one is most likely to experience the "exigency of transcendence," including in the workplace. Experiences of radical self-overcoming, self-mastery, and self-transformation of the "renewal of being" emanate from genuine experiences of intersubjectivity (i.e., dialogical partnership), ultra-meaningful relational experiences that point to the "eternal and absolute thou [God] that is the heart of all communion" (Gallagher, 1962, p. 95)—that is, communion as the emotional and spiritual closeness that is evoked in any relationship characterized by other-directed, other-regarding, and other-serving forms of fellowship. In more straightforward psychological terms, I am referring to the important role of the previously described emotional creativity in generating the psychological and moral conditions for entering into the dimension of the spirit that tends to potentiate the experience of a for-the-other transcendence. By way of concluding this chapter, I want to briefly suggest a few ways that emotional creativity, the spiritualizing of passions, is an important precursor, if not psychological prerequisite, for the experience of Marcelian- (and to a large extent Buberian-) conceived transcendence or for flourishing in the workplace.

Emotional creativity, as I use the term,[10] refers to the human capacity for using one's emotions, both positive and negative, to fashion more aesthetically pleasing, meaningful, coherent, and inspired contexts for inventive everyday living. Emotional creativity—for example, transforming one's anger, grief, or sexual desire into something original, imaginative, and life-affirming, such as assertiveness, joy, and love—is a form of sublimation that psychoanalysts have aptly described. As Averill points out, for emotions to be conceived as creative products, they must express three interrelated qualities: 1) they must be novel, something new, or different; 2) they must be effective and have a desired or intended result; and 3) they must be authentic and animated by one's dearly held beliefs and values (2009, pp. 251–253). Needless to say, there are a wide range of individual differences to emotional creativity—from those who suffer from alexithymia (extreme difficulty in feeling, describing, and expressing emotions, like the Holocaust survivor in the novel *The Pawnbroker*) or from inhibitions and other forms of neurosis, to those capable of expressing and actualizing deep and wide love (think of the great writer/poet Goethe, who was also a humane person in his everyday life). Likewise, there are a wide range of individual differences in terms of the childhood experiences and developmental influences that account for a particular person's capacity for emotional creativity. Indeed, the question whether there are patterns of emotions experienced by most creative individuals, and understanding exactly how such people apply and transform varied emotional experiences to facilitate creativity, is a widely researched but still debated one.

Indeed, both Marcel and Buber point to the disadvantages of misplaced emotion and, in particular, to the inordinately narcissistically driven subjectivity that is its underpinning. Instead, they advocate cultivating a different outlook, a way of being in which one sees and respects things as they are, as "thou," without the undue interference of our narcissistically driven strivings. By "thou," Marcel means "that which I can invoke rather than that which I judge to be able to answer me" (1952, p. 200); and for Buber, "The primary word *I-Thou* can only be spoken with the whole being" to the radically other (1958, p. 3). It is from this psychological and existential context that one is better able to engage in "creative testimony," in other words, to recognize, honor, and serve the other and the otherness of life, in love, faith, and hope, the very basis and expression of felt and lived transcendence. As Marcel noted, "The term *transcendence* taken in its full metaphysical sense seems essentially to denote an otherness, and even an absolute otherness" (2001a, p. 48). And for Buber, transcendence only occurs in dialogical meeting between an I and Thou, which is incapable of being described. Most importantly, following Marcel and Buber, I have argued that creation as we have been discussing it, as "creative testimony," does not inevitably refer to something external to the person; it is not mainly to produce an object like a work of art. What Marcel and Buber are affirming is that a most worthwhile goal for each of us, including the analysand, is to be a creator, to bear witness to a creation, especially through our "for the other" relationships, what is called prosocial motivation in vocational psychology and "generative altruism" in psychoanalytic theory. Generative altruism "is the ability to experience conflict-free pleasure in fostering the success and/or pleasure of another" (Seelig & Rosof, 2001, p. 947). Such people, few as they may be, observes Marcel, stand out "by the radiance of charity and love shining from their being." It is through their numinous and creative presence that they add a most "positive contribution to the invisible work which gives the human adventure the only meaning which can justify it" (2001a, p. 48). Put differently, to the extent that psychoanalysis can potentiate in the analysand the will and ability to engage his work as a sacred activity—one that points to "something more," "something higher," and "something better" and that requires an other-directed, other-regarding, and other-serving outlook and behavior—the chances of his experiencing work as a calling are greatly enhanced. Such a person is quite likely to feel the lived reality of dwelling in a different dimension of being, the realm of the spirit, where receptivity, emotional attunement, and dialogue are what matter most.

Notes

1 As Sweetman noted about Marcel, character development was always his main concern: "It is the type of person one is that will be decisive in ethical situations, not how one analyzes the situation, is clearly evocative of the notion of character formation by means of habitual virtuous activity that is the heart of traditional ethics" (Sweetman, 2008, p. 66).

2 It should be noted that there is a down side to a calling, that is, it can foster negative outcomes such as job idolization, workaholism, and exploitation. As Marcel would surely agree, humility, conceived as an organizational value can function as a mitigating frame against these negative outcomes (Molloy, Dik, Davis and Duffy, 2019).

3 While these three "transcendentals" comprising "properties of being," as philosophers have traditionally called them, involve value judgements, Richard Gardner (2012) has reframed them in a way that is plausible and thoughtful for our postmodern age. Beauty, Truth and Goodness are not to be taken as Platonic ideals, but are meant to point to a set of worthwhile valuative attachments that are context-dependent and setting-specific in terms of their instantiation.

4 I am aware that not all routine is detrimental, for without certain routines we would not be able to function in our everyday life (e.g., imagine what one's morning would feel like if we always put our toothbrush in a different place the night before and had to remember where we put it!), nor would we feel the crucial sense of ontological security that, as sociologist Anthony Giddens noted, routine helps us feel.

5 Early on his teaching career, Buber was "a rather clumsy teacher … his initial steps as a teacher were faltering and uncertain, particularly in leading seminars." Ernst Simon, a close associate, wrote a "scathing critique of the manner in which he conducted a seminar on Hasidism" (Mendes-Flohr, 2019, pp. 137–138).

6 One wonders if Giametti and Buber would agree with Freud (at least with the spirit of his comment), that teaching was one of the "'impossibe' professions" (psychoanalysis and governing were the other two). Freud believed that "unsatisfying results" were innevitable. He was alluding to the tremendous unconscious resistance that analysands and students have to making personal changes and learning (Freud, 1937, p. 248). This being said, in the *Standard Edition* translation Freud used the word "education" 222 times, and the words, "educator, educative" etcetera another

94 times. "Education to reality," the goal of analysis meant that a person cannot stay a child forever (Phillips, 2004, p. 786). Indeed, Marcel noted, "The truly wise man, whose wisdom is his heroism, is not afraid to look the world in the face" (1965b, p. 203).

7 For Buber, in contrast to an "individual," that is, a self-existing being who puts his needs and desires into the center of his actions and relates to the world in an I-It manner, a "person" wholly enters into a relationship with a Thou, affirming the other as an equal partner, while also assuming a personal bearing (Kramer & Gawlick, 2003, pp. 203, 204).

8 In this claim, Buber is reiterating a well-known Hindu claim that accounts for its general tolerance of other religious pathways to God. Says the Rig Veda, "Truth is one, but the wise speak of it many ways" (Marcus, 2003, p. 30). Buber was probably familiar with the Rig Veda, as he had explored Eastern philosophy early on in his career.

9 From what I can discern, Buber held to objectively valid and absolute values, as did Marcel, quasi-grounding their claims in Biblical and humanistic ethics, and their own and other testimonials.

10 I am largely drawing from Averill's (2009) work on emotional creativity in this section.

References

Akhtar, S. (2009). *Comprehensive dictionary of psychoanalysis*. London: Karnac.

Averill, J. R. (2009). Emotional creativity: Toward "spiritualizing the passions." In S. L. Lopez & C. R. Snyder (Eds.), *Oxford handbook of positive psychology* (pp. 249–258). Oxford: Oxford University Press.

Barnes, B. (1983). *T.S. Kuhn and social science*. New York: Columbia University Press.

Bellah, R. N., Madsen, R., Sullivan, W. M., Swidler, A., & Tipton, S. M. (1986). *Habits of the heart: Individualism and commitment in American life*. New York: Harper & Row.

Berg, J. M., Grant, A. G., & Johnson, V. (2010). When callings are calling: Crafting work and leisure in pursuit of unanswered occupational callings. *Organization Science, 21*(5), 973–994.

Biswas, G. (1996). Martin Buber's concept of art as dialogue. In M. Friedman (Ed.), *Martin Buber and the human sciences* (pp. 223–236). Albany: State University of New York Press.

Buber, M. (1958). *I and thou* (R. G. Smith, Trans.). New York: Scribner.

Buber, M. (1965). *Between man and man* (R.G. Smith, Trans.). New York: Macmillan.

Buber, M. (1973). *On Zion: The history of an idea* (S. Godman, Trans.). Syracuse, NY: Syracuse University Press.

Cain, S. (1963). *Gabriel Marcel*. South Bend, IN: Regnery/Gateway.

Cain, S. (1995). *Gabriel Marcel's theory of religious experience*. New York: Peter Lang.

Carroll, S. T. (2013). Addressing religion and spirituality in the workplace. In K. I. Pargament, A. Mahoney, & E. P. Shafranske (Eds.), *APA handbook of psychology, religion, and spirituality, volume 2* (pp. 595–612). Washington, DC: American Psychological Association.

Compton, W. C., & Hoffman, E. (2020). *Positive psychology: The science of happiness and flourishing*. Los Angeles: Sage.

Dik, B. J., & Duffy, R. D. (2009). Calling and vocation at work: Definitions and prospects for research and practice. *Counseling Psychologist, 37*(3), 424–450.

Dutton, J. E., Roberts, L. M. & Bednar, J. (2011). Prosocial practices, positive identity, and flourishing at work. In S. I. Donaldson, M. Csikszentmihalyi, & J. Nakamura (Eds.), *Applied positive psychology: Improving everyday life, health, schools, work, and society* (pp. 155–170). New York: Routledge.

Ehrenberg, D. H. (1992). *The intimate edge: Extending the reach of psychoanalytic interaction*. New York: Norton.

Eliot, G. (1882). *The wit and wisdom of George Eliot*. Boston: Roberts Brothers.

Erikson, E. H. (1959). *Identity and the life cycle: Selected papers* (Psychological Issues, Vol. 1, No. 1, Monograph 1). New York: International Universities Press.

Freud, S. (1895 [1985]). *The complete letters of Sigmund Freud to Wilhelm Fliess*, 1887–1904 (J. Masson, Ed.). Cambridge, MA: Harvard University Press.

Freud, S. (1937). Analysis Terminable and Interminable. In J. Stratchey (Ed. & Trans.), *The Standard Edition of the Complete Psychological Works of Sigmund Freud* (Vol. 23), pp. 209–254. London: Hogarth Press.

Friedman, M. S. (2002). *Martin Buber: The life of dialogue* (4th ed.). London: Routledge.

Fromm, E. (1947). *Man for himself. An inquiry into the psychology of ethics*. New York: Rinehart & Company.

Gallagher, K. T. (1962). *The philosophy of Gabriel Marcel*. New York: Fordham University Press.

Gardner, R. (2012). *Truth, beauty, and goodness reframed*. New York: Basic Books.

Gilbert, D. L. (1981). *Oxygen and living processes: An interdisciplinary approach*. Berlin: Springer-Verlag.

Hagmaier, T., & Abele A. E. (2014). When reality meets ideal: Investigating the relation between calling and life satisfaction. *Journal of Career Assessment. 23*, 367–382. https://doi.org/10.1177/1069072714547164

Hall, D. T., & Chandler, D. E. (2005). Psychological success: When the career is a calling. *Journal of Organizational Behavior, 26*, 155–176.

Hodes, A. (1971). *Martin Buber: An intimate portrait*. New York: Viking.

Johnson, A. G. (1995). *The Blackwell dictionary of sociology: A user's guide to sociological language*. Oxford: Oxford University Press.

Kernberg, O. (1979). Regression in organizational leadership. *Psychiatry, 42*, 24–39.

Kramer, K. P., & Gawlick, M. (2003). *Martin Buber's I and thou: Practicing living dialogue*. New York: Paulist Press.

Levi, P. (1996). *Survival in Auschwitz*. New York: Touchstone.

Levinas, E. (1969). *Totality and infinity*. Pittsburgh: Duquesne University Press.

Levine, H. (1997). Men at work: Work, ego and identity in the analysis of adult Men. In C. W. Socarides & S. Kramer (Eds.), *Work and its inhibitions: Psychoanalytic essays* (pp. 143–157). Madison, CT: International Universities Press.

Lilius, J. M., Kanov, J., Dutton, J. E., Warline, M. C., & Maitlis, S. (2012). Compassion revealed: What we know about compassion at work (and where we need to know more). In K. S. Cameron & G. M. Spreitzer (Eds.), *The Oxford handbook of positive organizational scholarship* (pp. 273–287). Oxford: Oxford University Press.

Love, P. G. (2019). Differentiating spirituality from religion. https://characterclearinghouse.fsu.edu; retrieved 12/29/19.

Love, P. G., & Talbot, D. (1999). Defining spiritual development: A missing consideration for student affairs. *NASPA Journal, 37*(1), 361–375.
Malikow, M. (2010). *Being human: Philosophical reflections on psychological issues*. Lanham, MD: Hamilton Books.
Marcel, G. (1952). *Metaphysical journal* (B. Wall, Trans.). Chicago: Henry Regnery.
Marcel, G. (1963). *The Existential background of human dignity*. Cambridge, MA: Harvard University Press.
Marcel, G. (1964). *Creative fidelity* (R. Rosthal, Trans.). New York: Farrar, Straus and Giroux.
Marcel, G. (1965a). *Homo viator: Introduction to a metaphysic of hope* (E. Crauford, Trans.). New York: Harper and Row.
Marcel, G. (1965b). *Being and having: An existentialist's diary* (K. Farrer, Trans.). New York: Harper and Row.
Marcel, G. (1973). *Tragic wisdom and beyond*. Evanston, IL: Northwestern University Press.
Marcel, G. (1995). *The philosophy of existentialism*. New York: Carol Publishing.
Marcel, G. (2001a). *The mystery of being: Volume I: Reflection and mystery*. South Bend, IN: St. Augustine's Press.
Marcel, G. (2001b). *The mystery of Being: Volume 2: Faith and reality*. South Bend, IN: St. Augustine's Press.
Marcel, G. (2005). *Music and philosophy* (S. Maddux & R. E. Wood, Trans.). Milwaukee, WI: Marquette University Press.
Marcel, G. (2008). *Man against mass society*. South Bend, IN: St. Augustine's Press.
Marcus, P. (2003). *Ancient religious wisdom, spirituality, and psychoanalysis*. Westport, CT: Praeger.
Marcus, P. (2017). *The psychoanalysis of career choice, job performance, and satisfaction: How to flourish in the workplace*. London: Routledge.
Marianetti, O., & Passmore, J. (2010). Mindfulness at work: Paying attention to enhance well-being and performance. In P. A. Linley, S. Harrington, & N. Garcea (Eds.), *Oxford handbook of positive psychology and work* (pp. 189–200). Oxford: Oxford University Press.
Meissner, W. W. (1997). The self and the principle of work. In C. W. Socarides & S. Kramer (Eds.), *Work and its inhibitions: Psychoanalytic essays* (pp. 35–60). Madison, WI: International Universities Press.
Mendes-Flohr, P. (2019). *Martin Buber. A life of faith and dissent*. New Haven, CT: Yale University Press.
Miceli, V. P. (1965). *Ascent to being: Gabriel Marcel's philosophy of communion*. New York: Desclee.
Molloy, K. A., Dik, B. J., Davis, D. E. & Duffy, R. D. (2019). Work calling and humility: framing for job idolization, workaholism, and exploitation. *Journal of Management, Spirituality & Religion*, 16, 428–444.
Nakamura, J., & Csikszentmihalyi, M. (2009). Flow theory and research. In S. L. Lopez & C. R. Snyder (Eds.), *Oxford handbook of positive psychology* (pp. 195–206). Oxford: Oxford University Press.
Phillips, A. (2004). Psychoanalysis as education. *Psychoanalytic Review*, 91(6), 779–799.
Reik, T. (1983). *Listening with the third ear*. New York: Farrar, Straus and Giroux.
Rockenbach, A. B., & Townsend, T. (2013). Addressing religion and spirituality in educational settings. In K. I. Pargament (Ed.), *APA handbook of psychology, religion, and spirituality, Vol. 2: An applied psychology of religion and spirituality* (pp. 577–593). Washington, DC: American Psychological Association.

Rodwick, D. W. (2013). Gabriel Marcel and American philosophy. *Faculty Scholarship. Paper 2*. www.exhibit.xavier.edu/philosphy_faculty/2

Rorty, R. (1990). *Objectivity, relativism, and truth*. New York: Cambridge University Press.

Rose, N. (1996). *Inventing our selves: Psychology, power, and personhood*. Cambridge: Cambridge University Press.

Rothbard, N. P., & Patil, S.V. (2012). Being there: Work engagement and positive organizational scholarship. In K. S. Cameron & G. M. Spreitzer (Eds.), *The Oxford handbook of positive organizational scholarship* (pp. 56–68). Oxford: Oxford University Press.

Seelig, B. J. & Rosof, L. S. (2001). Normal and pathological altruism. *Journal of the American Psychoanalytic Association, 49*, 933–959.

Silberstein, L. J. (1989). *Martin Buber's social and religious thought. alienation and the quest for meaning*. New York: New York University Press.

Simon, E. (1967). Martin Buber, the educator. In P. A. Schilpp & M. Friedman (Eds.), *The philosophy of Martin Buber* (The Library of Living Philosophers, vol. 12, pp. 543–576). La Salle, IL: Open Court.

Stairs, M., & Galpin, M. (2010). Positive engagement: From employee engagement to workplace happiness. In P. A. Linley, S. Harrington, & N. Garcea (Eds.), *Oxford handbook of positive psychology and work* (pp. 155–172). Oxford: Oxford University Press.

Sweetman, B. (2008). *The vision of Gabriel Marcel: Epistemology, human person, the transcendent*. Amsterdam: Rodopi.

Todd, S. (2003). *Levinas, psychoanalysis, and ethical possibilities in education*. Albany, NY: SUNY Press.

Wrzesniewski, A. (2012). Callings. In K. S. Cameron & G. M. Spreitzer (Eds.), *The Oxford handbook of positive organizational scholarship* (pp. 45–55). Oxford: Oxford University Press.

Zlotnick, R. https://twentytwowords.com › incredibly-inspiring-mr-rogers-quotes-that-will improve your whole day; retrieved 12/18/19.

Chapter 4

The spirit of faith

Faith is one of those evocative terms that stir great passion, whether to a secularist (e.g., faith in life) or religious believer (e.g., faith in God). It has been generically defined in the *Cambridge English Dictionary* as "great trust or confidence in something or someone," a definition that certainly points to an essential aspect at the heart of the faith structure in its various manifestations (https://dictionary.cambridge.org › dictionary › english › faith retrieved 1/8/20).

Freud, of course, was a devout atheist; he claimed religious faith was an ill-conceived, ill-advised, and ill-fated manifestation of infantile wish-fulfillment, and instead, he aligned himself with secular faith in scientific rationality. That is, Freud claimed that science was the singular truth, and that all phenomena must be tested in a scientific manner, even if, in some ways, science is not always reliable. For Freud, religious faith is the mistaken belief in an unevidenced, unseen, and therefore unreasonable God-image projection. For the most part, psychoanalysis has taken Freud as their lead, though as I will discuss shortly there have been notable exceptions who regard religious faith, at least some versions of it, as having a life-affirming ripple effect in the spiritual aspirant's everyday existence. In contrast to Freud and others who have discredited religious faith, Buber steadfastly affirmed that faith was the living and enlivening relationship between God and the believer: "The fundamental experience of faith itself," said Buber, "may be regarded as the highest intensification of the reality of meeting" (Buber, 1967b, p. 121). Marcel, too, believed that faith strongly pointed to a form of living that was enacted before the face of God, a divine/human encounter. As Cain notes, Marcel clearly believed that "absolute engagement *is* faith," that is, faith can be characterized, in Marcel's words, as "perpetual witness" to a transcendent realm or reality (Cain, 1995, p. 83). Thus, as I will later detail, for both Buber and Marcel, somewhat differently but still, faith was intimately linked with meeting, with person-to-person encounter, I-Thou relation (and Marcel's creative fidelity), that pointed to "something more," "something higher," and "something better," what they called God (the eternal Thou/absolute Thou, respectively). In this view, the trace of an I-Thou encounter transformed the existential orientation of the spiritual aspirant in a manner that was identity-defining and life-affirming, toward the ultimate goal, a "holy" way of being-in-the-world (roughly *imitatio dei*). Being-in-the-world was mindfully animated by the transcendent virtues, the valuative attachments of Beauty, Truth, and Goodness, the touchstones for fashioning a flourishing life.[1] What Levinas (who studied Buber, Rosenzweig, and Marcel) said more radically and extensively could also be said of Buber and Marcel, namely, that holiness (or saintliness) was always his main interest; "this holiness ... the supreme perfection ... which cedes one's place to the other" was what best characterized "humanity" (Levinas, 2001, p. 183). For Marcel, such holy people were "creators," they were discernible "by the radiance of charity and love shining from their being, they add a positive contribution to the invisible work which gives the human adventure the only meaning which can justify it. Only the blind may say with the suggestion of a sneer that they have produced nothing" (2001, p. 45). Likewise, for Buber, holiness meant enacting in the concrete situation we find ourselves an open, receptive dialogue with God, that is, "hallowing the everyday," hallowing one's life through efforts to make himself responsible to what is holy (Friedman, 1986, p. 131). Indeed, as Katz ((2006) noted, Buber (and Marcel) emphasized that the I-Thou encounter summoned one to ontic and fundamental moral obligations to the other: "Responsibility presupposes one who addresses me primarily, that is, from a realm independent of myself, and to whom I am answerable" (Buber, 1965, p. 17). Psychoanalysis has had almost no interest in using holiness as a viable concept in the clinical context, though I believe this may be a notion worth judiciously integrating into its theory and technique.[2]

In this chapter I am going to briefly review some of the more interesting psychoanalytic formulations of the psychology of faith, mainly religious (as Buber and Marcel were believers), less so secular, in order to illustrate in what manner analysts view how faith can operate positively in the real life of the spiritual aspirant. Next, I will present Buber and Marcel's views on faith, which, in part because of their dialogical personalist approach, can enhance how analysts understand the role of religious (and less secular) faith in the analysand's life and in the analytic dialogue. I should point out from the onset that I am not weighing in on whether it is reasonable or unreasonable to believe in God or a transcendent reality; that is for each individual to decide, including its implication for them in their real life. As the great Catholic theologian Thomas Aquinas famously said, "To one who has faith [in God], no explanation is necessary. To one without faith, no explanation is possible." Moreover, I am not trying to convert the reader to Judaism or Catholicism, qua Buber and Marcel, respectively, or for that matter to any other religious belief system (and as we shall see, for Marcel, conviction and faith are not exactly the same). Rather, I will suggest that psychoanalysis conceived as a spiritual discipline can be enhanced by exploiting Buber and Marcel's understanding of faith and its operations in everyday life, whether one is a believer or a non-believer, for they provide a phenomenology of religious faith (or a spiritually animated faith, as Marcel might say) that is significantly useful, as psychoanalysis tries to help the analysand live a more flourishing life. Similar to psychoanalytic ethos at its best, such a faith-driven outlook and behavior rejects "false moralism," "hyperintellectualism," and "rigid legalism" and opts for creating the conditions of possibility for a spiritual aspirant (and analysand) to will and choose, to become a poet of his life, as Nietzsche called it (Biemann, 2006, p. 108).

It needs to be stressed that engaging Buber and Marcel, qua religious believers, entails an empathic immersion in their "symbolic world," in their outlook, their "particular manner of construing the world" (Geertz, 1973, p. 110). Religion, politics, and psychoanalysis can operate as symbolic worlds. A symbolic world is a total system of beliefs, values, morals, and knowledge, which for the believer are usually extremely abstract and appear far above ordinary life, yet palpably intrude themselves on everyday life in their ability to inspire or to infuse meaning to individual or collective activity, to delegitimate other activity, and to wield social control (Wuthnow, Hunter, Bergesen, & Kurzweil, 1984, pp. 37, 75). Symbolic worlds provide a significant ordering impulse to social affairs and to collective outlooks of the world. Most importantly for this chapter, for hybrid believers like Buber and Marcel, these socially structured, taken-for-granted meanings have a stability originating from more powerful, otherworld sources, usually called God, than the historical labors of human beings and contribute therefore to the creation of ultimately powerful and meaningful notions of reality ("sacred cosmoi"). A symbolic world thus provides a framework of ultimate meaning and concerns (Berger, 1967, pp. 35, 36). Most importantly, while the study of the symbolic world of believers is essentially focused on what constitutes such a world as real and how it both forms and penetrates ordinary life, which is our characterization of the believer's world, the believer (even at the sophisticated level of a Buber and Marcel) may simply regard his world as the "real" world.

My claim, in short, is that without faith, minimally described by Buber and Marcel as existential openness and trust, it is difficult for the analysand to derive not only the strength, equanimity, and perspective that faith often provides (especially in making suffering sufferable, see next chapter), but perhaps even more importantly, as one Marcelian scholar aptly noted, it forecloses, or at least impedes, one's access to being or "the unity of experience" (Sweetman, 2011, p. 6) to embrace without reserve the Beauty, Truth, and Goodness in oneself, in others, and beyond (e.g., animals/objects). By using the words "being" or "unity of experience," I am pointing to the self's relative unity and organization, the consequence of its aptitude to sieve through and internalize an ever-increasing number of multifaceted desires, feelings, and experiences (Ruti, 2009, p. 23) that are often correlated with transcendence-pointing Beauty, Truth, and Goodness.

A pragmatic working definition of faith

Before getting to the heart of this chapter, I want to provide a more-or-less serviceable definition of the rather amorphous and ambiguous term *faith*, at least as I will be mainly discussing it. The definition comes from the pathbreaking study of the six stages of faith development formulated by J. W. Fowler (1981, updated 1995), a professor of theology and human development and a minister in the United Methodist Church. Fowler's stage theory, one that draws from Piaget's theory of cognitive development, Lawrence Kohlberg's stages of moral development, and Erik Erikson's psychosocial developmental theory, among other influences, has received considerable empirical support, though there have been methodological criticisms too (Coyle, 2011). Fowler's definition should be viewed as a "placeholder" for this chapter, for what constitutes faith is hardly agreed upon by philosophers/theologians and psychologists/ psychoanalysts. Faith is a

> Human universal ... an orientation of the personality, to oneself, to one's neighbor, to the universe; a total response; a way of seeing whatever one sees and of handling whatever one handles; a capacity to live at a more than mundane level; to see, to feel, to act in terms of a transcendent dimension.
>
> (Fowler, 1981, p. 11)

Thus, for Fowler, and to a large extent for Buber and Marcel, faith is a mode of finding/creating meaning and coherence in one's life. This involves embracing a "master narrative" to answer, if only provisionally, such basic questions as "What is the point of life?" (the problem of meaning), "Who is running things?" (is anyone? is God?), and "How do I live a praiseworthy life?" (an ethically animated flourishing life). As Marcel asked, "Who or what am I?" and "What am I worth?" (Anderson, 2006, pp. 60, 69). Thus, faith can be conceived of as how we existentially respond to whatever has transcendent significance and value to us; it is a way of being-in-the-world, that is, of trusting, committing to, and relating to others (and to ourselves). Of course, what differentiates so-called "healthy" or "mature" versus "unhealthy" or "immature" faith is hard to judge, but for Fowler it has a lot to do with the level of sophistication of cognitive processes applied to challenging moral dilemmas, calling to mind the great ancient religious and spiritual wisdom traditions (Compton & Hoffman, 2020, p. 341). However, the latter wisdom traditions always recognized that cognitive knowledge was not nearly enough (Marcus, 2003). In addition, mastery of the passions was essential via greater self-awareness, self-understanding, self-mastery, and self-overcoming, and always animated by a transcendence-pointing, other-directed, other-regarding, and other-serving existential/ethical orientation (Marcus, 2019). Buber and Marcel, at least broadly speaking, are lodged in this axial sensibility, the ancient religious "spirituality" and "wisdom" that flowered during that "pivotal age" from 800 to 200 BCE when the spiritual foundations of our current society were established by, for example, Confucius, Lao Tse, Upanishads, Buddha, Zarathustra, the Hebrew prophets, Homer, Plato, etcetera (Jaspers, 2011, pp. 51–60).

Fowler's stages of development are worth briefly summarizing, for they have some correlation with psychoanalytic formulations and because they point to what Buber and Marcel were getting at:[3] (1) *Intuitive-Projective*: This is the world of preschool children when fantasy and reality are frequently entwined and the child's most fundamental notions about God are usually appropriated from parents, teachers, and society. (2) *Mythic-Literal*: At school age, children begin comprehending the world in a more logical/rational manner. Typically, they appropriate the stories told to them by their faith community but are inclined to comprehend them in decidedly literal ways. Some people never develop beyond this stage. (3) *Synthetic-Conventional*: When children become teenagers, life significantly consists of a variety of social networks, and there is a need/desire to integrate them in terms of their social identity. When this unifying process occurs, the teenager usually embraces some kind of all-inclusive belief system (that functions similar to a faith structure). Moreover, they are inclined to resist thoughtfully considering other perspectives, and they believe that their way of seeing is the only one that is reasonable and acceptable. Often, authority is assigned to individuals or groups that represent the teenagers' strongly held beliefs. Many people, says Fowler, remain lodged in this stage throughout their life. (4) *Individual-Reflective*: In young adulthood, people begin thoughtfully considering other perspectives and realize that their angle of vision is only one among many alternatives. Such young adults tend to critically evaluate their beliefs and frequently become disenchanted with their prior faith. Paradoxically, the Stage 3 teenagers often think that Stage 4 young adults have become apostate-like or have "jumped ship," when in truth they have simply progressed forward and embraced a different, preferred perspective. (5) *Conjunctive Faith*: This is the usually midlife moment when people begin to reflectively acknowledge the limitations of logic/rationality and begin to come to terms with the paradoxical nature of life. They tend to perceive life as an unfathomable mystery, and often revisit sacred books and symbols but with a different sensibility, that is, without being trapped in a theological cage. (6) *Universalizing Faith*: Few people achieve this stage, and if they do, they too are in midlife, or even older. Such people assume an existential orientation that is other-directed, other-regarding, and other-serving, lodged in universal principles of love and justice, and comprehending people as part of a universal human community to which one responds with deep and abiding compassion. Such were the great religious teachers, sages, humanitarians, and saints, which comprised the Axial Age, as well as their contemporary counter-parts[4] (www.psychologycharts.com › james-fowler-stages-of-faith retrieved 1/21/20). Psychoanalysis has aptly described some of the so-called "lower" forms of religious/spiritual cognition/affect, but much less so in terms of what is potentially positive about so-called "higher" faith manifestations, Fowler's stages 5 and 6 appear to depict many of these characteristics, including those that Buber and Marcel touch on.

PSYCHOANALYTIC REFLECTIONS ON FAITH

D.W. Winnicott

Throughout his adult life, Winnicott (1896–1971) always had a "lingering [Christian] religiosity" (Goldman, 1993, p. 115); in fact, he wrote to his sister trying to clarify what psychoanalysis was by saying, "I shall probably be accused of blasphemy if I say that Christ was a leading psychotherapist" (Rodman, 2003, p. 43). Winnicott's biographer further noted, "From at least the mid-1940's to the mid-1960's, Jesus Christ was clearly a figure with whom he identified" (ibid., p. 291).[5]

Winnicott famously believed that faith as religious beliefs were "transitional phenomena." By this he meant an affect-integrating, meaning-giving, action-guiding experience that was largely subjectively created, lived in the immediacy of the moment, was thoroughly enjoyed, and was neither challenged nor unchallenged in terms of evidence and proof. Along with play/games, creativity/poetry, love, and certain types of spiritual/religious experiences, faith can be said to be a transitional phenomenon. "Transitional phenomenon" has been technically defined as "a process, relationship or activity" (in contradistinction to an inanimate object), "used as a symbolic representation of an important object," such as the mother or primary parental caregiver, "for the purposes of counteracting painful feelings in relationship to that object, particularly related to the object's absence" (Person, Cooper, & Gabbard, 2005, p. 561). Such adult manifestations of these processes, relationships, and activities are analogous to childhood "transitional objects," like the blanket or teddy bear a toddler relates to (Winnicott, 1953). The transitional object is said to reside in external reality (reality is conceived as being objectively present versus perception is reality) and, yet, is highly endowed with unconscious fantasy, in the service of the child's emotional growth and development. What the transitional object is said to do is to maintain the illusion of the comforting, soothing mother/parental caregiver, the psychological parent who symbolizes nurturing and stability, who is not in the child's field of vision and/or available to him in his real-life experience. As a result of this relationship to the transitional object, the child's autonomy and integration are enhanced because the blanket or teddy bear is under his command and control. "Transitional space" is the hypothetical area of the psyche where reality and unreality, co-occur and co-mingle, an intermediate realm of experience that is the birthplace of the imagination, in which paradox is central and taken for granted. For Winnicott, transitional space is the site of cultural experience as a whole, including adult faith in God.[6]

A few points about Winnicott's formulation are worth emphasizing (Jones, 1991). First, Winnicott's theory is less about the nature of the object, blankets and teddy bears; rather, it focuses on a particular kind of interpersonal experience. Thus, when a particular blanket or teddy bear retreats into the psychological background, there remains the trace of the creativity that motivates the spiritual aspirant to create faith in God (or other cultural products). Second, a key point about transitional processes, relationships, and activities, particularly as they relate to faith, is they involve the creation of an intermediate area of emotionally impactful experience that calls to mind the infant's experiences. In this context, the anxiety/disconnect between objectivity and subjectivity is transiently surmounted and inner and outer realities are bonded. As Winnicott summarizes his formulation:

> I have tried to draw attention to the importance both in theory and in practice of a third area, that of play, which expands into creative living and the whole cultural life of man. The third area has been contrasted with inner or personal psychic reality and with the actual world in which the individual lives, which can be objectively perceived. I have located this important area of experience in the potential space between the individual and the environments ... it is here that the individual experiences creative living.
>
> (1971, pp. 102–103)

> It is in playing and only in playing that the individual child or adult is able to be creative and to use the whole personality, and it is only in being creative that the individual discovers the self.
>
> (ibid., p. 54)

"Creative living" and "discover[ing] the self" for Winnicott can include religious feeling and faith in God, though Winnicott does not describe in much detail how such faith in God can positively animate how a person, thinks, feels, and acts in his effort at artful living, my main focus. However, similar to how the mother or parental caregiver's felt presence generates an experience of silent/gentle relatedness, one that makes the child feel safe and secure, there is a religious correlation in adulthood: "The capacity to be alone in the felt presence of the mother—parallels the traditional idea of the Presence of God as being both intimate and ultimate" (Goldman, 1993, p. 123).[7] In this view, God can be experienced as similar to a "holding environment" (the totality of the emotionally containing environmental circumstances), as "good enough mothering" (the devoted, empathic, emotionally modulating parent) or the "facilitating environment" (one that promotes the child's growth and development), such that the adult's way of experiencing his God is as loving and infinitely gracious in the bounty and plenitude directed towards the spiritual aspirant, as he gratefully perceives it (Hoffman, 2011, p. 141). For example, in mystical experience, Winnicott suggests focusing on "the mystic's retreat to a position in which he can communicate secretly with subjective objects and phenomena, the loss of contact with the world of shared reality being counterbalanced by a gain in terms of feeling real" (Winnicott, 1965, pp. 185–186). The main problem with Winnicott's formulation is that while he beautifully describes the infancy-emanating intrapsychic analogues to adult religious faith, he does not distinguish between a faith experience and its behavioral correlates that can be life-affirming versus life-destroying, Mother Theresa versus Osama bin Laden. Nor does he put forth any workable criteria for making such moral distinctions, admittedly a thorny philosophical and psychological problem that does not have any easy answers.

W. R. Bion

Bion (1897–1979) came from a rigorously religious family in India in which the family motto was, "Without God there is no purpose"; thus, he was raised in an environment in which "religious education and discipline were the family standard" (Hoffman, 2011, p. 70). He went to the Christian Bishop's Storford College prep school in England, where he unhappily (he claimed) attended compulsory Christian education, prayers, and church services. His feelings about all of this "wavered between fear of unknown spiritual forces and an absolute detesting of religion" (ibid.). This being said, Bion had a life-long interest in mysticism (he often used mystical metaphors in his theorizing and clinical practice, for example, drawing from Meister Eckhart and St. John of the Cross), even stating to Bionian-inspired psychoanalyst Michael Eigen who saw him for two sessions while Bion was visiting in New York in 1977, two years before he died: "Do you know the Kabbalah? *The Zohar*? … I use the Kabbalah as a framework for psychoanalysis" (Eigen, 2014, pp. 17–18). Taking his lead from Bion, Eigen noted that Kabbalah and psychoanalysis are focused on catastrophe (i.e., traumatic psychic reality) and faith. Mainly conceived as intuitive openness to the unknown, both are focused on infinity (i.e., the intimations of the undifferentiated core of a person) and the intensity of personal experience, both are focused on shatter (e.g., imploding) and the possibility of enduring and evolving the kind of mind that can metabolize the dimensions of the spirit that receptiveness accesses, and finally, both are focused on the ontological ramifications of the unknown (e.g., mystery) and the centrality of how one negotiates, if not nurtures, the upsurge of emotions within the totality of circumstances that one finds oneself in (Eigen, 2012, p. x).

Bion's views on faith revolve around the term "O." O denotes that "The fundamental reality is 'infinity,' the unknown, the situation for which there is no language—not even one borrowed by the artist or the religious—which gets anywhere near describing it" (Bion, 1994, p. 372). O is thus described as the "ultimate reality, absolute truth, the godhead, the infinite, the thing-in-itself" (Bion, 1970, p. 26). Unlike Kant, where the thing-in-itself was a transcendent idea, for Bion it referred to "both an idea and the existing unknown reality-in-itself" (Vermote, 2019, p. 30). In psychoanalysis, says Eigen, O is equated with "emotional reality," that which is evoked in the intersubjective context (Eigen, 2014, p. 38). O was thus hypothesized as the unknowable reality behind the mental representations, the unknowable emotional experience coming forth/

evolving during a session (Vermote, 2019, p. 122). What Bion seems to be claiming is that the truth resides in the external world, "out there," waiting to be embraced by a receptive mind and responsive heart (e.g., what ideally transpires between the analyst/analysand), one that has emptied itself of memory, desire, understanding, and coherence, in short, intellectual/emotional preconceptions (this is an ideal *tabula rasa*, not one that is actually attainable, hence self-awareness of these psychic processes is what really matters). The Oedipus complex, for example, is a truth that existed prior to Freud discovering it. While obtained knowledge can prime the existential base from which the leap to faith is implemented, in fact it is through abandoning knowledge and experience (perhaps an "un-selving" or "trans-selving"-like process) that enacts a movement in the direction of O. Faith involves bracketing knowledge and experience, and permitting oneself to perceive the truth of the movement, the emotional reality during a session as it exists, unfolds and is transformed (Akhtar, 2009, p. 192). Faith, says Bion, is the mental attitude behind an analysand's representations that facilitates meaningful contact (i.e., thinking as the psychological processing of affects) with this unknowable reality, O, that has not yet been metabolized and taken shape as a representation (Bion, 1970). Transformation of the truth of O, the undifferentiated psychic functioning into usable, creative psychic experience is the goal (or at least a goal). "At-one-ment," growth with O involves the analysand's willingness and ability to experience the massive Unknown, such that thoughts may evolve out of the infinity and nothingness (Vermote, 2019, pp. 172–173). Paraphrasing James Grotstein, Vermote notes, the analyst's job is to assist the training analysand "to become a competent mystic" via experiencing O (ibid., p. 167). It is worth noting that Bion did not equate his version of faith with religious faith:

> An act of Faith is peculiar to scientific procedure and must be distinguished from the religious meaning with which it is in conversational usage .... For me 'faith' [and "awe"] is a scientific state of mind and should be recognized as such. But it must be faith unstained by any element of memory or desire.
> (Bion, 1970, pp. 32, 34–35)

This is the very opposite of Buber and Marcel's notions of faith, who believed that it is the ultimate expression of memory that is of promise-making, and the desire to be faithful to a moment, of symbolic revelation of the other that points to God.

As Eigen notes,

> a lot of therapy is about the slow recovery of faith (2014, p. 118) ... faith is the vehicle that radically opens experiencing and plays a role in building tolerance for experience ... it is germane to the fervour and possibility of existence, tension, and struggle, with roots in grace. Faith rooted in

> profound grace deeper than catastrophe [traumatic emotional reality], a sense that has impact on the flavor of our lives.
>
> (ibid., p. 124)

Moreover, says Eigen, such faith, which is more profound than conscious belief (that is suffused with preconceptions), as in conventional religion, implies a spiritual or emotional sensitivity, "sensitivity to another person and to yourself with another person. How are you affecting the other person? That is the realm of spiritualty I am most interested in" (ibid., p. 95). Needless to say, Buber and Marcel have a somewhat different notion of grace in their oeuvre, but what Eigen is saying resonates, at least in general terms, with a Buberian/Marcelian spiritual sensibility.

It is hard to disagree with Eigen's gloss on Bion, including the valuative attachments he embraces, such as sensitivity to others and oneself. This being said, Civitarese (2019, p. 388), claims that O represents Bion's "Pseudo-Mystical Path," one that mistakenly inaugurates "a 'mystical' psychoanalysis" that he wants to "refute," for it has given "rise to the most disconcerting interpretations and many misunderstandings" (a rather presumptuous, if not arrogant judgment). In fact, Civitarese says that O is not only "very difficult to define," but it is "dangerously close to nonsense" (ibid.). Civitarese does, however, acknowledge Bion's devotion to help the analysand "grow" via "emotional *at-one-ment*," "the meeting of minds involved in digesting [transforming] reality (O)" (p. 391), in which unconscious experience as it is enacted in treatment is truthfully faced/metabolized in the here-and-now (truth is a pragmatic, intersubjectively agreed upon notion between the analysand/analyst). "O as the Godhead thus becomes" Bion's "theory of humanity, and his conception of what it means to become more human or to grow one's mind" (p. 293) in order "to gain emotional competence" (p. 399). While emotional competence surely matters for Bion, his view of faith does plausibly appear to include "variants of mystical participation" in the world (Eigen, 2014). As Grotstein notes about the main thrust of psychoanalysis, "the capacity to experience O is the privilege of the ineffable subject of psychoanalysis … the 'Man of Achievement,'" this sure sounds like more than emotional competence (2007, p. 127).

E. H. Erikson

Erik Erikson (1902–1994) was born out of wedlock to a Danish/Jewish mother who separated from his non-Jewish father during pregnancy (not much is known about him). Erikson was then adopted by his Jewish stepfather (his treating pediatrician), hence the "H" in his name (Homburger). Erikson never knew until late in life that his stepfather was not his biological father, a deception that troubled him for the rest of his life. As Erik looked Danish but was raised Jewish, he was teased by his peers from both directions (actually, anti-Semitically mocked by his Danish peers), this became one of the important factors in his identity conflicts. He married a non-Jew (the daughter of an Episcopalian minister) and converted to Christianity and was buried in the First Congregational Church Cemetery in Harwich, Massachusetts.

For Erikson, the earliest sense of identity embraced by an infant emanates from his relationship with his mother (or main parental caregiver) in the context of the feeding experience. When the mother has been willing and able to respond lovingly, reliably (e.g., with reasonable consistency, continuity, and sameness), and in a rapidly attuned manner to the infant's demands and distress, the infant gradually develops a self-assured expectation, "basic trust." As Erikson notes, basic trust is not only having the conviction that the external world is trustworthy, "but also that one may trust oneself and the capacity of one's own organs to cope with urges; and that one is able to consider oneself trustworthy enough so that the providers will not need to be on guard lest they be nipped" (Erikson, 1950, p. 248). For the infant who experiences himself and the world as trustworthy, the ego "virtue" (i.e., strength) that emerges is hope: "Hope is the enduring belief in the attainability of fervent wishes, in spite of the dark urges and rages which mark the beginning of existence" (Erikson, 1964, p. 113). When the child has appropriated mutual recognition and affirmation of the mother and child bond, he experiences the mother as a numinous presence (i.e., awe-inspiring, holy, powerful), repeatedly affirmed by her familiar, comforting, empowered, empowering facial expression, voice quality (it is through hearing that the infant/child first learns the seeds of virtue), and feel of her touch. This thoroughly validating and uplifting felt presence takes place, then, in the context of the infant's need for biological survival and the ritualized loving devotion that facilitates emotional survival. Over time, the aforementioned caring matrix potentiates a sense in the child of an autonomous identity that also assists him in surmounting his nameless dread associated with aloneness and separateness (Monte, 1980, pp. 246–247).

One can see that there is a potential correlation between basic trust and the development of hope and faith in Erikson's formulation, especially when one considers his perspective from the point of view of the infant/child leaning into the adult future. That is, conscious and unconscious hope gives the infant/child and, most importantly, the adult a sense of realistic/reasonable optimism that his needs and desires to love, work, and meaningfully participate in community will be gratified, and he can effectively master challenges, if not overcome adversity. Thus, for Erikson faith emanates from the aforementioned psychological context, in which the adult's hope that all will be well for him in love, work, and community gets bracketed, and with deep and abiding desire, anticipation, even love, this hope is applied to humanity in general, to societies prosocial institutions, to nature, and to subsequent generations. As Erikson notes, one important aspect of ego-integrity, the last stage of the life-cycle in his theory, is the acceptance of the fact that my life in all of its richness and fullness (including its victories, defeats, and unrealized dreams) was one life-cycle in the larger movement of history. The ego virtue of "wisdom" is in fact defined by Erikson as a faithful affirmation: "informed and detached concern with life itself, in the face of death itself" (Erikson, 1964, p. 134).

There have been other thoughtful psychoanalytic contributions to understanding the psychology of religion, including aspects of faith, though most of them follow the aforementioned themes first developed by Freud and, more recently, Winnicott, Bion, and Erikson. Rizzutto (1979), Meissner (1984), Leavy (1988), Loewald (1988), Jones, (1991) and Eigen (2014), for example, imply that religion can have an adaptive, identity-defining, life-affirming role in a person's life, that faith can be an affect-integrating, meaning-giving, and action-guiding way of positively being-in-the-world. Likewise, there have been a few analysts that have correlated certain Buddhist (Molino, 2013) and other Eastern spiritual/religious notions with psychoanalysis (Vaidyanathan & Kripal, 2002) that touch upon the faith experience. What Buber and Marcel add to the conversation on what constitutes the best of a religiously animated faith experience has been underappreciated by the psychoanalytic community, and it is to this subject that I now turn.

BUBER AND MARCEL ON FAITH

Buber

Buber (and Marcel) view the faith experience from highly personalized religious points of view, though many of their insights have application for the non-believing spiritual aspirant. It is worth mentioning that Buber had an initial interest in mystical ways of being-in-the-world before he became a dialogical philosopher that emphasized interhuman (roughly intersubjective) relations. In fact, he venerated the mystic as one who accomplishes integration/unity by living one's life (*Erlebnis*, "life experience") with the fullness of his being without it being linked to space/time/social coordinates, the goal being an integration/unification of the inner self and the cosmic spirit. Buber's devotion to mysticism motivated him to initially support World War I, mainly because he romantically believed that soldiers on both sides would be propelled to great heroism that would lead to a revelation of the Absolute or Unconditioned Divine. However, after accepting the ongoing criticism of one of his friends, the social anarchist/pacifist Gustav Landauer, in 1916 Buber understood that the dreadfulness and disaster of the war could not be legitimated by mystical or metaphysical angles of vision (Moore, 1996a, p. 200). Buber called this transformation of his being, of outlook and sensibility, "*one* great experience of faith." By this he meant, "an experience that transports a person in all his component parts, his capacity for thought certainly included, so that, all the doors springing open, the storm blows through all the chambers" (Buber, 1967a, pp. 690–691). Concretely, this meant that Buber went from a belief in the Absolute or Unconditioned Divine of Eastern mystical thought to the Biblical God of the burning bush (when

Moses asked God his name and received a *koan*-like response, see below) that he described as the eternal Thou (Moore, 1996a, p. 202). Revelation was now conceived as neither objective truth nor inspired subjective experience, but rather "address and response, hearing and responding [the 'between'] to the" cosmic "voice that speaks to man out of creation and history" (Friedman, 1986, p. 44). As Paul Mendes-Flohr noted, there was a transition "from mysticism to dialogue" in Buber's thought, beginning with *I and Thou,* that took Buber to the end of his life (Zank, 2006, p. 64).[8]

Friedman aptly describes what he called the "essence of faith" from a Buberian point of view.

> Not only does our world of It experience ever new creation through the flaming forth of the Thou, but each new Thou renews in all presentness the past experiences ofThou. It is this which is the essence of faith: not the past deadening the present, but the present recalling the past to life so that the moments of the past and the moment of the present become simultaneously present and joined in living unity.
>
> (Friedman, 2002, p. 292)

What Friedman is saying is that when Moses asked God his name at the burning bush, and God responded "I am that I am" as the Hebrew (Ex.3:14) is typically translated (i.e., the self-existent, unified, spiritual, and Everlasting God), Buber in line with his philosophy of dialogue translated God's response differently, "I shall be there as I shall be there." In other words, while "God promises that He will always be present," He will not manifest Himself in any known or anticipated form. Rather, "He identifies himself only as the Presence [a presence as Power] which comes and departs, as the imageless God who hides and reveals Himself" (ibid.). In this context, the spiritual aspirant is left in a state of ambiguity and mystery about God per se, though it evokes in his mind and heart a fundamental obligation of doing God's work to repair this imperfect world: "All the Lord has spoken we will do, and obey" (Ex.24:7), said the ancient Israelites when they received the Law via Moses at Mount Sinai (Levinas views this biblical passage as the key to his ethics as first philosophy, for it suggests instinct-like obligation to the other before conscious understanding).

For Buber, faith is not conceived as belief per se, that is, belief in the veracity of propositions that cannot be logically and rationally verified (e.g., they are unevidenced and unseen), but are assumed to be true, such as Moses was appointed by God to lead the Israelites out of Egypt to the Promised Land, or that Jesus was directed by God to save humanity (Silberstein, 1989, p. 216). For Buber, and for biblical and rabbinic Judaism in general, belief does not mean merely a cognitive belief in the existence of God (this was assumed to be true in the same way as one's neighbor exists). Rather, following biblical/rabbinic Judaism, for Buber faith was a way of being-in-the-world, one that reflected an existential orientation that was infused with emotion that expressed unconditional deep trust (*emunah*) in God.[9] Thus, for Buber, to be a believer meant to trust and be faithful to God.[10] Most importantly, this trust/faith is only enacted in the interhuman relationship: "Faith is a factual event, lived life in dialogue" (Buber, 1967b, p. 133). The believer is addressed by the dialogical partner "in word and sign," and chooses to respond in kind (Silberstein, 1989, p. 217). For Buber, "the essence of religiosity," of faith, begins with the unqualified human act of decision-making that ruptures the human condition of spiritual apathy and strives to actualize divine *Gestalt*. In other words, a righteous action below impacts action above. It exploits the human capability "to imitate God, intensify His reality, and redeem His presence" (Braiterman, 2006, p. 114).

Buber's unorthodox religious faith—"I do not accept any absolute formulas for living," his openness to "absolute discovery … to the adventure in heightened awareness in living"—was aptly expressed in a debate with a religious dogmatist in 1919:

> O you secure and safe one's you who hide yourselves behind the ramparts of the law so that you will not have to look into God's abyss! Yes, you have secure ground under your feet, while we hang suspended looking out over the endless deeps. But we would not change our dizzy insecurity and poverty for your security and abundance.
>
> (Hodes, 1971, p. 56)

What Buber was promoting was the person of faith's commitment to a way of being-in-the-world in which he walked on the "narrow ridge" of "holy insecurity." By narrow ridge Buber meant,

> On the far side of the subjective, on the side of the objective, on the narrow ["rocky"] ridge where an *I and Thou* meet, there is the realm of the "between." … Here the genuine third alternative is indicated, the knowledge of which will help to bring about the genuine person again and to establish genuine community.
>
> (Buber, 1965, p. 204)

What Buber was pointing to was not, say, the value of the golden mean of the Greek ideal, but rather a more daring leap to faith: "You can think of the narrow ridge as a region within yourself where you cannot be touched [roughly an "inner citadel called the soul" says Marcel (Sweetman, 2011, p. 72)]. Because there you have found yourself and so you are not vulnerable" (Hodes, 1971, p. 57). Clarifying his definition of the narrow ridge in terms of interhuman relations, Buber added,

> the narrow ridge is the meeting place of the We. This is where man can meet man in community. And only men who are capable of truly saying "Thou" to one another can truly say "We" with one another. If each

> guards the narrow ridge within himself and keeps it intact, this meeting can take place.
>
> (ibid.)[11]

Buber is emphasizing that the faith experience occurs within the context of "the between," that relational space where mutual presence of human relationships miraculously happens. However, to be able to say Thou requires an inner center of gravity such that one can make the leap into the common ground of the between of subjectivity and objectivity, transcending the separateness, a realm that is neither imagined or constructed (Kramer & Galwich, 2003, p. 78).

It was in the context of his study of Hasidism and biblical prophecy that Buber developed his evocative notion of "holy insecurity," a sensibility already intimated in Buber's aforementioned response to the religious dogmatist. The prophets of Israel, says Buber,

> always aimed to shatter all security and to proclaim in the opened abyss of the final insecurity the unwished-for God who demands that His human creatures become real, they become human, and confounds all who imagine that they can take refuge in the certainty that the temple of God is in their midst.
>
> (Buber, 1957, p. 73)

It is in part, for this reason, when one's world is assaulted (from external and/or internal sources), when it begins to implode for reasons and in ways that are beyond intelligibility, that the person of faith embraces his fate as God's will, or at least as God-given. This does not mean that he does not aggressively question his fate, or doesn't try to make things better (indeed, some believers maintain that the darkening of one's world is dialectically meant to provoke the spiritual aspirant's creation of light). This means he accepts his concrete situatedness as having a divine directedness and/or significance, in part meant to bring out the best in him. In Biblical context, this means "fear of God" (perhaps best understood as "grateful reverence" or "loving fear" of God) (Hertz, 1960, p. 790). As Friedman notes, "the 'fear of God' is the essence of 'holy insecurity,'" for as Buber claims, "it comes when our existence becomes incomprehensible and uncanny, when all security is shattered through the mystery" (Friedman, 2002, p. 159). The mystery is not about that which is not yet known, the undiscovered, but rather points to God's "undefinable and unfathomable" behavior (Buber, 1957, p. 50). This being said, "holy insecurity" can be defined as "life lived in the face of God." It is life in which one learns to be a quiet and clear truth-teller, regardless if one is speaking to a group or individual, even though, or maybe because, one has been through hellish experience and returned to the light of day again, to affirm life lived in relation to God (Friedman, 2002, p. 158).

In the next chapter I will discuss Buber's (and Marcel's) views on making suffering sufferable, which, of course, is a key collateral concern for the person of faith. However, for now, what is important is that faith for Buber involves walking the "narrow ridge" in a condition of "holy insecurity," what Buber (and Marcel) would probably call grace. In this context, grace means that Buber, qua man of faith, was spontaneously immersed with the fullness of his whole being in the present moment, and always aimed to actualize unrealized potential for individuals and groups to access God-given, or at least God-inspired, Beauty, Truth and Goodness (i.e., "finding God in all things," as Buber said)—for example, as manifested in his biblical-animated philosophical anthropology (i.e., how one comprehends the person as such). Grace also involves a reprieve from suffering. As Buber stated, "'Faith' is not a feeling in the soul of man but an entrance into reality, and entrance in the whole reality without reduction and curtailment" (Buber, 1967c, p. 27).

Thus, Buber never put forth a systematic philosophy of faith, at least not as conventionally understood (though he did write a comparative study of Judaism and Christianity in 2003). He was quite clear about this not being his intention, which speaks to the heart of this personalist philosopher of dialogue:

> I must say it once again: I have no teaching. I only point to something... I point to something in reality that had not or had too little been seen. I take him who listens to me by the hand and lead him to the window. I open the window and point to what is outside. I have no teaching, but I carry on conversation.
>
> (Buber, 1967a, p. 693)

Moreover, while this conversation was mainly interhuman, it also included speaking with God "out there." Buber defined God (a symbol for the eternal Thou, the reality of the "between") in *I and Thou* as "the Being that is directly, most nearly, and lastingly, over against us, that may properly only be addressed and not expressed" (Friedman, 1986, p. 15, 43). Reflecting on a moment of self-talk, Buber declares:

> If I believe in God means to be able to talk about him in the third person, then I do not believe in God. If to believe in him means to be able to talk to him, then I believe in God ... The God to whom Daniel [the prophet] prays in his suffering is my God and the God of all.
>
> (1967c, pp. 24–25)

We can now summarize some of the essential aspects of Buberian faith. A life of faith is one willfully lived with the fullness of one's whole being before the face of God, a life characterized by unqualified openness and trust to the Thou of one's life (remember, every Thou points to the eternal Thou) (Moore, 1996b,

p. 100). Kaufman has aptly characterized the renewing activity of Buberian faith in greater detail:

> It is an absolute trust that holds fast to the hope *(esperance)* that is above all hope (*espoir*); to the meaning that seems to be lost in meaninglessness of this world; to the unifying power of healing and of hallowing that reaches through disunion and doubt and carries us over the abyss of despair. It is the devoted giving of self that demands commitment and makes possible acceptance; the truth to give oneself up for the sake of future possibilities; it is the vicarious sacrifice of the "servant of God," in whose mystery Buber has again and again become absorbed. In faith, and only in faith—and just in the faith of which Buber speaks—suffering becomes the sacrament presented to us and that we take to ourselves. He who is capable of this is made by it not only richer and deeper; in suffering there also is unveiled to him the countenance of God.
>
> (Kaufmann, 1967, p. 232)

For Buber then, a person of faith is one who has the will and ability to engage in mutual knowing that emanates from genuine meeting, from free, flowing and unrestrained presence to the other, and to the Holy Other, the eternal Thou. As Buber repeatedly noted, "the I-Thou relation to God and the I-Thou relation to one's fellow man are at bottom related to each other" (Buber, 1964, p. 99). In other words, "our faith has our humanity as its foundation and our humanity has our faith as its foundation" (Buber, 1967b, 117).[12] And again, Buber's affirmation of "my faith in the meaningfulness of creation and its completion," *Zion* is not a divine-based security but "a God-given chance" (Buber, 1967a, pp. 702, 705). In this context, there is no certainty on the narrow rocky ridge, that is, no philosophical or theological perspective of objective truths that can help one creatively and effectively navigate the treacherous terrain and abysses. There is "only the certainty of meeting what remains undisclosed" (Buber, 1965, p. 184).

Marcel

When Buber described Jesus as his "great brother" and declared that "a great place belongs to him in Israel's history of faith," one "that cannot be described by any of the usual categories" (2003, pp. 12–13), he might as well have been pointing to the spirit of Jesus as manifested in the believing humanism of Marcel. For Marcel, qua Christian, Jesus and the "the great truths of Christianity" have an "essential agreement" with "human nature" (1964, p. 79) (Buber felt likewise about Judaism). For example, psychologically speaking, the Jesus paradigm is a portrayal we all can relate to, "of coming through fully, murdered, abandoned, resurrected, supported" (Eigen, 2014, p. 35). Indeed, Marcel believed that there is a domain of experience that reflects mystery, not so much because it is unknowable, but that it can best be phenomenologically approached via secondary reflection (personally engaged contemplation that presences the mystery of being) as opposed to primary reflection (detached analysis of problem-solving cognition). Love, hope, fidelity, and faith, some of the ways of accessing the plenitude of being, fall into this category. Marcel converted to Catholicism at age 40, in part, at the invitation of Francois Muriac (a Noble Prize–winning novelist), and he gives us a sense of his ambivalent struggle before his faith-driven conversion experience:

> It seemed to me that he [Muriac] was but a spokesman and that the call came from much higher up. It was as though a more than human voice were questioning me and putting me into my own presence. "Can you really persevere indefinitely in that equivocal position of yours?" this voice asked me. "Is it even honest to continue to think and to speak like someone who believes in the faith of others and who is convinced that this faith is everything but illusion, but who nevertheless does not resolve to take it unto himself"? It seemed to me that I could only reply to this last interrogative with an assent.
>
> (Marcel, 1984, p. 29)

While Marcel's conversion did not radically alter his philosophy, it did lead him to focus more on the role of transcendence in his general oeuvre, including "the mystery of faith, and the search for the transcendence in human life" (Sweetman, 2008, pp. 54, 75). For Marcel (similar to Buber), transcendence is a form of reaching out of oneself toward the intersubjective character of existence, a reaching out which is a constituent aspect of human being-in-the-world, and without which we are never existentially fulfilled. Such a transcendent experience often evokes an affirmation of God, and in fact, says Marcel, it necessitates the existence of God for its ultimate justification, regardless of whether a specific person references God. Moreover, the experience of transcendence involves freedom, since the person is free to affirm or to decline the experience of the transcendent, and grace, because the experience emanates from the outside, that is, it cannot be fully cognitively grasped and made into propositional knowledge (ibid., pp. 6, 88). As Keen notes, "Marcel never gives the word *faith* an adequate definition," and Marcel doubts whether it is even possible to assert a "general theistic position." This being said, a serviceable definition of Marcelian faith, says Keen, is "a relationship to an absolute Thou who is the creator of the world and who places us under ethical obligation to our neighbors" (Keen, 1984, p. 120).[13] For example, it is the Christian notion of the indwelling of Christ in the person who is utterly faithful to Him, or conceptualizing the relationship between the faithful and living God, as "fatherhood in its purity" (Marcel, 2001, p. 140).

Take a real-life example, such as a faith-driven whistleblower. For Marcel, the capacity to act morally courageously is not simply, or rather I would prefer to say not only, a matter of maintaining deep inner convictions, that is, a belief or opinion that is held firmly. In fact, Marcel has a lot of trouble with the word "conviction" and distinguishes it from "belief" or faith, which he maintains is the deeper and "higher" animating existential basis for courageous actions, especially what he claims is the ultimate expression of courage, self-sacrifice, as in martyrdom. For Marcel, the problem with "conviction" is that it "appears as an unshakeable position, definitive, without the power to justify these characteristics."[14] In contrast, faith represents "movement from the closed ... to the open." In other words, "to believe," to have faith "is not to believe *that* [e.g., being persuaded or convinced that], but to believe *in*, that is, to open a credit [to be "available," *disponibilité*] in the favor of, to place oneself at the disposal of" (Marcel, 2001, p. vi). Where a conviction is a strictly cognitive/intellectual judgment about some kind of propositional "truth" on so-called "objective" reality (what people typically mean by belief), faith is a creative testimonial, an existential attestation of believing in, of trusting and being confident in another person or supra-personal reality. As Marcel notes, a person may *have* an opinion or conviction, but he *is* his belief: "Belief in the strong sense of the term—not in the sense of believing that, i.e., assuming that—is always belief in a *thou,* i.e., in a reality, whether personal or supra-personal, which is able to be invoked, and which is as it were, situated beyond any judgment referring to an objective datum" (Marcel, 1964, pp. 266–267). Marcel is here making an important distinction, namely, that the "down" side of conviction is that it represents a fixed and definite perspective on something that is not open to change, revision, or correction; it claims to "arrest time" suggesting being closed (ibid., pp. 131, 133). Faith, on the other hand, not only believes that something is true, but it requires giving oneself up to an "other," to someone or something that one deeply cherishes. It is out of this fecund faith consciousness that the courage of the whistleblower, and indeed courage in all of its glorious forms, is nurtured and unfolds.

In Chapter 2 (The spirit of love), I have discussed Marcel's notion of "creative fidelity" in some detail—"the hold the other being has over us" (Marcel, 1965b, p. 46)—that is, the human tendency to make profound unconditional commitments such as to a spouse or significant other, or as evidenced say in the phenomenology of hope, presence, and intersubjectivity, and which cultivates an ethical approach to others (though avoids ethical formalism and ethical individualism) (Sweetman, 2008, p. 69). For Marcel, these common human experiences are not adequately grasped in an objective, abstract manner (i.e., primary reflection); rather, they are best articulated with reference to an absolute, transcendent reality, the absolute Thou. In creative fidelity, "my behavior will be completely colored by this act [of promise-making] embodying the decision that the commitment will not again be questioned" (Marcel, 1964, p. 162). In other words, creative fidelity means donating ourselves (or maybe the "core" of ourselves) to others, which is accomplished by mutually partaking in love and friendship, or engaging in the creative, performing, and fine arts (Marcel was a well-regarded dramatist and music lover). Creative fidelity connects us to others, affirming the other's separate, unique subjectivity while affirming our own. Creative fidelity is the resolute, continuous desire to expound who we are, in part, in order to have an enhanced sense of being. Similar to Buber, we become creatively faithful when we transcend the space or breach between ourselves and others in the process of making ourselves available, that is, present to them.

For Marcel, as fidelity necessitates an absolute promise, an unconditional commitment, it necessitates the same to an absolute Thou (i.e., to the Absolute Personal Being, to God).[15] That is, the *homo viator* who makes such an unconditional commitment to another person provides witness to the absolute Thou, and this may involve not enouncing this witness (a so-called "wordless witness," as Christians say): "One might say that conditional pledges are only possible in a world from which God is absent. Unconditionality is the true sign of God's presence" (Marcel, 1950, p. 40). In other words, somewhat similar to Buber and Levinas, absent religious faith of some sort, absolute, unconditional commitment cannot be affirmed: "Fidelity can never be unconditional except when it is Faith, but we must add, however, that it aspires to unconditionality" (Marcel, 1965a, p. 133). What Marcel is saying is that for the spiritually animated person who creatively lives his fidelity, the "inwardly consecrated soul," as Marcel calls him, fidelity "reveals its true nature, which is to be an evidence, a testimony," about that which is both "Absolute [eternal] in us" and in the loved other (ibid., p. 134).

A few general points about Marcel's description of faith may be helpful before closing this section. First, for faith to have a strong interpretive grip on one's outlook and behavior it must overpower the *homo viator*, that is, it must profoundly emotionally impact the heart of his existence ("being incarnate," that is, embodied, or bodying-forth in Marcelian language, which disseminates radiance). Second, faith is a relation that involves the totality of one's being, the whole self, or at a minimum, something vitally real in oneself, something which feels that to reject it would mean rejecting the whole self (i.e., the totality of circumstances that constitute who one believes one is). Third, even though the faith commitment may feel true to the believer, it always disavows certainty. That is, since faith is a free act (a "leap" with no guarantees), it resides in (or at least has proximity to) a realm of ambiguity, ambivalence, and doubt. Marcel detested fanaticism: "I assert without a shadow of hesitation—the first duty of the philosopher of our world today is to fight against fanaticism *under whatever guise it may appear*" (Hernandez, 2011, p. 107). Fourth, faith is not merely a personal affirmation (not a projection of one's inner world though it correlates to it) but is, in addition, something that involves divine grace. That is, for Marcel, faith without grace is not conceivable because it objectifies the divine gift experience within the subject, implying there is no "genuine existence of an absolute of non-human origin" (i.e., "no living presence of God") (Selzer, 1988, p. xviii). Rather, faith is always co-mingled with grace, divine gift-giving, as it is for Buber and Levinas. Indeed, Marcel felt similar to

Buber, who in the latter's reply to Carl Jung noted that psychology and psychoanalysis are not "authorized to make a distinction," a definitive judgment "between psychic statements to which a super-psychic reality corresponds and to psychic statements to which none corresponds" (i.e., "Whether God can exist independent of man") (Buber, 1988, p. 135). What grace allows us to do is to glimpse the divine nature, to feel His transforming healing presence without being able to adequately account for why we have received this mysterious gift: "We are again in the order of what can be found and taken in account rather than what can be understood" (Marcel, 2001, p. 181). In a word, for Marcel, grace can be conceived as the transcendent and nonobjectifiable assumption of the act of faith (Marcus, 2013, p. 69).

Implications for treatment

Faith is one of those summoning notions that is prone to "loose use" in that it has different meanings to different people, with little consensus about scholars and laypersons. Similar to God, it is beyond representation, and can only be evocatively pointed to. This being said, analysts have provided observations and formulations that resonate with Buber's and Marcel's rendering of this challenging philosophical, theological, and psychological subject. As religious scholar Huston Smith (1979, p. 11) noted, faith reflects the human tendency "to see, to feel, to act in terms of a transcendent dimension," to sense meaning and significance that is more than ordinary and commonplace. Paul Tillich has a similar perspective; he called faith "an act of a finite being who is grasped by, and turned to, the infinite." Moreover, Tillich says, "Faith consists in being vitally concerned with the ultimate reality to which I give the symbolical name of God" (Tillich, 1958, p. 18). Both Buber and Marcel would most likely agree with the main thrust of Smith's and Tillich's definitions, but what do Buber and Marcel contribute to the faith conversation that has some positive bearing on psychoanalysis conceived as an art of living a flourishing life? Four points come to mind.

First, what is especially noteworthy is that these two religiously animated personalist dialogical philosophers make the love relationship, poetically rendered as I-Thou and creative fidelity, respectively, the most robust port of entry into the faith moment that always implies a relationship with the eternal/absolute Thou (or perhaps its secular transcendent equivalent). In other words, the heart of faith for Buber and Marcel is faithfulness to a moment, fidelity to a self- and other-consecrating event, to a transforming response between two people that reveals the awesome, mysterious, ineffable transcendence-pointing goodness of the other, the basis for trust in the future (Heschel, 1955, pp. 132, 155). Faith, says Buber, is a "binding oneself to something, an involvement of one's person, an immeasurably binding venture" (1967b, p. 126). Put in familiar psychological language, faith, Buber and Marcel suggest, is vital to a love relationship and living, for it provides "coherence and direction," it connects one to "shared trusts and loyalties," it existentially "grounds" one's "personal stances and loyalties in a sense of relatedness to a larger frame of reference" (e.g., God-animated, biblical-based ethicality), and it helps people to cope adequately with the "limit conditions" and inevitable suffering of existence, all by using compelling psychological resources that have a sense of "ultimacy" and transcendence (Shafranske, 1996, p. 168).

Second, Buber and Marcel were probably aware that while faith may begin at the mother's breast, and morphs into faith in ourselves and in others, even to humanity as a whole, and to God for the believer, in whatever form it takes, it seems to be something that we need and/or desire to live a flourishing life. As Fowler has noted, humanity appears to have "evolved with prepotentiated capacities that underlie the structuring activities of faith and that equip people for their ontological callings to relatedness and partnership with God" (Fowler, 1994, pp. 182–183; Jeeves & Brown, 2009). This being said, Buber and Marcel were mainly focused on faith as an existential orientation that reflects an inner center of gravity, such that the specific object, whether called God or its secular equivalent, was of secondary importance in terms of living a flourishing life. This is faith conceived as a character trait, a way of being-in-the-world as opposed to say only a set of conscious beliefs/postulates that one is loyal to (Fromm, 1947, p. 199). Such beliefs can enhance faith, but they can also close it down because they are estranged from ongoing originary intimations related to the unknown that faith is in part rooted in (Eigen, 2012, p. 43). As Buber and Marcel were believing humanists, they saw earthly and celestial existence as always co-mingled and co-potentiating; I-Thou and creative fidelity always pointed to "something more," "something higher," and "something better." Faith in God and faith in man were inseparable.

Third, for Buber and Marcel (and Levinas), forms of mysticism (perhaps including Bion/Eigen/Grotstein's psychoanalytic musings) were not their preferred context to grasp faith affirmations as they conceived it. In fact, they were somewhat mistrustful of aspects of mysticism as an overall existential orientation, for it focused too much on actualizing some "big" transformational insight/realization, such as unity with God/Divine, or striving to directly experience the ultimate reality. Rather, faith was mainly an action-orientation that was best expressed in concrete, situated behavior that was other-directed, other-regarding, and other-serving, that emanated from a commanding or, at least, summoning God. Faith in the living God required aspiring to holiness or goodness (mainly using a biblical ethical calculus), which was best accessed through one's being-for-the-other, especially before oneself as Levinas emphasized. Marcel's rendering of love, hope, fidelity, and faith make this point especially clear.

Fourth, both Buber and Marcel were well aware that faith that was based on mere acceptance of authority (e.g., fear of God's power/punishment) was not credible. Rather, they put forth a rational version of faith that demanded robust intellectual reckonings and emotional metabolism. Their faith was anchored in their own independent productive experience, including intense emotional processing, and in their relative assuredness in their power of thought, observation, and judgment (Fromm, 1947). Such faith is perhaps less a belief in something, even the Divine conceived as "out there," than it is a manifestation of believing in the ultimate value of promise-making, creative fidelity as Marcel called it. That is, faith in God is a direction not a substance or endpoint, and said Buber quoting Rabbi Mendel of Korzk, this means "not to make an idol even of the command of God" (Moore, 1996a, p. 28). For such an inner attitude expresses faith in oneself (e.g., to have the will and ability to vigorously pursue holiness/goodness), in others (e.g., that they too have holiness/goodness that can be actualized and we can help bring forth), and in God (e.g., that we can grow in our ethical potential if we work at it and learn from our failings). Playing off Levinas's "religion for adults," Buber and Marcel are putting forth a difficult wisdom, a "faith for adults."

I am well aware that the aforementioned four points are not earth-shattering or even entirely new, especially for someone who is familiar with the glorious insights of the great Axial sages, religious teachers, and philosophers. But Buber and Marcel have graced us with oeuvres that have put into sharp focus a phenomenology of faith in a most summoning manner, that is, a faith that can contribute to the art of living a flourishing life. Indeed, as positive psychologists Compton & Hoffman (2020, p. 306) summarize, much of what Buber and Marcel are pointing to has been reasonably supported by scientific researchers. For example, greater faith (i.e., religiousness and spirituality) has been fairly reliably linked to better mental health and higher subjective well-being. One study interestingly reported that a person's perceived nearness to God (remember for Buber/Marcel, a life of faith is one willfully lived with the fullness of one's whole being before the face of God) was the sole biggest predictor of life satisfaction across all age ranges. Moreover, people who are more behaviorally religious/spiritual tend to display better emotional well-being and lower rates of delinquency, alcoholism, drug abuse, and social problems. Not only do such faith-animated *homo viators* have greater happiness and life satisfaction (the latter only somewhat) compared to those without religious faith, but for those who can cultivate such faith-animated religious/spiritual practices, they can increase positive emotional states such as joy, hope, optimism, and compassion as well as promote positive virtues like self-control. One wonders if this is what Bionian-inspired analyst Civitarese had in mind when he said that the goal of analysis is "to gain emotional competence" (2019, p. 399).

Of course, it is not the psychoanalyst's role to try and convince the analysand to embrace any religious or spiritual outlook or practices, for that would be an imposition of a crude moralism, which all analysts find repugnant. However, what Buber and Marcel beautifully put forth is a mode of sacred attunement, an affect-integrating, meaning-giving, action-guiding existential positioning that is thoroughly lodged in apperception of the impossible-to-pin-down eternal/absolute Thou, though who one feels summoned to respond to as one engages in other-directed, other-regarding, and other-directed actions meant to potentiate and actualize the best in oneself and others.

Final comment

What Buber and Marcel are pointing to in their reflections on religious faith is the birth of a new spiritual horizon (or a reclaiming of an old one, with some profound modification, but calling to mind an Axial sensibility). Indeed, Buber and Marcel put into sharp focus a dimension of the spirit that most psychoanalysts and others have not adequately noticed, let alone embraced in their theory and practice. That is, most of the time analysts view faith as mainly an intrapsychic phenomenon as a way of relating to and being open to the vicissitudes of one's barely hinged mind. No doubt the ability to metabolize the upsurge of strong emotions, however they are induced, is one of the key conditions of possibility for Buberian/Marcelian faith. However, as Marcel aptly put it, "the only religion [and psychoanalysis?] that can count for me is that which opens to us another world where the miserable barriers that separate beings of flesh vanish in love" (Marcel, 1967, p. 229). Put differently, the enactment in everyday life of Buberian/Marcelian faith includes not only the intuitive opening to the unknown possibilities of psychic reality, a kind of facing the catastrophe of living that Bionian-inspired analysts have described (Eigen, 2014), but even more importantly, it suggests an originary, divinely inspired, if not commanded, ethical/moral obligation to the human/divine other. To quote Marcel again, "What is not done for love and by love is done against love," and it is such a love-derived faith-affirmation that represents the "royal road" to hope (Hernandez, 2011, p. 117). Indeed, Buber and Marcel would probably agree that love is the starting point for grasping the mysteries that faith and psychoanalysis strive to encounter. For love is the example par excellence of mystery, when "the distinction between what is *in me* and what is only *before me* can break down"; when I am not able to place myself outside it or before it, a faith-animated total engagement in the encounter that envelops me and understands me, even if I don't understand it (Marcel, 1949, p. 20).

Notes

1 I capitalize the terms because, following Buber and Marcel (and Levinas who wrote that goodness was his only "absolute value" about "absolute" alterity, and responsibility as an a priori fundamental obligation etc.), they believed that there were "eternal values" and the "eternal norm" (and elsewhere, "true human life," "conscience" and "ultimate truth") as Buber called them (Buber, 1965, p. 116). While these virtues/values/norms were impossible, or near-impossible, to objectively prove, let alone universalize, as there is no "god's-eye" evaluative standard (e.g., these virtues/values/norms could have a dangerous potential depending on how they were instantiated, such as by religious extremists), they could be positively pointed

towards, calling to mind Heidegger's phenomenological investigatory procedure of "formal indication." This being said, while Buber for example used the aforementioned essentialist/foundational terms from time to time, some scholars believe that he did not believe in "a transhistorical essence of the human being beyond the structure or form of fundamental relationality" (Batnitzky, 2006, p. 155), nor did he "start from some external, absolutely valid ethical code" that one enacted in the move from I-It to I-Thou, but rather the unfolding concrete situation. For Buber, the "good" is not an objective condition or an internal feeling, but rather the dialogue that occurs between man and man and man and God (Friedman, 1986, pp. 60, 63). Likewise, Marcel, used the term "universal values" not in terms of a form of Platonism, "the Idea of the good or the true," but rather to affirm that "their living scope and actual relations that confer on human existence … its proper dignity" (Sweetman, 2011, p. 124).

2 Eigen (2012) briefly mentions his personal experience of the holy. He notes, "A sense of the Good, Beauty, Holy, Justice intertwined, opposed to, fused with destruction. That we recoil at this notion indicates that we are afraid to let in fully our experiential capacity" (p. 74). Marcus (2008) applies Levinas's notion of holiness, being-for-the-other, especially before oneself, to psychoanalytic theory and technique.

3 For a simplified version of Fowler's theory, see Peck (1987).

4 There have been other interesting empirically verified stage-based theories of religious/spiritual development. See, for example, Day (2017).

5 I am grateful to Hoffman (2011) for some of my cited biographical information.

6 Winnicott's notion of "use of an object" or "object usage" is important in all of this, namely, that it is only after the fantasized destruction of the good object (e.g., the caregiving parent or the analyst), and her/his subsequent survival of the onslaught, that an infant (and later, an adult) can in fact "use" the object. That is, relate to the other without a need or desire for omnipotent control, thus honoring the other's independence and alterity. Such a psychic achievement facilitates divergent and enhanced ways of experiencing the self (e.g., as more real/authentic) and the other, including in the faith realm.

7 *Presence* is hardly an unambiguous term. For Marcel, the word *presence* suggests more than "being there," as in "within the patient's experiential world," such as "patient-analyst connectedness" (a kind of witnessing presence) as many analysts conceptualize it (Eshel, 2019, p. 1). In addition, it "is a reality; it is a kind of influx," a "kind of interior accretion, of accretion from within, which comes into being as soon as presence is effective," that is "grounded in the realm of total spiritual availability (*disponibilité*); that is to say, of pure charity" (incidentally, Buber also uses the words "influx of the message" (Friedman, 1986, p. 64). For example, "presence is something which reveals itself immediately and unmistakably in a look, a smile, an intonation or a handshake" (Marcel, 1949, pp. 24, 26). Buber defines presence as both "being fully 'there'" without holding oneself back, and "being fully 'open,'" willing and able to enter into evolving dialogue with others. His definition clearly resonates with the aforementioned "being there" (Kramer & Gawlick, 2003, p. 204).

8 This being said, Friedman noted that "until his death" Buber "remained actively concerned with comparative mysticism." His study of Taoism, Hasidism, and Zen, for example, "was an integral part of his path, of his being" (1986, p. 102). However, Buber made it clear about say Lao-Tzu, "I see the reality of being entirely otherwise than he" (1964, p. 17).

9 In contrast to *emunah,* Buber (2003) suggests that *pistis*, a word first used in Greek mythology, was embraced by Christianity and translated/defined as "faith." In this account, faith is mainly a cognitive assertion in which the person has a knowledge-base of the proposition, in this instance about God, and willingly concurs with its truth validity. *Pistis* is faith in the notion that redemption will arrive at some future time; however, *emunah* emphasizes trust in the ultimate oneness of God in the world and His ability to elevate and sanctify all things material—that is, trust that the world, anything can be meaning-giving, can potentially be addressed as Thou (Friedman, 1986, p. 35). In today's "enlightened" theological/psychological world, faith is regarded as both an emotional and cognitive experience, reflecting the fact that the person of faith is a way of being-in the-world (qua Heidegger, as an integrated entity of thought/feeling/behavior).

10 Buber's faith/trust in the eternal Thou is exemplified in his reflection on death: "The genuine faith speaks: I know nothing of death, but I know that God is eternity, and I know this, too, that he is my God. Whether what we call time remains to us beyond our death becomes quite unimportant to us next to this knowing, that we are God's—who is not immortal, but eternal. Instead of imagining ourselves living instead of dead, we shall prepare ourselves for a real death which is perhaps the final limit of time but which, if that is the case is surely the threshold of eternity" (1967b, p. 231).

11 Marcel also used a language similar to Buber's when he was speaking about spiritual availability and presence: "Between these two [dogmatism and mystery] I believe that there exists a middle way—a narrow, difficult and dangerous path which I have tried to discover" (1949, p. 29); And again, Marcel noted before his conversion to Christianity, "I might also say that I walked a tight rope for a long time, that at a certain moment I needed some outside intervention, that of Muriac" (Sweetman, 2008, p. 150). Finally, he noted, "I consider myself as having always been a philosopher of the threshold, a philosopher who kept himself in rather uncomfortable fashion on a line midway between believers and nonbelievers so he could somehow stand with believers, with the Christian religion, the Catholic religion, but also speak to nonbelievers, make himself understood by them and perhaps to help them" (ibid., 152).

12 I am grateful to Moore (1996b, p. 94) for these two quotations.

13 Buber, too, believed that, "Always it is the religious which bestows, the ethical which receives" (1988, p. 95).

14 For a somewhat different view of the positive role of strong inner convictions, one that to some extent challenges Marcel's view, see my *Autonomy in the Extreme Situation. Bruno Bettelheim, the Nazi Concentration Camps and the Mass Society* (1999). In my book, I claim that strong inner convictions decisively helped many "believing" concentration camp inmates (e.g., religious Jews, Catholics, Jehovah's Witnesses) to maintain their autonomy, integration, and humanity, especially compared to their "non-believing" fellow inmates.

15 Buber also spoke about God as the Absolute Person, who, while not a person per se, was one who gradually became known and loved as he interacts with God. This is the paradox of the transcendent and immanent God, eternal and yet who enters into direct relationship with us (Friedman, 1986, p. 24)

References

Akhtar, S. (2009). *Comprehensive dictionary of psychoanalysis*. London: Karnac.
Anderson, T. C. (2006). *A commentary on Gabriel Marcel's* The mystery of being. Milwaukee, WI: Marquette University Press.
Batnitzky, L. (2006). Revelation and *neues denken*—Rethinking Buber and Rosenzweig on the law. In M. Zank (Ed.), *New perspectives on Martin Buber* (pp. 149–174). Tubingen: Mohr Siebeck.
Berger, P. (1967). *The sacred canopy: Elements of a sociological theory of religion*. New York: Anchor.
Biemann, A. D. (2006). Aesthetic education in Martin Buber: Jewish Renaissance and the artist. In M. Zank (Ed.), *New perspectives on Martin Buber* (pp. 85–110). Tubingen: Mohr Siebeck.
Bion, W. R. (1970). *Attention and interpretation*. London: Tavistock.
Bion, W. R. (1994). (Ed. F. Bion). *Cogitations*. London: Karnac.
Braiterman, Z. (2006). Martin Buber and the art of ritual. In M. Zank (Ed.), *New perspectives on Martin Buber* (pp. 111–124). Tubingen: Mohr Siebeck.
Buber, M. (1957). (Trans. M. Friedman). *Eclipse of God: Studies in the relation between religion and philosophy*. New York: Harper Torchbooks.
Buber, M. (1964). *Philosophical interrogations*. S. Rome & B. Rome (Eds.). New York: Holt, Rinehart and Winston
Buber, M. (1965). (Trans. R. G. Smith). *Between man and man*. New York: Macmillan.
Buber, M. (1967a). Replies to my critics. In P. A. Schilpp & M. Friedman (Eds.), *The philosophy of Martin Buber* (The Library of Living Philosophers, vol. 12, pp. 689–744). La Salle, IL: Open Court.
Buber, M. (1967b). (Trans. M. Freedman). *A believing humanism—My testament, 1902–1965*. New York: Simon & Schuster.
Buber, M. (1967c). Autobiographical fragments. In P. A. Schilpp & M. Friedman (Eds.), *The philosophy of Martin Buber* (The Library of Living Philosophers, vol. 12, pp. 3–39). La Salle, IL: Open Court.
Buber, M. (1988). (Introduction by R. M. Selzer. Translation of *Gottesfinsternis*). *Eclipse of God: Studies in the relation between religion and philosophy*. Atlantic Highlands: Humanities Press.
Buber, M. (2003). *Two types of faith*. Syracuse: Syracuse University Press. Originally published 1950.
Cain, S. (1995). *Gabriel Marcel's theory of religious experience*. New York: Peter Lang.
Civitarese, G. (2019). Bion's O and his pseudo-mystical path. *Psychoanalytic Dialogues, 29*, 388–403.
Compton, W. C., & Hoffman, E. (2020). *Positive psychology: The science of happiness and flourishing*. Los Angeles: Sage.
Coyle, A. (2011). Critical responses to faith development theory: a useful agenda for change? *Archive for the Psychology of Religion, 33*(3), 281–298.
Day, J. (2017). Religion and human development in adulthood: Well-being, prosocial behavior, and religious and spiritual development. *Behavioral Development Bulletin, 22*, 298–313.
Eigen, M. (2012). *Kabbalah and psychoanalysis*. London: Routledge.
Eigen, M. (2014). *Faith*. London: Karnac.
Erikson, E. H. (1950). *Childhood and society*. New York: Norton.

Erikson, E. H. (1964). *Insight and responsibility*. New York: Norton.
Eshel, O. (2019). *The emergence of analytic oneness: Into the heart of psychoanalysis*. New York: Routledge.
Fowler, J. W. (1994). Pluralism and oneness in religious experience: William James and faith development theory. *Psychology of Religion Newsletter, 19*, 182–183.
Fowler, J. W. (1995). *Stages of faith: The psychology of human development and the quest for meaning*. New York: HarperOne.
Friedman, M. S. (1986). *Martin Buber and the eternal*. New York: Human Sciences Press.
Friedman, M. S. (2002). *Martin Buber: The life of dialogue* (4th ed.). London: Routledge.
Fromm, E. (1947). *Man for himself. An inquiry into the psychology of ethics*. New York: Rinehart & Company.
Geertz, C. (1973). *The interpretation of cultures*. New York: Basic Books.
Goldman, D. (1993). *In search of the real: The origins and originality of D. W. Winnicott*. Northvale: Jason Aronson.
Grotstein, J. (2007). *A beam of intense darkness*. London: Karnac.
Hernandez, J. G. (2011) *Gabriel Marcel's ethics of hope. evil, God and virtue*. London: Bloomsbury.
Hertz, J. H. (Ed.) (1960). *The Pentateuch and Haftorahs*. London: Soncino Press.
Heschel, A. J. (1955). *God in search of man: A philosophy of Judaism*. New York: Farrar, Straus and Giroux.
Hodes, A. (1971). *Martin Buber: An intimate portrait*. New York: Viking Press.
Hoffman, M.T. (2011). *Toward mutual recognition. Relational psychoanalysis and the Christian narrative*. London: Routledge.
Jaspers, K. (2011). *The origins and goal of history*. London: Routledge. (Original work published 1953).
Jeeves, M., & Brown, W. S. (2009). *Neuroscience, psychology, and religion. illusions, delusions, and realities in human nature*. West Conshohocken: Templeton Press.
Jones, J. W. (1991). *Contemporary psychoanalysis & religion: Transference and transcendence*. New Haven: Yale University Press.
Katz, S. (2006). Martin Buber in retrospect. In M. Zank (Ed.), *New perspectives on Martin Buber* (pp. 255–266). Tubingen: More Siebeck.
Kaufmann, F. (1967). Martin Buber's philosophy of religion. In P. A. Schilpp & M. Friedman (Eds.), *The philosophy of Martin Buber* (The Library of Living Philosophers, vol. 12, pp. 201–233). La Salle, IL: Open Court.
Keen, S. (1984). The development of the idea of being in Marcel's thought. In P. A. Schilpp & L. E. Hahn (Eds.), *The philosophy of Gabriel Marcel* (The Library of Living Philosophers, vol. 17, pp. 99–120). La Salle, IL: Open Court.
Kramer, K. P., & Gawlick, M. (2003). *Martin Buber's I and Thou: Practicing living dialogue*. New York: Paulist Press.
Leavy, S. (1988). *In the image of God*. New Haven: Yale University Press.
Levinas, E. (2001). (Ed. J. Robbins). *Is it righteous to be? Interviews with Emanuel Levinas*. Stanford: Stanford University Press.
Loewald, H. (1988). *Sublimation*. New Haven: Yale University Press.
Marcel, G. (1949). (Trans. M. Harari). *The philosophy of existence*. New York: Philosophical Library.
Marcel, G. (1950). Theism and personal relationships, *Cross Currents, 1*(1), 38–45.
Marcel, G. (1964). (Trans. R. Rosthal). *Creative fidelity*. New York: Noonday Press.

Marcel, G. (1965a). (Trans. E. Crauford). *Homo viator: Introduction to a metaphysic of hope.* New York: Harper and Row.
Marcel, G. (1965b). (Trans. K. Farrer). *Being and having: An existentialist diary.* New York: Harper & Row.
Marcel, G. (1967). (Transl. M. Machado). *Metaphysical journal*, 1938–1943. Pittsburgh: Duquesne University Press.
Marcel, G. (1984). An autobiographical essay. In P. A. Schilpp & L. E. Hahn (Eds.), *The philosophy of Gabriel Marcel* (pp. 1–68). La Salle, IL: Open Court.
Marcel, G. (2001 [1951]). *Mystery of being. Volume II. Faith and reality.* South Bend, IN: St. Augustine's Press.
Marcus, P. (1999). *Autonomy in the extreme situation: Bruno Bettelheim, the Nazi concentration camps and the mass society.* Westport, CT: Praeger.
Marcus, P. (2003). *Ancient religious wisdom, spirituality, and psychoanalysis.* Westport, CT: Praeger.
Marcus, P. (2008). *Being for the other: Emmanuel Levinas, ethical living and psychoanalysis.* Milwaukee: Marquette University Press.
Marcus, P. (2013). *In search of the spiritual: Gabriel Marcel, psychoanalysis, and the sacred.* London: Karnac.
Marcus, P. (2019). *The psychoanalysis of overcoming suffering: Flourishing despite pain.* London: Routledge.
Meissner, W. W. (1984). *Psychoanalysis and religious experience.* New Haven: Yale University Press.
Molino, A. (Ed.) (2013). (Eds. R. Carnevali, A. Giannandrea, & D. Yang). *Crossroads in psychoanalysis, Buddhism, and mindfulness: The word and breath.* Lanham: Jason Aronson.
Monte, C. F. (1980). *Beneath the mask: An introduction to theories of personality*, 2nd ed. New York: Holt, Rinehart & Winston.
Moore, D. J. (1996a). *Martin Buber. Prophet of religious secularism.* New York: Fordham University Press.
Moore, D. J. (1996b). Martin Buber and Christian theology. In M. Friedman (Ed.), *Martin Buber and the human sciences* (pp. 93–106). Albany: State University of New York Press.
Peck, M. S. (1987). *The different drum: Community making and peace.* New York: Simon & Schuster.
Person, E. S., Cooper, A. M., & Gabbard, G. O. (Eds.). (2005). *Textbook of psychoanalysis.* Washington, DC: American Psychiatric Association.
Rizzutto, A. M. (1979). *The birth of the living God.* Chicago: University of Chicago Press.
Rodman, F. R. (2003). *Winnicott: Life and work.* Cambridge: Perseus.
Ruti, M. (2009). *A world of fragile thing: Psychoanalysis and the art of living.* Albany: State University of New York Press.
Selzer, R. M. (1988). Introduction. In M. Buber, *Eclipse of God: Studies in the relation between religion and philosophy* (pp. ix–xxii). Atlantic Highlands: Humanities Press International.
Shafranske, E. P. (Ed.). (1996). *Religion and the clinical practice of psychology.* Washington, DC: American Psychological Association.
Silberstein, L. J. (1989). *Martin Buber's social and religious thought: Alienation and the quest for meaning.* New York: New York University Press.
Smith, H. (1979). *Forgotten truth: The primordial tradition.* New York: Harper & Row.
Sweetman, B. (2008). *The vision of Gabriel Marcel: Epistemology, human person, the transcendent.* Amsterdam: Rodopi.

Sweetman, B. (Ed.) (2011). *A Gabriel Marcel reader.* South Bend: St. Augustine's Press.
Tillich, P. (1958). *The dynamics of faith.* New York: HarperCollins.
Vaidyanathan, J. G., & Kripal, J (Eds.). (2002). *Vishnu on Freud's desk. A reader in psychoanalysis and Hinduism.* Oxford: Oxford University Press.
Vermote, R. (2019). *Reading Bion.* London: Routledge.
Winnicott, D. W. (1965). *The maturation process and the facilitating environment.* London: Karnac.
Winnicott, D. W. (1971). *Playing and reality.* London: Routledge.
Winnicott, D. W. (1953). Transitional objects and transitional phenomena: A study of the first not-me possession. *International Journal of Psychoanalysis, 34,* 89–97.
Wuthnow, R., Hunter, J. D., Bergesen, A., & Kurzweil, E. (1984). *Cultural analysis.* Boston: Routledge & Kegan Paul.
Zank, M. (2006). Buber and *Religionswissenschaft*: The case of his studies on biblical faith. In M. Zank (Ed.), *New perspectives on Martin Buber* (pp. 61–82). Tubingen: Mohr Siebeck.

Chapter 5

The spirit of suffering

If ever there was a huge impediment to fashioning a flourishing life, the fact of personal suffering surely is it. Regardless of whether the suffering emanates from a partially or fully unhinged mind, as in neurosis or psychosis, respectively, or from other forms of so-called "mental illness," or an external event, like the premature death of a significant other, a tornado that obliterates one's home and community, or unlawful internment in prison, it is undeniable that such mental distress, especially when it is long-term and feels undeserved ("when bad things happen to good people"), cuts very deeply into a person's ego, self or soul. For some individuals, such suffering often paralyzes or near paralyzes their will and ability to press on, to make things better, at least initially, while for others, it is an interminable condition of helplessness, hopelessness, and haplessness, in short, despair. In a letter that aptly expresses a dark sentiment that most people have felt from time to time, the elderly Church Father St. Augustine wrote, "Everyone should realize the misery which is part of human life extends from the tears of the newly born to the last breath of the soon to die" (Burt, 1999, p. 417). Indeed, this gloomy statement calls to mind Freud's tragicomic line (Marcus, 2013) in *Studies on Hysteria* that the purpose of analysis is "transforming your hysterical [neurotic] misery into common [normal] unhappiness" (Breuer & Freud, 1955, p. 305). Freud was well aware that a modicum of mental distress or psychic pain was the necessary precondition for differentiation and individuation and the ability to experience the object (i.e., a significant other) as separate and independent. What St. Augustine and Freud are getting at is that life is a distress-filled existence from the cradle to the grave (Buddha's first "noble truth" of suffering, in contemporary psychological parlance, is that everyone has challenging "problems in living"). Indeed, there are "limit-situations," as philosopher Karl Jaspers called them, existential "givens," like suffering, struggle, guilt and death, which one cannot avoid, let alone permanently resolve or transcend (Cooper, 2015 p. 22). In fact, all suffering is a foretaste of death in the sense of feeling impotent or passive, a kind of psychological materialization that calls to mind a corpse (Lingis, 2015, p. 237). The upsurge of awareness of our vulnerability, finitude, and mortality is particularly ego-chilling. As psychoanalyst

D. W. Winnicott quipped, "Death is a disaster which you have to put up with, because you're human" (Neve, 1992, p. 176).

In this chapter I want to discuss how psychoanalysis views a particular form of suffering that mainly emanates from the external world as opposed to the internal one, like an alleged organically driven depression, psychosis or certain type of severe neurosis. So-called internal (i.e., subjectivity) and external worlds (i.e., culture/situational forces) are in fact always interrelated, interdependent, and interactive; they co-mingle and co-potentiate each other.[1] I am referring to life in extremity: the struggle to maintain one's autonomy, integration, and humanity in the Nazi concentration camps. What matters most, however, is how a person socially constructs his world, and this centrally includes how he metabolizes his perceived suffering within the totality of his life circumstances as he construes them. For perception is reality, as the often-cited sociological Thomas theorem affirms: "If men define situations as real, they are real in their consequences" (Marcus, 2020, p. 43). This means that how you behave largely depends on your perspective on your situation, including your ordeal of suffering, and whether you can make your suffering "sufferable" (Geertz, 1973, p. 104) and, perhaps, surmount it, and even learn from it. In this sense, Aeschylus put his finger on the aforementioned critical points in a manner that resonates with the best of psychoanalysis conceived as a spiritual discipline: In *The Orestia* he wrote, "We must suffer, suffer into truth," and in *Agamemnon* he noted, "Wisdom comes alone through suffering" (Marcus, 2019, pp. 260, 1). Most sensible or, more accurately, wise people learn important usable truths about artful living from their suffering, though as Bion noted, many in fact have neither the will nor the ability to do so: Individuals have a "hatred of learning from experience," roughly a "hatred of a process of development" (1961 pp. 7, 77).

I have chosen to focus on one admittedly extreme paradigmatic example of suffering, for it puts into sharp focus some of the troubling limitations of "mainstream" psychoanalysis, conceived as a "symbolic world," a "particular way of looking at life" (Geertz, 1973, p. 110), one that not only has bearing on understanding life in extremity but also, in a lesser manner, managing the harshness of life as Freud called it, including serious problems in living (i.e., life really hurts). In addition, the Nazi concentration camp example allows us to reasonably exploit some of the insights of Buber and Marcel's religiously animated dialogical personalism that support my claim that psychoanalysis would be a more robust "technology of the self" (what Foucault called "self-steering mechanisms" (Rose, 1996, p. 29)) that can help analysands make their suffering sufferable, if it conceived itself and was implemented both inside and outside of the consultation room, as a spiritual discipline.

Specifically, I am referring to the differences between how the typical secular intellectual and/or humanist camp inmates, the so-called "non-believers," like Bruno Bettelheim (and other analysts),[2] struggled to "remain human"[3] in the Nazi concentration camps, compared to the "believers," like religious Jews and Christians and staunch communists and Zionists. These two groups (henceforth, the psychoanalytic intellectuals and the believers) had very different ways of understanding and managing their extreme ordeal of suffering, and I believe we can learn something important about making suffering sufferable from considering these contrasting outlooks and behavior, especially when glossed through the insights of Buber and Marcel. For while Buber and Marcel were both steeped in a broadly conceived Judeo-Christian outlook, they developed their ideas in highly personal, yet existentially relevant ways that can expand and deepen how psychoanalysis, conceived as a spiritual discipline understands, the analysand's suffering and its alleviation. I will conclude this chapter by suggesting some of the positive implications of Buber and Marcel's reflections on making suffering sufferable that may have bearing on the clinical context.

Definitions of suffering, reality, symbolic world, intellectual and believer

Suffering

While I will not engage in any detail with the philosophically and psychologically murky issue of defining the difference between pain and suffering, given that this chapter is about suffering and not pain, I will provide what I regard as a rudimentary and serviceable way of thinking about what distinguishes one from the other. Indian American author Deepak Chopra has succinctly described a central difference between pain and suffering,

> Pain is not the same as suffering. Left to itself, the body discharges pain spontaneously, letting go of it the moment that the underlying cause is healed. Suffering is pain that we hold on to. It comes from the mind's mysterious instinct to believe that pain is good, or that it cannot be escaped, or that the person deserves it.
>
> (2004, pp. 65–66)

Another related way of distinguishing pain from suffering is to view it as the average person literally speaks about it in everyday life: pain tends to be described as a physical happening, like a toothache or backache, while suffering tends to be situated in the emotional realm, like when a love relationship abruptly ends or one gets fired and can't find another job and has a family to take care of. It is worth noting that pain can morph into suffering, such as when debilitating chronic physical pain becomes the basis for feeling hopeless, and suffering can morph into pain, like when one has successfully mourned a loved one and then their birthday is remembered, which leads to an upsurge of searing feelings. While all of these distinctions are debatable, the reader understands that I am mainly interested in the suffering associated with some existentially compelling aspects of life that are not easily remedied by traditional "pain management," such as via prescription medication, physical rehabilitation or going to a medical doctor. Certainly, imprisonment in a Nazi concentration camp constitutes the worst kind of suffering; though it was infused with pain every inch of the way.

Reality

Drawing from this example of life in extremity, that is, prisoner behavior in the Nazi concentration camp, where the "shattering of the self was one of the deepest forms of damage" (Appelfeld, 1994, p. 22), I want to first briefly suggest how under-theorized the environment (i.e., the external world) has been, and still is, in psychoanalytic theory. Most importantly, such a theoretical neglect of the role of the environment in understanding behavior has constraining consequences for how psychoanalysis understands itself and, therefore, how it views suffering, including the mental anguish among inmates, and how best to help analysands better manage, if not make good strides in mastering their mental anguish. While there has been progress in theorizing the environment in psychoanalytic studies recently, what former president of the American Psychoanalytic Association Robert Wallerstein said in 1973 in many ways is still true today, that the study of so-called "reality" has been "relatively neglected or taken for granted in usual psychoanalytic discourse" (Kabatznick & Marcus, 1986, p. 121). He believed that this neglect is implicit in the long-standing belief of a fixed world "out there" of an unvarying "average expectable environment" (ibid.). Indeed, in general, as Erik Erikson believed, psychoanalysis has regarded the introspective subjective, the metasubjective, and the intersubjective as more important than the objective (Hoare, 2002, p. 86), while Loewald noted, "objectivity, rationality, and reality themselves are not what we thought them to be" (1979, p. 773). "By 'reality,' psychoanalysis means what is actually out there, can be objectively perceived and consensually agreed upon" (Akhtar, 2009, p. 240); however, what the brilliant "classic" social psychologists have persuasively demonstrated is that this foundational assumption of psychoanalysis about what is "out there" and how the world hangs together is mistaken, that reality is perception, it is not fixed (Marcus, 2020).[4]

More recently, psychodynamic psychologist Tamara McClintock Greenberg noted, "within mainstream psychoanalysis, there has been relatively little emphasis on 'real events,' including the effects of adult-onset trauma," such as illness in old age (2016, p. 43). Moreover, "reality," or at least "certain kinds of external or practical concerns," has "not been integrated very well into [psychoanalytic] theory" (ibid., p. 9). For example, three famous experimental social psychological studies that are pertinent to "moral psychology"—Solomon Asch's classic experiment on social pressure/conformity (i.e., telling the truth vs. lying), the "bystander" experiments by Bibb Latané and John Darley on altruism versus self-interest, and Stanley Milgram's study of obeying or refusing authority—all challenge psychoanalysis to generate a more robust psychology of "everyday" situational behavior that gives greater consideration to the role of reality (i.e., situational forces) alongside fantasy and wish in understanding vitally important types of human behavior (Marcus, 2020). For as the celebrated Israeli novelist/Holocaust survivor Aharon Appelfeld told Philip Roth in an interview, "Reality, as you know, is always stronger than the human imagination. Not only that, reality can permit itself to be unbelievable, inexplicable, out of all proportion. The created work [i.e., fantasy/imagination], to my regret, cannot permit itself all that" (1994, p. 68) without suffering serious, "real-life" consequences. This being said, it is important to remember that while man is a context-dependent and setting-specific being, he also imaginatively hungers to transcend context and setting, leaning into the future, desiring something "more," "higher," and "better."

It was Bruno Bettelheim, a Holocaust survivor, who argued in *The Informed Heart* (1960) that psychoanalytic theory (i.e., classical theory) was inadequate in explaining "what constitutes a well integrated personality" in the radically extreme social environment of the camps, or "which behavior is preferable, or which personality more adequate" (ibid., p. 20). Bettelheim observed that some of the prisoners who maintained their "old personality structure, stuck to their values in the face of extreme hardships, and as persons were hardly touched by the camp experience"; they were people whom psychoanalysts would have viewed "as extremely neurotic or plainly delusional, and therefore apt to fall apart, as persons, under stress" (ibid.). Such were the Jehovah's Witnesses (and others with strong religious/political moral convictions) "who not only showed unusual heights of human dignity and moral behavior, but seemed protected against the same camp experience that soon destroyed persons considered very well integrated by my psychoanalytic friends and myself" (ibid.).[5] Those persons who, according to psychoanalytic theory, should have stood up best under the harshness of the camp experience, such as the secular "intellectuals, the liberals, the humanists, the professors of sociology, and the like," as Elie Wiesel described them (1974, p. 273), were often the first to cave in to the extreme stress. They became regressed, that is, depressed, anxious and most importantly, morally corrupted, as they identified with Nazi values. Behavior in the camps could not be explained based on past life history and former personality, or on those aspects of personality that at the time seemed significant in the then current psychoanalytic thinking. Bettelheim points out that this conclusion emanated, in part, from his own personal experience of disappointment with psychoanalysis as a self-sustaining frame of reference in the camps. Bettelheim writes,

> Most surprising of all, psychoanalysis which I had come to view as the best key to all human problems offered no suggestion or help toward the solution of how to survive and survive halfway decently in the camps. For that I had to fall back on qualities that in my psychoanalytic experience and thinking were of little importance, if not of negative valence, while those qualities I had learned to stress were often as much of a hindrance as a help.
> (1960, pp. 15–16)

What Bettelheim ultimately showed in both his early and later studies on the concentration camp experience was that psychoanalysis, which included various post-Freudian versions as self-psychologists/Holocaust survivors Paul and Anna Ornstein told me (personal communication, 1989), was inadequate to explain why and how inmates maintained their autonomy, integration and, most importantly, their humanity during their horrendous ordeal. Bettelheim argued that this theoretical and practical deficit was because psychoanalysis did not give enough theoretical importance to the powerful influence of the social environment in changing the individual. He came to realize that psychoanalysis, as a treatment modality, was not the most potent influence to bring about personality change. Rather, an extreme environment such as the camps could more swiftly and invasively shape the person for better or worse. Says Bettelheim, "The impact of the concentration camp ... within a few weeks, did for me what years of useful and quite successful analysis had not done" (1960, p. 12). Psychoanalyst Franz Alexander, one of the originators of psychoanalytic psychosomatic medicine and criminology, has noted that Bettelheim "recognized that psychoanalysis was conceived in times of stability and did not pay sufficient attention to the environmental influences on shaping personality" (1961, p. 42). He thus asserted that psychoanalytic theory needed to be changed.

According to Bettelheim, what was necessary to help reshape psychoanalytic theory to effectively illuminate situations of extremity, which arguably includes a seriously depressed/anxious person who views himself as in an "extreme" situation, was the development of a theory that took the powerful role of the social environment into consideration along with the vicissitudes of the sexual and aggressive drives and early life history. Says Bettelheim,

> I only wish to suggest that the psychoanalytic theory of personality is deficient in suggesting what makes for a "desirable," well integrated personality; and this because it overstresses the importance of the inner life to the neglect of the total man as he deals with his human and social environment.
> (1960, p. 21)

Even more to the point, Bettelheim noted, "What psychoanalysis has already achieved for the personality within a stable social context must now be done for personality and social context in their interaction, when both of them are changing" (ibid., p. 37), like in the concentration camp. Bettelheim thus seemed to recognize deficiencies in psychoanalytic personality theory that, as he intimates, forced him to try to modify his psychoanalytic perspective with insights from the field of social psychology (e.g., the role of the social environment in changing personality). What Bettelheim was identifying as problematic in psychoanalytic theory is still a theoretical, clinical, and practical conundrum that has not been adequately addressed by the psychoanalytic community. Psychoanalysis has not drawn from social psychology and sociology in a sophisticated way to develop a theory that can make better sense out of behavior in radically unstable social environments, including how specific social/situational forces shape, even determine behavior (Marcus, 2020). While most of us have mercifully not endured concentration camps or other such extreme situations, the conditions of possibility that tend to bring about depression/anxiety are often correlated with the real and imagined utter "outrageousness" of an external world (e.g., to a lesser extent but still, the pandemic of 2020) that radically subverts one's autonomy, integration and humanity. To better grasp how such people consciously and unconsciously build their private "concentration camp" for themselves (Appelfeld, 1994, p. 17) requires that we have a better understanding of the role of powerfully toxic "real" environments in propelling them into their depressive abyss.[6]

Symbolic world

A symbolic world is roughly equivalent to a perspective, "a particular manner of construing the world" (Geertz, 1973, p. 110). Religion, politics, and psychoanalysis can operate as symbolic worlds. Psychoanalysis, for example, as a life-narrative, has its own version of the human condition and its own idea of what the "good life" (or flourishing one) is and how to achieve it (and different theories of psychoanalysis have divergent versions of the human condition, what constitutes psychopathology and treatment). Perhaps most important, psychoanalysis has its own notions about how to effectively assimilate the emotionally dissonant experiences of life, including suffering and death, "into a comprehensive explanation of reality and human destiny" (Berger & Berger, 1972, p. 352). In a certain sense, those who seek out psychoanalysis are attracted to its "vision of reality," to the system of meaning and metaphor that it promulgates (Schafer, 1976, p. 22). Sounding somewhat like an Evangelical Christian who has "seen Jesus," Michael Eigen declared in his book *Faith*, "For me, psychoanalysis breathes. I am a psychoanalytic person … [Regarding Guntrip's work] I felt a positive sense of shared values and vision enabled enough to happen to make it more than worthwhile—a gift to us" (2014, p. 40, 39).

Extreme situation

In an extreme situation, especially as it applies to concentration camp inmates, an individual feels deprived of any close, affirming, and need-gratifying personal relationships. Deprived of hope, he feels utterly powerless in relation to those in authority, and fears that the extreme situation is inescapable and interminable (Bettelheim, 1979, pp. 112–126). In other words, the extreme situation can be equated with the radical subversion of a person as a consequence of the loss of his world. For Buber, suffering is also equated with the loss of one's world, that is, it can be an agonizing, insoluble riddle of life for the believer in a living God: "When God seems to withdraw himself utterly from the earth and no longer participates in existence," when "the space of history is full of noise but empty of divine breath," this "eclipse of God," this sustained hiddenness, makes living nearly impossible (Friedman, 1986, p. 150). What is impossible, says Buber, is the feeling of "radical forlornness" rooted in a felt "distance from God, a void of God, this being the "anthropomorphic image" only "granted to us" (speaking about rather than to God) (Lawritson, 1996, pp. 302, 305). Marcel, too, viewed suffering as a radical subversion of one's world: "In all suffering, I risk becoming self-centered and thus locking myself up in despair" (1984, p. 201). Moreover, "suffering and evil" "resists all attempts at integration or absorption into an intelligible system," thus leaving the person feeling the utter thrownness of existence (ibid. p. 368). It is this "impossibility of retreat" and "being cut off from every living spring" that characterizes suffering, especially physical suffering, says Levinas (1969, p. 238).[7] Many analysands frequently feel as if they are in something of an extreme situation, real or imagined.

Intellectual and believer

Tentative definitions of an intellectual as it applies to the death camp,[8] Auschwitz in particular, are offered by Jean Améry and Primo Levi. About the person with an "intellectual background and intellectual basic disposition," Améry writes:

> An intellectual, as I would like it to be understood here, is a man who lives within what is a spiritual frame of reference in the widest sense. His realm of thought is an essentially humanistic one, that of the liberal arts. He has a well-developed esthetic consciousness.
>
> (Améry, 1980, p. 2)

Most psychoanalysts and psychoanalytically oriented intellectuals can be included in this broadly conceived skeptic-humanistic category. For those psychoanalytic intellectuals who are religious or political believers,[9] ideological commitments, along with the concomitant potential benefits, tend to be somewhat blunted by their skeptical psychoanalytical intellectualism. These analysts may have religious beliefs, but their commitment to their faith lacks the passionate emotional commitment and absolute leap of faith of the "true believer." They tend to be more ambivalent, critical, and questioning of their faith and more angst-ridden, reducing the belief's psychological usefulness and possibility of transcendence in extreme situations and life in general.

My claim, following Buber and Marcel (and further developed by Levinas), is that those people who are best able to sustain themselves as persons inside the camps (and perhaps, also in "normal" life) are those who are steeped in a form of life characterized by strongly felt, flexibly and creatively applied, transcendent-pointing moral beliefs and values that are primarily other-directed, other-regarding, and other-serving (e.g., "lone wolves" who attempted to survive at any price in the camps not only lost their humanity, but rarely physically survived). Whether the intellectual was a man of letters, a philosopher of science, a naturalist, a sociologist, a mathematician or, I would add, a psychoanalyst, these intellectuals were more vulnerable to the Nazi assault than the believers. My hope is that this "thought experiment," this comparison between the psychoanalytic intellectual and the religious believer, will put into sharp focus what is possibly missing in psychoanalytic accounts of how people can best "manage" their suffering. By identifying and describing some of those personal qualities, beliefs, values, and group affiliations that were most helpful to them as they faced the extreme situation, I hope to shed some light on how other painful and distressing experiences in life can be better borne, made more sufferable. More generally, perhaps, the mode of practicing and acting upon the world of the "believers," with their strongly felt, flexibly and creatively applied, transcendent-pointing moral beliefs and values that are primarily other-directed, other-regarding and other-serving, can provide some new insights into the human condition and human potential at its best.

I will focus my discussion mainly on a broadly-based Freudian psychoanalysis, although much of what I will discuss has some bearing on other psychoanalytic perspectives that have different assumptions about what constitutes the human condition, psychopathology and treatment (e.g., relational psychoanalysis; Marcus & Rosenberg, 1988). I do this because the only existing systematic discussion of survival in a concentration camp written by a psychoanalytic intellectual is that of Bruno Bettelheim, who was lodged in a broadly-based Freudian outlook, as were most of the survivor psychoanalysts I have spoken to. The "believers" I will be describing are mainly devout Jews. This is because they are both the most written-about group in the pertinent Holocaust literature and the group of survivors I have had the most personal and clinical contact with.

Sustaining the self, ego, and soul in the camps

My focus is on the problem of sustaining the self in the extreme situation from the point of view of those who were less capable of surviving as "human beings" (Bettelheim, 1960, p. 16) in the camps, the intellectuals, the psychoanalytic intellectual in particular. There is considerable support for this claim, including from three famous Auschwitz survivors, Jean Améry, Elie Wiesel, and Primo Levi (Levi, 1986, pp. 145–146).

As Améry writes:

> One way or the other, in the decisive moments their political or religious belief was an inestimable help to them, while we skeptical and humanistic intellectuals took recourse, in vain, to our literary, philosophical, and artistic household gods. Their belief or their ideology gave them the firm foothold in the world from which they spiritually unhinged the SS state. Under conditions that defy the imagination they conducted Mass, and as

> Orthodox Jews they fasted on the Day of Atonement although they actually lived the entire year in a condition of raging hunger. They survived better or died with more dignity than their irreligious or intellectual comrades, who often were infinitely better educated and more practiced in exact thinking.
>
> (1980, p. 13)

Wiesel writes:

> Within the system of the concentration camp ... the first to give in, the first to collaborate—to save their lives—were the intellectuals, the liberals, the humanists, the professors of sociology, and the like ... Very few Communists gave in ... They were the resisters ... Even fewer to give in were the Catholic priests ... yet there were exceptions. But you could not have found one single rabbi—I dare you—among all the *kapos* or among any of the others who held positions of power in the camps.
>
> (1974, p. 273)[10]

Most important for this chapter, it was Bettelheim (who was incarcerated in Dachau and Buchenwald in 1938–1939), who at the time of his imprisonment could reasonably be described as a psychoanalytically oriented intellectual (see below) and who devalued the role of psychoanalytic experience and thinking in helping him survive as a "person" halfway decently in the camps. It was his aforementioned quoted testimonial that prompted my interest in comparing the psychoanalytic intellectual and the religious believer:

> It is a well-known fact of the concentration camps that those who had strong religious and. moral convictions managed life there much better than the rest. Their beliefs, including belief in an afterlife, gave them a strength to endure which was far above that of most others. Deeply religious persons often helped others, and some voluntarily sacrificed themselves—many more of them than of the average prisoners.
>
> (1979, p. 296)

What Bettelheim is stressing is that his psychoanalytic perspective did not significantly help him maintain his autonomy, integration, and humanity in the concentration camps. Bettelheim's psychoanalytic experience and thinking did not help him achieve his goal:

> If I should try to sum up in one sentence what my main problem was during the whole time I spent in the camps, it would be: to protect my inner self in such a way that if, by good fortune, I should regain my liberty, I would be approximately the same person I was when deprived of liberty.
>
> (ibid., p. 126)

Bettelheim writes that his psychoanalytic perspective "strangely enough, and to my sharp disappointment, did not help me in any specific ways to protect myself from that danger [i.e. personality disintegration], nor to understand why those who stood up well under the experience were able to do so" (ibid., p. 24).

Why then was psychoanalysis, which can be conceptualized as a symbolic world, a master narrative with a particular angle of vision on life, including its own way of assimilating the painful and frightening experiences of life, and even death itself, so unsuited for helping individuals to sustain themselves as "human beings" in the extreme situation?

To help answer this question, and to suggest what moral and other resources a believer could use to "remain human," including making his suffering sufferable, resources that were generally not available to the psychoanalyst, I will further discuss the one existing "classic" concentration camp narrative written by a psychoanalytic intellectual, Bettelheim's *The Informed Heart*.

Bettelheim's ambivalence toward the helpfulness of his Freudian psychoanalytic outlook in the concentration camp

It is appropriate to begin with the ambivalent reflections of Bettelheim, the only psychoanalytic thinker/survivor that I am aware of who directly raises the issue under investigation in this chapter. Bettelheim struggles with the limitations of psychoanalysis in helping him and other inmates "survive as human beings" in the camps (1960, p. 16). Moreover, Bettelheim has been regarded by many as the embodiment of the "European intellectual." He received a classical education at the University of Vienna and was well-versed in literature, history, sociology, mythology, and the humanities of Freud (Fischer, 1991, p. 163).[11]

In *The Informed Heart*, Bettelheim defines psychoanalysis before he indicates which aspects of his psychoanalytic framework were useful to him while incarcerated at Dachau and Buchenwald. He notes that technically

> psychoanalysis is really at least three different things: a method of observation, a therapy, and a body of theories on human behavior and personality structure. They are valid in descending order, the theory of personality being the weakest link of a system quite in need of revision.
>
> (1960, p. 19)

Bettelheim further points out that as a personal method of observation, psychoanalysis:

> more than proved its value and was most helpful to me. It gave me a deeper understanding of what may have gone on in the unconscious of prisoners and guards, an understanding that on one occasion may have saved my life, and on other occasions let me be of help to some of my fellow prisoners,

> where it counted (ibid., pp. 19–20). Without the understanding gained from psychoanalysis I would not have been able to comprehend what the concentration camp did to people, nor why.
>
> (1979, p. 107)

Such understanding was "psychologically reconstructive" for Bettelheim in the camps, in that part of his "old psychoanalytic system of mastery" was saved, his "belief in the value of rational examination" (1979, p. 13). For Bettelheim, the strength of psychoanalysis in the concentration camp was as an "instrument of understanding": "The explanatory value of psychoanalysis is beyond question, always" (Fisher, 1991, p. 167).

In contrast, however, Bettelheim also has serious reservations about psychoanalysis as a body of theories explaining human behavior and a personality structure that could adequately comprehend inmate behavior in the camps. He makes the point that psychoanalytic theory and the views on personality that derive from it were "inadequate to explain fully what happened to the prisoners" (1960, pp. 18–19). Bettelheim reasons that "outside of its particular frame of reference"—the uniquely controlled context of the analyst's consultation room—psychoanalysis cannot explain human behavior unless it is modified to take into consideration radically changing social environments. Thus, Bettelheim believes that psychoanalysis "distorted" the meaning of the ways in which individuals survived and maintained their humanity amidst the radically changing social environment of the concentration camps (ibid.).

In contrast to the aforementioned example of the Jehovah's Witnesses, who were supposedly "extremely neurotic or plainly delusional," those persons who, according to psychoanalytic theory, should have endured best under the severity of the camp experience were often the first to succumb to the extreme stress. Behavior in the camps could not be explained by an inmate's personal history and his previous personality, by "those aspects of personality" that, at the time, seemed important in then-current "psychoanalytic thinking" (1960, p. 17). Bettelheim points out that this conclusion emanates from his own disappointment with psychoanalysis as a self-sustaining frame of reference in the camps. "Other aspects of psychoanalysis, the introspection, the self-criticism, are not very useful in an extreme situation" (Fisher, 1991, p. 167).

There seems to be a tension in Bettelheim's relationship to his psychoanalytic framework, especially as it relates to the question of its usefulness to him in his struggle to survive and "remain human" in the camps, to make his suffering sufferable. On the one hand, as already quoted, Bettelheim says that psychoanalysis "proved its value and was most helpful" to him, "that on one occasion [it] may have saved" his life. On the other hand, he says that it offered "no suggestion or help toward the solution of how to survive and survive halfway decently in the camps." Perhaps Bettelheim's comments refer to his earlier distinction between psychoanalysis as a method of observation, as he calls it, and a theory of human behavior and personality structure. For example, Bettelheim's psychoanalytic training and mode of understanding may have helped him maneuver effectively against an individual prison guard, but as a general theoretical framework for understanding his overall predicament and how to survive and "remain human" in the camps, it may have been largely unhelpful. Similarly, Bettelheim may have found aspects of his psychoanalytic framework helpful in observing the behavior of his fellow inmates, but the theory, as a master narrative, as the "key to all human problems," as he described it, he found severely lacking.

One important reason Bettelheim felt that classical psychoanalysis was inadequate to explain what had happened to the camp inmates was that it did not give enough theoretical importance to the powerful influence of the social environment in changing the individual. Eventually, he did realize that psychoanalysis as a treatment modality is not the most potent influence in fostering personality change. Rather, an extreme environment, such as the camps, could more invasively and swiftly shape the person, for better or worse. Further, this realization dramatically altered his previous view that only personal changes in man, in his subjectivity, can effect changes in society. He explains:

> My experience in the camps taught me, almost within days, that I had gone much too far in believing that only changes in man could create changes in society. I had to accept that the environment could, as it were, turn personality upside down, and not just in the small child, but in the mature adult too. If I wanted to keep it from happening to me, I had to accept this potentiality of the environment to decide where and where not to adjust, and how far. Psychoanalysis, as I understood it, was of no help in this all important decision ... We should never again be satisfied to see personality change as proceeding independent from the social context.
>
> (1960, pp. 15, 37)[12]

For Bettelheim, psychoanalysis could not adequately address the dramatic influence of the environment on an inmate's personality, and psychoanalytic theories were inadequate to explain what constituted a well-integrated personality within the camps. Nor was what would have been considered a well-integrated personality by psychoanalytic criteria be predictive of who could withstand or adapt to the onslaught of the camp environment and remain human.

Bettelheim believes that the main reason a psychoanalytic frame of reference was not helpful in his struggle to remain human in the camps was because of its emphasis on "what ... [goes] wrong in people's lives" and on "what can be done to correct the mishaps." He further says that this has always been the domain of psychoanalysis and notes that this is entirely appropriate. However, psychoanalysis "does not offer a theory of personality giving positive guidance toward the good life" (ibid., p. 25).

Psychoanalysis emphasizes the pathological and tends to neglect the positive (after all, most people come to analysis and other forms of psychotherapy because they are experiencing mental distress). In the camps, the issue was not how to rid oneself of one's distorted pathology, but rather how to identify and draw from one's strengths in order to behave in a manner that enhanced physical and spiritual survival. If pathology is one's frame of reference for human action, the camp inmate had little direction in helping him determine what to do. Bettelheim says:

> Psychoanalysis is the best method for uncovering and understanding the hidden in man, but by no means an especially good tool for understanding man in his entirety, least of all for understanding what makes for "goodness" or "greatness" in him. The conclusion then seems warranted that while psychoanalysis can explain the psychological upheaval, the pathology that got something started, it is much less successful in explaining why and how, from such starts, positive developments take place.
>
> (1960, p. 27)[13]

What this could have meant for a camp inmate is that if he were lodged in a psychoanalytic perspective, his ability to sustain himself as a person would have been strained, since his frame of reference offered very little helpful direction on how to behave. In the camps, the way a man acted, rather than why he acted a certain way, became of prime importance. It also altered how the inmate saw himself and acted throughout his ordeal. Bettelheim observes:

> Only dimly at first, but with even greater clarity, did I also come to see that soon how a man acts can alter what he is. Those who stood up well in the camps became better men, those who acted badly soon became bad men; and this, or at least so it seemed, independent of their past life history and their former personality make-up, or at least those aspects of personality that seemed significant in psychoanalytic thinking.
>
> (ibid., pp. 16–17)

Further, in the camps, the psychoanalytic view that the unconscious processes underlying an action were equal in importance to the overt behavior was not tenable. As Bettelheim indicates:

> It just would not do under conditions prevailing in the camps to view courageous, life-endangering actions as an outgrowth of the death instinct, aggression turned against the self, testing the indestructibility of the body, megalomaniac denial of danger, histrionic feeding of one's narcissism or whatever category the action would have to be viewed from in psychoanalysis. These and many other interpretations have validity in terms of depth psychology or the psychology of the unconscious, and they certainly did apply. Only viewing courageous behavior by a prisoner within the spectrum of depth analysis seemed ludicrously beside the point. So while

> psychoanalysis lost nothing as far as it went, it went unexpectedly, and in terms of my expectations, shockingly short of the mark.
>
> (1960, p. 17)

Bettelheim thus highlights what he thinks are the deficiencies of Freudian-based psychoanalysis in terms of what it does not or cannot adequately take into account, chiefly the social world and the individual's strengths and positive attributes. In the next section, by contrasting the believers, mainly devout Jews, and the psychoanalytic intellectual, I hope to illuminate what individual and group resources, in particular, what resources rooted in believers used to remain human, especially strongly felt, flexibly and creatively applied, transcendent-pointing moral beliefs and values that are primarily other-directed, other-regarding and other-serving, to make their suffering sufferable, resources that were in most instances not accessible to the psychoanalyst. Indeed, Buber and Marcel's believing humanism resonates with much that is in the next section, including their stated and implied criticisms of psychoanalysis, qua symbolic world.

Some differences between the psychoanalytic intellectual and the believer in response to the Nazi assault[14]

Self-transcendence in the face of suffering and death

In his masterpiece, *At the Mind's Limits*, subtitled "Contemplations by a Survivor of Auschwitz and Its Realities," Jean Améry writes:

> Whoever is, in the broadest sense, a believing person, whether his belief be metaphysical or bound to concrete reality, transcends himself. He is not captive of his individuality; rather he is part of a spiritual continuity that is interrupted nowhere, not even in Auschwitz.
>
> (1980, p. 14)

Primo Levi elaborated on this point when he described "the saving force" of the believer's faith:

> Their universe was vaster than ours, more extended in space and time, above all more comprehendible, they had a key and point of leverage, a millennial tomorrow so that there might be a sense to sacrificing themselves, a place in heaven or on earth where justice and compassion had won, or would win in a perhaps remote but certain future: Moscow, or the celestial or terrestrial Jerusalem. Their hunger was different from ours. It was a Divine punishment or expiation, or votive offering [consecrated in accomplishment of a vow], or the fruit of capitalist putrefaction. Sorrow,

> in them or around them, was decipherable and therefore did not overflow into despair.
>
> (1986, p. 146)

As I will elaborate shortly, for the devout Jew, his self-transcending belief had a very specific form, as it was lodged in a passionately felt, direct relation to the eternal/Absolute Thou, to God (for Buber and Marcel, the symbol of the eternal/Absolute Thou respectively). His God evoked devotion and worship, and perhaps, most importantly, He commanded ethical conduct, responsibility for the other, as prescribed in the sacred texts. Moreover, the devout Jew's suffering was to be understood and responded to in terms of his love and awe of God, who was characterized by inexhaustible mystery and sacredness, radical alterity, compassion, and justice. This point was expressed by the Hassidic Rabbi Levi Yitzhak of Berditchev (cited in Buber, 1963, pp. 81–82), whose words convey this animating feature of the devout Jew's capacity to make his suffering sufferable via his heartfelt, dialogic relation to the eternal/Absolute Thou: "Master of the universe. I do not know what questions to ask. I do not expect You to reveal Your secrets to me. All I ask is that You show me one thing—what this moment means to me and what You demand of me. I do not ask why I suffer. I ask only this: Do I suffer for Your sake?" (Rabinowicz, 1982, p. 94).

For the devout Jew, at the deepest level of the self, God was an intimate presence, an exemplary other, a partner in the never-to-be finished work of creation and *tikkun olam* (repairing the world). Though at times the eternal/Absolute Thou was experienced as enigmatic and ambiguous, the Holy and Blessed One participated in the pain and suffering of His creatures, of Israel and of individual Jews (Buber emphasized this point in his biblical studies, and Marcel also described divine empathy, the fact that the Absolute Thou suffers in human suffering, perhaps the most, as it says in Psalms 91:15: "I will be with him in trouble"). This dialogical partnership in suffering, in which God is concerned and implicated in the fate of His people, is injured by their pain and suffering and is liberated by their redemption, in part, constituted the divine pathos as Heschel called it, from which the devout Jew experienced, understood and, to some extent, transcended his particular suffering (Wolf, 2004, pp. 303–304). As Eigen noted, "God lacks us as we lack God. We seek each other, not only to fill up, but to live the lacks we are" (1998, p. 239).

Does the psychoanalytic intellectual have a similar ability to transcend the extreme situation by virtue of his psychoanalytic thinking and experience? First, it should be noted that Freudian psychoanalysis (and all other schools of thought) claims to be anti-ideological; it sees itself as not having its own distinct *Weltanschauung* (worldview). As Alan Bass has indicated, for Freud, to seek out or create a *Weltanschauung* is anti-psychoanalytic,[15] it goes against the basic thrust of psychoanalysis, in that for Bass, following Freud, it cannot be systematic. Philosophers, theologians, and psychotics, according to Freud, strive towards systematicity, but psychoanalysis should not, in part because it fundamentally concerns itself with "unconscious energic processes" that by definition are contradictory, paradoxical and ambiguous, and therefore must challenge our habitual conscious patterns of organizing data. For Bass, like Freud, to seek out or create a *Weltanschauung* is to succumb to an "illusory wish fulfillment" (Bass, 1998, p. 412). Buber and Marcel's belief that thematization and conceptualization suppress and possess the other, including the otherness of the eternal/ Absolute Thou, and their non-systematic philosophies that emphasize "situated involvement" (i.e., "the human subject is a being-in-a-situation" (Sweetman, 2008, pp. 33, 32)) and their highly personal writing styles, are to some extent in harmony with the anti-systematicity of psychoanalysis.

The implications of such a psychoanalytic viewpoint could be catastrophic for the camp inmate, for it rejects the very notion of the desirability of an "all-embracing," coherent "fabric of meaning[s]" "that comprehends him and all of his experiences" and by its very nature involves "a transcendence of individuality" (Berger, 1967, p. 54). Without an ideologically informed overarching universe of meaning, including strongly felt, flexibly, and creatively applied, transcendent-pointing moral beliefs and values (that are primarily other-directed, other-regarding and other-serving) that are meant to guide a person and are believed by the individual to be absolute, psychoanalytic inmates were seriously limited in their ability to make sense of and endure their nightmarish situation. Améry remarks that, for the believer, "the grip of the horror reality was weaker where from the start reality had been placed in the framework of an unalterable idea. Hunger was not hunger as such, but the necessary consequence of atheism or capitalist decay. A beating or death in the gas chamber was the renewed sufferings of the Lord or a natural political martyrdom" (Améry, 1980, p. 13).

In contrast, psychoanalysts have no transcending concepts that can transport them to a different dimension of the spirit, or that can protect them from the extreme situation by radically altering the meaning of their suffering. To the psychoanalyst, religion and politics, at least the type that we are referring to as they relate to the camp inmates, are an "admirable and redeeming illusion, but an illusion nonetheless" (Hanly, 1993, p. 17).[16] As Charles Hanly points out, "Psychoanalysis finds itself at odds with ideologies because they are governed by visionary ideas and values that are exempted from critical investigation" (ibid.). From the point of view of Buber and Marcel, this is a self-serving overstatement, for there are those that hold the aforementioned "illusions" and "visionary ideas and values," such as religious ones, but do so in a non-ideological manner, as typically understood, that continually demand rigorous analysis and reasoned argumentation on the way to a leap to faith and a way of life linked to sacred realms and forces. Moreover, an ideology can be judged as bad or good, it is "a set of cultural beliefs, values and attitudes that underlie and thereby to some degree justify and legitimate either the status quo or movements to change" (e.g., White racism and gender oppression versus the

Green movement and radical feminism) (Johnson, 1995, p. 137).[17] Finally, both Buber and Marcel would regard Hanly's comments as a questionable form of "psychologism," for he does not deal with the ontic realm of human existence and therefore, reduces cosmic phenomena to purely psychic ones. This is based on Hanly believing that his perspective has epistemic superiority on such matters.

While psychoanalysis has certain ideological aspects, such as its orthodoxies, dogmatic creeds, and worldviews that put forth a version of the human condition, Hanly's view more closely approaches the core of psychoanalysis. For while there is greater tolerance for theoretical pluralism within psychoanalysis, there is distinct sense that the different theories or schools of thought represent radically different perspectives that have their staunch ideologues, in part, because as Greenberg and Mitchell noted, "Psychoanalytic models rest upon … irreconcilable claims concerning the human condition" (and therefore psychopathology and treatment) (1983, p. 404). Thus, psychoanalysts could not generate their own enduring and enabling "illusions" by drawing from the psychoanalytic framework. Not even the immortal unconscious could redeem them, for they were too tied to "reality" as they construed it. This particular way of constructing reality is one that is, according to Améry, decidedly different from that of the believer. In the camps, he implies, this may have made the difference between sustaining oneself as a person and surrendering to Nazi barbarism. Says Améry,

> He [the believer] is both estranged from reality and closer to it than the unbelieving comrade. Further from reality because in his Finalistic attitude he ignores the given contents of material phenomenon and fixes his sight on a nearer or more distant future; but he is also closer to reality because for just this reason he does not allow himself to be overwhelmed by the conditions around him and thus can strongly influence them. For the unbelieving person, reality, under adverse circumstances, is a force to which he submits; under favorable ones it is material for analysis. For the believer, reality is clay that molds, a problem that he solves.
>
> (1980, p. 14)

As Geertz points out in another context (1973), in contrast to the believer the psychoanalytic intellectual "questions the realities of everyday life out of an institutionalized skepticism which dissolves the world's givenness into a swirl of probabilistic hypotheses" (p. 112). However, says Geertz, the religious perspective questions everyday reality in terms of a "wider, non-hypothetical" truth (ibid.). "Detachment" and "analysis," the watchwords of the psychoanalytic intellectual, are replaced by "commitment" and "encounter," if you will, subjectivity (ibid.). It is "the imbuing of a certain specific complex of symbols—of the metaphysic they formulate and the style of life they recommend—with a persuasive authority which, from an analytic point of view, is the essence of religious action" (ibid.). In the camps, this meant that religious inmates had the symbolic capacity to transform their reality, at least to some extent and episodically, into something other than the dehumanizing reality. Through their faith, including the rituals that they participated in, frequently in a communal context, they had the ability to move beyond the realities of everyday life to more transcendent realities that, says Geertz, corrected and completed the painful realities of the camp.

In contrast, psychoanalytic intellectuals were lodged in a more commonsense mode of experiencing the world. This, says Geertz, involves "a simple acceptance of the world, its objects, and its processes as being just what they seem to be," even after they are coated with a psychoanalytic gloss (ibid., p. 111). Such a view, with its "pragmatic motive," that is, "the wish to act upon the world so as to bend it to one's practical purposes, to master it, or when that proves impossible, to adjust to it," does not allow psychoanalytic intellectuals to fuse together "the world as lived and the world as imagined" into one world under "a single set of symbolic forms" (as a religious person does by means of religious ritual), thus transforming their consciousness into another mode of existence (ibid., p. 112). Unlike religious inmates, the psychoanalytic intellectuals did not have the symbolic capacity to place the proximate acts in ultimate meaning-giving, affect-integrating, and action-guiding contexts and, in so doing, decisively alter the Nazi landscape. Devout Jews viewed Nazi brutality against the background of The Fall of Jerusalem and other Jewish calamities which, though it does not adequately explain the brutality, at least places it in a moral, cognitive, and affective context. The devout Jews' beliefs tended to render their experience intelligible and within cognitive understanding, at least to some degree. Indeed, Buber and Marcel would agree with Sartre, that "a lucid view of the darkest situation is already, in itself, an act of optimism," for it suggests that the situation is thinkable (1965, p. 289).

For example, Améry notes that in the camps the believers and non-believers had very little or nothing to do with one another. Religious and political comrades, says Améry, "paid no attention to us, be it in tolerance, in the willingness to help, or in anger. 'You must realize one thing,' a practicing Jew once told me, 'that here your intelligence and your education are worthless. But I have the certainty that our God will avenge us'" (1980, p. 14). The point is that such inmates, mainly through their meaning-giving, affect-integrating, and action-guiding relationship with the eternal/Absolute Thou, "transcended themselves and projected themselves into the future. They were no windowless monads; they stood open, wide open onto a world that was not the world of Auschwitz" (ibid.). Psychoanalytic intellectuals could not derive a similar conceptual capacity from their psychoanalytic thinking and experience.

For the Freudian, and most other psychoanalysts lodged in different versions of psychoanalysis, life has a tragic dimension. Hostility, aggression, and self-destructiveness are inevitable, as is death. In fact, Freud indicates in his formulation of the death instinct that the purpose of life is death. For Freud, death is absolute. Since the individual knows for sure that he or she is going to die one day, the crucial question becomes how one relates to the inevitability of one's death. Does one face up to it or does one seek cover inside a form from this existential fact? How that is to be accomplished is difficult to imagine, but I think that for the skeptical psychoanalytic intellectual, accepting the inevitability of one's death entails recognizing that this world is all we have and that our only reasonable option is to make the best use of the time we do have. This results from viewing the world as a wall rather than a gate, which is the view of the devout Jew.

The approach has its obvious limitations within the context of the concentration camp in that it does not allow psychoanalytic intellectual inmates to "lose themselves" in a meaning-giving, affect-integrating and action-guiding transcending symbolic world. Thus, their terror can be overwhelming. That is, if the terrifying circumstances one is in are unthinkable, if we feel we are lost in a sudden, massive and decisive maze of grotesque happenings, and we cannot dissociate ourselves from it, at least in our mind, and maintain some kind of observational stance, we are not able to transcend the grotesque happenings and become resolute about how to respond, even if the decisions we face are desperate (Sartre, 1965, p. 289).

The situation was quite different for the devout Jew. For example, a religious Jew could draw comfort from the doctrine of *Kiddush Hashem*, the sanctification of the Divine Name, often through martyrdom. This notion and behavioral instruction acted as a guide for Jewish responses to crisis and catastrophe (Huberband, Gurock, & Hirt, 1987). In the camps, the belief that one's death in some way sanctified God served to diminish the inmate's death panic by giving an other-worldly meaning and focus to his or her death. The belief that he would be rewarded in the world-to-come for his sacrifice and that there would be some kind of Divine retribution against his enemies reassured and comforted the devout Jew in the face of his death. Such religious Jews did not feel that they were merely passive victims in the face of Nazi assault. They did not wish to die, but their capacity to interpret their death as a holy act of *Kiddush Hashem*, as the ultimate expression of their responsibility to their beloved God, indicates choice and action. They were able to will meaning into their suffering and death. By anchoring their identity in a cosmic reality, religious inmates were, to some extent, protected from the terror associated with anticipating and facing death. In contrast to psychoanalytic intellectuals, devout Jews and other religious inmates were better fortified against many of the dehumanizing Nazi realities. Buber and Marcel both had other-worldly aspects to their believing humanism, though the latter was always tied to a "situated involvement" (i.e., it is via an embodied context that the person is in contact with reality and enmeshed in it (Sweetman, 2008, pp. 33, 32)) that calls to mind Améry's description of the devout Jew's relationship to reality, he was "both estranged from reality and closer to it than the unbelieving comrade" (Améry, 1980, p. 14).

Sustaining a measure of dignity and self-respect amidst the Nazi assault

As Primo Levi points out, for a number of reasons the intellectual was more likely to feel tortured by a sharp sense of "humiliation" and "destitution" in both the death and concentration camps (1986, p. 132). Bettelheim indicates that without "a consistent philosophy, either moral, political, or social," non-believing inmates had no way to protect their integrity or to derive strength to stand up, even if only within themselves, against Nazism. Such inmates had few or "no resources to fall back on" when they faced the shock of incarceration. Their self-esteem and self-concept were mainly based on the "status and respect" that emanated from their professional position, their place as "head of a family," or similar outside factors (1960, pp. 120–121). Fromm also noted that without the "props" on which their self-esteem and self-identity rested, these non-religious, non-political middle-class inmates collapsed "morally like a deflatable balloon" (1973, p. 86).

The radical loss of self-respect played havoc with prisoners in relation both to their former social status and to their sense of personal worth. It should be noted that social status and a sense of personal worth that is confirmed by the social world are not unimportant to most people, including believers. However, to a deeply religious person, such as the Orthodox Jew, the social world as described above was frequently less significant. As Berkovitz says with regard to devout Eastern European Jews, "Ultimately, what really matters is what kind of Jew one is, that alone is the source of one's self-respect" (1979, p. 55). To the extent that the devout Jew lived a life of heartfelt and exacting responsibility—to God and tradition, the Jewish people, and to his fellow human beings—he viewed himself as worthwhile, dignified and deserving of God's blessings in this world or the world to come. As Buber noted in one of his biblical interpretations, "When man hallows himself in all his limbs and, spirit to spirit, cleaves to the Torah, he becomes himself a complete Torah," that is, he has embraced and enacted without reserve the "responsibility of a single one for the piece of world entrusted to him" (1960, pp. 237, 253).

However, without their social status, psychoanalytic intellectuals were unable to restore a connection with their past, and were thereby unable to rescue it "from oblivion" (Levi, 1986, p. 139). In contrast, the deeply religious or avidly political inmates' reliance on the outside world was less pronounced. They were more rooted inside themselves, in a realm of the spirit that was less susceptible to the influence of their unsure destiny of an outside reality (Berkovitz, 1979, p. 54). They were better able to sustain themselves as persons because, in their view, they did not fashion their identity primarily from the values and standards of the Christian, capitalist, Western society that was consuming them (ibid.). However, the world to which psychoanalytic intellectuals belonged plunged into moral and spiritual bankruptcy, and because their identity was so enmeshed in that world, they were left bereft of self-esteem and self-respect.

The role of group membership

Those inmates who were part of a community or group in the camp were also more likely to survive physically, sustain themselves psychologically and "remain human." The community was a crucial source of emotional sustenance, morale building, and practical help to its members. Such social support also allowed the inmate to sustain his counter-narrative to the dehumanizing Nazi reality. Believers were all able to recreate, usually in a highly modified form, their former communities. In the camps, these inmates stayed together and assisted each other. In the case of devout Jews, they participated in communal religious rituals, such as secretly meeting to pray together, observing the Sabbath and the holidays, lighting Hanukkah candles, keeping kosher, studying Torah, baking matzahs and "conducting" Passover seders (Landes, 1983).[18] Some Hasidim in Bergen-Belsen even made a sukkah (a hut in which observant Jews reside during the seven-day festival of Sukkot, commemorating God's providence over the Israelites in the desert). Straw from a torn and dirty mattress acted as a makeshift roof (Eliach, 1980).

It hardly needs to be restated that Buber and Marcel's believing humanism emphasized the need to realize Thou via community. Buber was a religious socialist, and community was defined as an organic unity, which has evolved from common beliefs, morals, possessions and/or work (Friedman, 2002, p. 52)). "Community is the overcoming of otherness in living unity" (Buber, 1957, p. 102). In Marcel's version of the ontological development in man, community was an extremely important vehicle through which a person struggling with adversity can create meaning: There "can be no hope which does not constitute itself through a *we* and for a *we*" (Marcel, 1973, p. 143). Both Buber and Marcel recognized that this often involved creating new ways of being together.

For the devout Jew (and Christian), the community was considered to have intrinsic spiritual value and meaning. The preservation of "mitzvah-based communities" (Landes, 1983 p. 265), upholding the precepts and commandments that God commanded, was a way of maintaining and expressing the Jew's deeply internalized values, which gave individual Jews the feeling that their pre-Holocaust sense of self was not completely destroyed. This aided the inmates' survival as it tended to help them reconstitute their ontological security, thereby defending themselves against the Nazi attempts at dehumanization and depersonalization. Sounding similar to Buber and Marcel, Auschwitz survivor/analyst Anna Ornstein points out (1985) that sustaining deeply internalized values within the camps indicated that the nuclear self more or less maintained its continuity in space and time regardless of the radical changes in one's body and disruptions in one's physical environment. In addition, she says that in the camps, "the creation of small groups provided an opportunity to experience and express aspects of the nuclear self, specifically related to the pole of ideals, and it provided the all-important empathic selfobject[19] matrix that reinforced a modicum of self-esteem" (p. 115).

For psychoanalytic intellectuals, however, the likelihood of their establishing a strong group membership was diminished not only because of practical considerations, such as a paucity of psychoanalytically oriented members, but also in part because their way of understanding their relationship to the community was influenced by their grim individualistic assumptions. For example, as Greenberg and Mitchell point out:

> The unit of study of [Freudian] psychoanalysis is the individual, viewed as a discrete entity. Man is not, in Aristotle's terms, a "political animal"; he does not require social organization to allow him to realize his true human potential. Society is imposed on an already complete individual for his protection, but at the cost of renunciation of many of his most important goals… It is thus possible and even necessary to speak of a person divorced from his interpersonal context.[20]
>
> (1983, p. 44)

The pre-incarceration mindset of the psychoanalytic inmate was not geared to seeing other people, in the communal context, as a resource. Rather, the Freudian version of the person hypothesizes an atomistic, autonomous, self-regarding individual more or less devoid of an intrinsic social or communal existence. Moreover, Freud portrays human society as fundamentally unstable, trying to control and fend off forces antagonistic, if not subverting, to its very existence. For Freud, the battle between primordial human instinct and civilization is inevitable. Aggressiveness is a deep and abiding feature of human nature. Such a view neither facilitates reaching out to others nor fosters community. Relational theories of psychoanalysis have to some extent revised the above-described cynical and gloomy Freudian version of the human condition, such as maintaining that individuals desire relationships with others for the inherent satisfaction of connectedness, and not merely to diminish drive energy. Thus, from the perspective of the relational/structural model of the mind, "there is no human nature outside society," and "human fulfillment is sought in the establishment and maintenance of relationship with others" (Greenberg & Mitchell, 1983, p. 403). This being said, the tendency of contemporary relational theorists to embrace a postmodern epistemology has created a whole series of problems for how it understands knowledge and truth (Govrin, 2016), let alone resiliency during life in extremity, such as the Nazi concentration camps. For as I have suggested, from the perspective of the believing inmate, the eternal/Absolute Thou, for example, was an objective reality and truth, though not necessarily one that was always accessible to reason (a mystery), but still a soul-saving basis for a leap to faith.

Finally, while psychoanalysis provides an intellectual orientation and a camaraderie with other analysts, it does not generate the same kind of communal loyalty and devotion that religion or a fundamentalist political ideology does. A psychoanalytic worldview does not confer upon the individual a spiritual membership in a community that, theoretically at least, has existed for thousands of years and is inspired by thought of contact with the eternal/Absolute Thou. Such membership, for the devout Jew and all such religious believers, is mainly brought about through living a life of selflessness, compassion and justice, that is, a life of responsibility for and to the other, a holy life.

Summary: why did religious believers fare better than the psychoanalytic intellectuals in sustaining themselves as persons in the camps?

Unlike the psychoanalytic intellectuals, the believers, in particular the devout Jews, had a symbolically mediated relation between themselves and the extreme situation that gave a specific meaning to their environment in the camps, one that was "symbolic of a transcendent" truth (Geertz, 1973, p. 98) and that gave them a more helpful general orientation through which to view the horror they were experiencing. This self-sustaining, transcendent-pointing truth was rooted in a deep-seated sense of responsibility for the other (i.e., fellow inmates and the eternal/Absolute Thou), a truth that to some extent made the devout Jew steadfast and immovable, maybe even serene, relatively speaking. As Geertz points out in a different context, for the devout Jew the extreme situation of the camps had a greater degree of "interpretability" (ibid., p. 100).

In contrast, psychoanalytic intellectuals felt utterly overwhelmed by a situation that was "at the limits of their analytic capacities, at the limits of their powers of endurance and at the limits of their moral insight" (ibid.). Geertz further says, if situations of "bafflement, suffering, and a sense of intractable ethical paradox" become intense enough or are endured long enough, they radically challenge people's ability to orient themselves effectively within them. Such situations threaten "to unhinge" one's mind (ibid.).

Thus, the psychoanalytic intellectual did not have the symbolic resources to make the extreme situation sufferable. However, devout Jews had religious symbols which provided "a cosmic guarantee not only for their ability to comprehend the world, but also, comprehending it, to give a precision to their feeling, a definition to their emotions" (ibid., p. 104) that enabled them to better endure the extreme situation. Intense, relentless brute pain could be endured "by placing it in a meaningful context, providing a mode of action through which it can be expressed, being expressed understood, and being understood, endured" (ibid., p. 105). Psychoanalytic intellectuals did not have such symbolic resources by virtue of their psychoanalytic thinking and experience.

It should be emphasized that the Nazi concentration camp was not only a situation to be suffered; as in intense neurotic conflict, it also threatened the inmates' ability to make moral judgments. The camps challenged the inmates' "resources to provide a workable set of ethical criteria, normative guides to govern" their actions in the face of radical evil (ibid., p. 106). For Buber and Marcel, qua believers, there was an absurdity to suffering—such that it could never be adequately explained or justified ("eclipse of God," and the realm of mystery, "despair ... that God has withdrawn himself from me," as described by Buber and Marcel, respectively). Nevertheless, it could be viewed as a "test" (Hordes, 1971, p. 34) or "trial" (Marcel, 1984, p. 370), a sacrament that is sent to us and that we are obligated to respond to with trust and hope, and guided by the best of our religiously animated moral and ethical ideals.

Unlike devout Jews, who could draw on what they viewed as a God-given sacred moral code to give direction to their actions, psychoanalytic intellectuals were faced "with [an] intractable ethical paradox, the disquieting sense that one's moral insight is inadequate to one's moral experience" (Geertz, 1973, p. 98). Such an ethical paradox is of course characteristic, to some degree, of how all analysands experience their serious problems in living, especially in the moral realms of love and other interhuman contexts. Psychoanalytic intellectuals were faced with the shattering sense that their intense pain lacked not only any manageable "emotional form," but that their life in the camps lacked any "moral coherence" (ibid., p. 108). Consequently, they were prone to experience a high degree of "analytic, emotional, and moral impotence" in the face of evil and suffering (ibid.).

Though devout Jews had their doubts, uncertainties and questions, and made protests to their God for their suffering and the evil they were facing, they did have the faith that, while elusive, there was a moral, intellectual, and emotional explanation for their encounter with evil. The certainty that there was a principle or explanation that could and maybe would, in this world or the next, eventually make their suffering intelligible and meaningful meant that they could sustain the moral structures of their world. The believing inmates thus maintained a sense of agency, efficacy, and control over their situation. As Erving Goffman writes, "Strong religious and political convictions have served to insulate the true believer against the assaults of a total institution" (1961, p. 66).

Making suffering sufferable: the challenge to psychoanalysis conceived as a spiritual discipline

Helping people to endure and possibly surmount their suffering is the heart of all versions of clinical psychoanalysis. By comparing the psychoanalytic intellectual and the believers, mainly devout Jews, in the extreme situation of the Nazi concentration camp, I have tried to demonstrate some of the limitations of psychoanalysis, as a symbolic world, in helping individuals to sustain themselves as persons, and to maintain their autonomy, integration, and humanity. These are the same goals all analysands have when they suffer, whether they are facing suffering caused by the external world, such as "when rocks fall from the sky," or suffering caused by others, or when faced by suffering in their internal world, such as neurotic misery. The testimonials of camp inmates and survivors of the concentration camps, of believers and non-believers, strongly suggest that something crucial is missing (or at least is underdeveloped) in the "mainstream" psychoanalytic "way of looking at life." Its "particular manner of construing the world," its "vision of reality" (and meaning and value), and the technology of self that it advocates, as it engages the problem of suffering, could benefit from spiritual expansion and deepening. My brief comments are meant to be suggestive, not definitive, of a future direction for our "under siege" discipline.

I should say from the onset that I am not going to concern myself with the abstract, theoretical theological/philosophical issues of divine justice and the problem of evil, including the various theodicies (and "antitheodicy" (Braiterman, 1998) that have been put forth. For example, from a Christian point of view, suffering conceived as part of a providential plan has been accounted for as punishment, refinement, judgment, opportunity, and suffering as a narrative that is not our own (Douthat, 2020, p. 9). Marcel believed that "Theodicy is atheism" since it views God as if He were an object, as someone "about whom" one can talk as if he were not present (speaking about God in this way is not speaking to God) (Gallagher, 1962, p. 126). Rather I want to focus on what, if anything, we psychoanalysts can learn from Buber and Marcel as they gloss the existential problem of meaning in terms of the problem of suffering in real-life circumstances. For, as I have repeatedly mentioned, Buber and Marcel were less concerned with philosophical and theological discourse than with understanding human behavior and experience within the context of situated participation. They were philosophers who personified what Hadot called "philosophy as a way of life," who embraced an "existential attitude" that consisted of choosing "how to live human reality" according to certain values that reflected practical wisdom, and a particular form of goodness (Hadot, 1995, pp. 30, 35).

For Buber and Marcel, the problem of personal suffering (roughly the problem of evil in theology/philosophy) is best understood in terms of their broadly conceived biblical perspective of existence as the dialogue between man and God, for it is within this context that transcendence (at least to some extent) is possible: "No salvation," says Buber, "is in sight for us, however, if we are not able again 'to stand before the face of God' in all reality as a We—as it is written in that faithful speech that once from Israel ... started on its way" (1998, p. 108). Marcel too notes that the word *transcendent* does "*not* mean 'transcending experience,' but on the contrary there must exist a possibility of having an experience of the transcendent as such," or else the word lacks intelligibility (2001a, p. 46). For Marcel, this summoning urge for transcendence reflects the pure desire that is open and receptive and infused with intelligibility (Anderson, 2006, p. 31).

Having said this, Buber and Marcel were well aware that there is no absolute answer to the problem of suffering (let alone in its diverse manifestations); it is an intractable if not eternal mystery of God (it is a mystery, not a problem, best approached through secondary rather than primary reflection in Marcel's language). Rather, what matters is how one responds to suffering, whether it propels one to live in a more godly or holy manner, especially in terms of the communal we. For example, Buber wrote about the Book of Job, and he seems to have credibly concluded that for the believer, "it is surrender, acceptance of the nearness of God, submission to God's demand of love at the expense of justice, and the right to question divine justice" that is the most existentially plausible response to the mystery of suffering (Palmer, 2006, p. 198): the response that helps the believer to sustain the meaning-giving, affect-integrating, and action-guiding character of his symbolic world in the face of the "eclipse of God" (his hiddenness, if not absence). In other words, the believer has to patiently wait for God, calling to mind Samuel Beckett's play *Waiting for Godot*, except Godot never arrives (Kaufman, 1985, p. 75). For Buber believed to the end of his life "in a transcendent being with whom he can communicate," who was experienced as "a higher power" but who was impossible to fully grasp (1998, p. 138).

One of Buber's main insights about suffering ought to be emphasized. Like Job (and the ancient Israelites), when God never gives him an adequate response to his accusations of undeserved suffering (and in a sense all suffering feels undeserved from the perspective of the sufferer), the most summoning response is to create the will and ability to maintain the dialogue between man and God in the here-and-now. That is, "Meaning is to be experienced in living action and suffering itself, in the unreduced immediacy of the moment .... He [the suffering person] is ready to confirm with his life the meaning which he has attained" (1988, p. 35). Put differently, the commanding Voice that emanates from suffering is saying not to just passively accept one's situation (one's earthly circumstances), but to continue questing after a found/created meaning to one's suffering, as the aforementioned quote from Rabbi Levi Yitzhak of Berditchev powerfully attests: bearing suffering for God's sake, a kind of "suffering love" (Buber, 1949, p. 232). Such a transcendent quest is not only likely to reduce one's suffering as it provides a context of intelligibility, but from Buber's point of view, it continues the dialogue, which is what really matters (i.e., with God, others and oneself), and thereby potentially opens up new life-affirming possibilities, maybe even for fashioning a more evolved self/other relation (i.e., one that points to greater beauty, truth and goodness). Redemption, whether historically (e.g., the Jewish people or humanity) or personally, whether a Heavenly Voice from the whirlwind like Job, or its silent/still aftermath, or the voice of conscience, always involves one's personal engagement and life experience, with the fullness of one's whole being, who can say to God (and others), Thou (Moore, 1996, p. 62). Thou points toward genuine relationship characterized by mutuality, uniqueness, and wholeness. Indeed, as Buber noted, it was Jesus (a prophet of Israel before he was Christianized/deified), "my great brother," who personified the "immediacy with God, the great devotion" (1960, pp. 251, 247), and who preached and enacted the "perfected living together of men, the true community in which God shall have direct rule" (Friedman, 2002, p. 50). In a word, for Buber, personal suffering was best metabolized in terms of the longstanding Jewish moral vision, its possibilities and limits, rooted and affirmed in the covenant (i.e., the ongoing dialogue) with the eternal Thou.[21]

And yet, when one suffers, one feels a degree of despair that is very difficult, if not impossible, to bear, let alone surmount. Despair, says Marcel, is "the shock felt by the mind when it meets with 'There is no more'" (1965a, p. 102). Or put differently, "Despair is in a certain sense the consciousness of time as closed or, more exactly still, of time as a prison" (1965b, p. 53). Despair, like depression, tends to be highly narcissistic (utterly self-absorbing and egocentric). As Marcel notes, "the essence of the act of despair" is "always capitulation before a certain *fatum* [literally "what has been spoken," fate] laid down by our judgment" (1965b, p. 37). In the words of Marcel qua believer, despair is "a declaration that God has withdrawn himself from me" (ibid, p. 47). Similar to Buber, Marcel's main concern is how one responds to despair, and he focuses on the phenomenology of hope, which is always entwined with faith and love (ibid., 46). While I previously discussed the phenomenology of hope in Chapter 2 (The spirit of love), I will only make a few additional comments as it relates to the existential experience of suffering. It should be mentioned from the onset that the French word *esperance* that Marcel uses for hope also means trust, and one Marcel scholar believes it is the more apt translation (Anderson, 2006, p. 170), calling to mind Buber's aforementioned emphasis on the traditional Jewish notion of *emunah* (the unconditional deep trust in God) in the face of suffering and the "eclipse of God."

For Marcel, hope is not what most psychoanalysts tend to think of it as, namely, "excessive hope as being pathological" (Akhtar, 2009, p. 133), such as an overindulged oral phase that leads to hyper-optimism. For Marcel, hope does not occur in the domain of "I myself" as does optimism, it is a form of communion (1965b, p. 38); hope is a defensive response against anxiety and sadness connected to castration fantasies; and hope is a manifestation of character armor that maintains reality testing. More positively, there is conscious hope that seeks the fulfillment of wishes and unconscious hope that is linked to the quest for object experiences that propel development forward (Akhtar, 2009, p. 133). While all of these formulations about hope have their benefit in certain clinical situations, they are not what Marcel was pointing towards. That is, hope is not merely subjective/psychological experience, but rather it reflects a person's spiritual life that can at best be faintly apprehended, as with any abiding mystery of being, like fidelity, faith, and love.

For Marcel, hope is a courageous, though humble affirmation, for it upsurges when one is in captivity, whether it is the captivity associated with, for example, a life-threatening illness, the inevitability of death, intractable depression and/or anxiety or imprisonment in a concentration camp. Hope is not merely wishing for a way out of the aforementioned, but goes a step further; to hope, "to trust is to carry within me the personal assurance that however black things may seem, my present intolerable situation cannot be final; there has to be some way out" (2001b, p. 160). For example, to some extent, the person, like the camp inmate who affirms that justice will ultimately prevail in the world, be he a believer (e.g., a Christian) or a non-believer (e.g., a Marxist), "proclaims that this world *shall come* into existence," and personifies the "prophetic nature of hope" (ibid., p. 159). In other words, while such hoping may seem like auto-suggestion or a self-fulfilling prophecy (and indeed, it sometimes has positive effects in terms of outcome, such as in illness), Marcel is suggesting something additional about the experience of hoping itself, namely, that unlike the closedness of auto-suggestion and a self-fulfilling prophecy (which is a "desire" often rooted in fear that aims for a particular outcome, like getting well or liberation), it is open to something "more," "higher" and "better" that is hard to pin down. As Marcel says, paradoxically, "the less life is experienced as a captivity the less the soul will be able to see the shining of that veiled, mysterious light, which we feel sure, without any analysis, illumines the very centre of hope's dwelling place" (ibid., p. 32).

Anderson (2006) puts forth the view that Marcelian hoping/trusting is not a dodging of reality as analysts may think, especially when they pathologize hoping, but rather that Marcel is suggesting "that trust is grounded in an experience of being (intrinsic eternal value) in human beings, and humans have intrinsic eternal value because they are gifts from God" (ibid., p. 172). Thus, hope/trust is not a dodging of reality, but rather "a penetration into its very depths where it discovers the presence of being" (ibid., p. 173). By claiming that hope is lodged in the presence of being, Marcel means the following, perhaps one of his clearest definitions of hope: Hope "consists in asserting that there is at the heart of being, beyond all data, beyond all inventories and all calculations, a mysterious principle [the absolute Thou] which is in connivance with me, which cannot but will that which I will, if what I will deserves to be willed and is, in fact, willed by the whole of my being" (Marcel, 1995, p. 28). Hope is always embedded in patience and humility, just as it is embedded in trust and love, that is, hope is communion ("I hope in thee for us" (Marcel, 1965b, p. 60)), it needs others, and tends to project itself far and wide, to everyone (Gallagher, 1962, pp. 74, 75).

As Anderson notes, in this view, despair is a form of betrayal of God and the moral vision of Christianity rooted in the imitation of Jesus, especially his emphasis on communal love. For it asserts that the loving God has abandoned me and I have lost trust that in this world, or the next one, I will be in eternal union with the Absolute Thou (e.g., via revelation, immortality). Similar to fidelity and love, there are people who trust, including amidst profound suffering, even death, that in the final analysis life is a meaningful gift that is not ended in death from an absolute Thou (Anderson, 2006, p. 174). Thus, the person, who in the face of despair hopes for "deliverance," appeals to the transcendent for deliverance since he apprehends that it is the Almighty who put this urge for being, for transcendence, inside him as part of our spiritual cast of mind: "Where despair denies that anything in reality is worthy of credit, hope affirms that reality will ultimately prove worthy of an infinite credit, the complete engagement and disposal of myself" (Treanor, 2006, p. 86). In other words, hope allows one to free oneself from the horror of the past and leans into a better future. As Marcel notes, to believe in this perspective is a choice; however, the beauty, truth, and goodness in the world and the richness of the universe that one apprehends through sacred attunement point towards the summoning nature of the unconditional experience of hoping in the grace of a loving God (ibid.). As Marcel literally ends his magisterial essay *A Metaphysic of Hope*, he provides a summarizing definition that integrates most of what I have attempted to convey about his formulation:

> We might say that hope is essentially the availability of a soul which has entered intimately enough into the experience of communion to accomplish in the teeth of will and knowledge the transcendent act—the act establishing the vital regeneration of which this experience affords both the pledge and the first fruits.
>
> (1965, p. 67)

Final comment

I realize that there is a lot of "god talk" in Buber and Marcel's formulations regarding life-affirming responding to suffering. And while for the believer, who at his best is a magician of allegories and symbolism (Bouretz, 2007, p. 182),[22] much of what has been referred to probably resonates with his outlook and behavior, the non-believer, which probably includes most analysands and analysts, may feel estranged from some of this material. Therefore, I want to end this chapter by emphasizing one of the take-home points regarding recasting psychoanalysis as a spiritual discipline as it engages the problem of helping the analysand, whether a believer or a non-believer, respond in a life-affirming manner to his personal suffering.

Extrapolating from the aforementioned discussion of the outlook and behavior of the believing and non-believing inmates in the Nazi concentration camps to ordinary life, it is reasonable to suggest that to the extent that the analysand can fashion strongly felt, flexibly and creatively applied, transcendent-pointing moral beliefs and values that are primarily other-directed, other-regarding, and other-serving, he is most likely to be willing and able to maintain his autonomy, integration and humanity, and thus endure and maybe even surmount his ordeal of suffering. These transcendent-pointing moral beliefs and values can be rooted in God (as with Buber and Marcel) or its secular equivalent, but what is important is that they be enacted in concrete behavior that regards responsibility for and to the other as primary, or at least as important as oneself. Moreover, such an existential comportment not only involves being willing and able to be receptive, responsive, and responsible to life and the world, but it simultaneously involves metabolizing the shocks of existence that must be borne to actualize the best one can be.

What do these ordinary people who behave in extraordinary ways look like in real life? Who are these people we can try to emulate, including their beliefs, values, and behavior, which we analysts, lodged in a sensibility that conceives of psychoanalysis as a spiritual discipline, may want to not only embrace, but transmit to our analysands? For psychoanalysis is a moral psychology, that is, a value-laden dialogue, and we analysts need to have the courage to acknowledge our commitments to such a moral vision. Drawing from the Holocaust literature, Bettelheim mentions these "righteous ones," who represent the "hope for humanity" (1990, pp. 19, 297) that Buber and Marcel would most assuredly so characterize: Father Kolbe, a Polish priest, who, while in Auschwitz, volunteered to die in place of a Polish political prisoner, allowing him to survive and return to his wife and children (the priest had no such family). He was starved to death by the Nazis:[23] Janusz Korczak, who steadfastly refused many offers to be saved from extermination in the death camps in order to stay with the orphaned children under his care, until they were all murdered by the Nazis; and Miep Giese, who at great personal risk provided Anne Frank and her family, and the others who hid out with them, with the essential food and supplies that kept them alive, and with the human companionship they required to endure their terrible isolation.

What shines through from the aforementioned stories of the "righteous ones" is that they epitomized what many would view as a praiseworthy form of life, one characterized by radical autonomy, integration, and humanity. Such an art of living (including dying) reflected their commitment to a transcendent-pointing morality as they conceived it, experienced as akin to a categorical imperative—being other-directed, other-regarding, and other-serving—as their motivating life principle. That is, as Bauman notes, such behavior was freely directed at the other's welfare, "it is uncalculated, natural, spontaneous and mostly unreflected-upon manifestation of humanity" (2008, p. 105). While Father Kolbe may have felt an inner command or Voice rooted in his faith in God, and Korczak and Giese had their own irrepressible voice of conscience and responsibility, the fact is that for these extraordinary people their moral actions were enacted for the other's best interests, with no stake in self-aggrandizement or psychological profit.[24] Their courageous and decent actions did not serve any purpose, had no ulterior motive, except to do good (ibid.). At the same time, their lives reflected an aesthetic outlook, a style of life (even in captivity), in which creativity and imagination (as Marcel has written about it), practical wisdom and striving towards personal excellence, especially moral excellence, were what mattered most (Kekes, 2002). Their epitaph might be, "Forgive me, all of you whom I could not help" (Bauman, 2008, p. 98).

Notes

1 This being said, internal and external are arbitrary though pedagogically useful categories (i.e., they are the result of primary reflection, as Marcel says) if one believes, as

I do, that following Heidegger, man is being-in-the-world. By being-in-the-world, I mean to emphasize that the human being is best conceptualized as an individual unity of thought, feeling/kinesthetic and action, engaged in the lived actuality of his everyday life (i.e., being; his behavior is context-dependent and setting-specific (Marcus, 2020).

2 I have also communicated on this and related subjects with other survivors who became analysts: Paul and Anna Ornstein, Dori Laub, Louis J. Michaels, Marion M. Oliner, Jack Terry and Fred Wolkenfeld. For a critical review of many of the other well-known psychologically based narratives of survival in the camps, see Marcus (1999).

3 I am aware that what it meant by "remain human" or surviving as "human beings" as I later refer to it, in the concentration camps, is a radically philosophical question whose answer depends on one's form of life, including one's theoretical perspective, valuative attachments and historical situatedness, that is, one's *episteme*, or socio-intellectual reality. It should be categorically stated that this chapter in no way attempts to judge the "truth claims" of psychoanalysis, religion or politics. Rather, my intention is to try to understand how "believers" and the mainly Freudian psychoanalytic framework were used by individuals and groups to help or hinder their psychological and spiritual survival, their ability to "remain human" in the extreme situation (i.e., to maintain their autonomy, integration and humanity).

4 Relational analysts have emphasized that "ordinary reality" can no longer be regarded as objective ("what is really there"), but is rather a construction that can be helpful or unhelpful depending on the circumstances (Mitchell, 2002, p. 107). However, they too, mainly opine on reality as it is manifest, co-produced in the clinical context and not in the aforementioned social psychological sense, in which one's behavior in the "real world" is significantly influenced, if not determined by impersonal social forces.

5 The Jehovah's Witnesses who were incarcerated in Buchenwald were particularly ideologically steadfast, especially in light of the fact that, according to Eugen Kogon, "On September 6, 1938, the SS offered them the chance to abjure their principles in writing, especially their refusal to swear oaths and render military service, and thus to purchase their liberty. Only a very few failed to withstand this temptation" (1958, p. 42).

6 While I am suggesting that "reality" has a huge influence on behavior, as I have noted in the text, I am aware that it is always mediated through a person's unique outlook and way of metabolizing experience. This includes drawing from conscious and unconscious resources. Hence, some people are more skillful at "managing" the more extreme aspects of toxic reality than others, what Erikson called "contextual mastery" (Hoare, 2002, p. 74).

7 Halpern (2002, p. 10) usefully criticizes Levinas for making a sharp distinction between physical pain and moral and psychological pain, the latter she says, Levinas mistakenly believed one can detach oneself from compared to physical pain which is inescapable in its suffering. I tend to agree with Halpern, that anyone who has treated a severely depressed or psychotic analysand understands that mental anguish can be as terrifying and inescapable as physical pain.

8 There are important differences between concentration camps (where Bettelheim was), work or labor camps, a prisoner of war camp (where Levinas was) and death camps (where Améry, Levi, and Wiesel were). It is beyond the scope of this chapter to detail all of this.

9 Ernst Federn, a psychoanalyst/survivor who had strong Marxist commitments when he was incarcerated in Buchenwald for many years, as far as I know never stressed in any of his writings on the subject that his Marxist background helped him to remain human or cope more effectively (in a psychological sense) with Nazi barbarism in the day-to-day grind of everyday life. Federn and Bettelheim were incarcerated together in Buchenwald in 1939 (Federn, 1980).

10 It is important to appreciate the context of Wiesel's remarks for, as far as I can tell, they have a somewhat rhetorical quality. Wiesel made his comments as part of his improvised reply to a controversial lecture given by Richard Rubenstein to the question of "What can be told, what can be written, where must silence be kept, what can be witnessed only by living?" (the quote is cited by the editors, p. 269).

11 Bettelheim has been accused by Richard Pollack (1996), his "vengeful biographer," as a *New York Times* book reviewer called him, of having been a brilliant charlatan. Pollack claims, for example, that Bettelheim was a lumber dealer who grandly reinvented himself by means of a forged set of academic credentials after emigrating to the United States in 1939. Whatever the facts are, in my view Bettelheim's many thoughtful, provocative, and at times brilliant books and essays indicate that he was an impressive and well-rounded intellectual. For a more balanced and sympathetic view of Bettelheim, see Nina Sutton (1996) and Theron Raines's (2002) biographies.

12 Bettelheim, like Erich Fromm and other early psychoanalytic writers, was in a certain sense ahead of his time. Contemporary psychoanalysis, in its relational and intersubjective versions, is more concerned with social context in the analyst/analysand interaction than in earlier theorizing. However, in my view, psychoanalysis has yet to develop a sophisticated social psychology that adequately integrates the external world, particularly impersonal situational forces, into its theorizing. This especially includes the seminal findings from experimental social psychology (Marcus, 2020).

13 Freud's answer to his question, "Why should analyzed men and women in fact be better than others?" is supportive of Bettelheim's observations, specifically about "goodness." According to Freud, "Analysis makes for integration but does not of itself make for goodness" (Hale, 1971, p. 188).

14 While I stress the "positive" aspects of the believer's mode of being and the limitations of the intellectual perspective in this chapter, I am aware that the matter is extremely complex. For example, in certain instances maintaining a strong religious conviction could diminish an inmate's chances of personal survival as well as threaten the lives of fellow inmates. Langer (1987, pp. 70–71) tells of a group of Hasidim who declined to work in a brush factory on Yom Kippur, deciding rather to pray. Other inmates "pleaded with them, fearing for their own safety if the Germans discovered that the output was less than expected." The Hasidim, however, refused. The SS became aware of the situation and shot the Hasidim, "and began beating and randomly executing some of the other inmates." It should also be pointed out that in some instances engaging in certain intellectual activity, such as remembering or discussing a poem, helped an inmate remain human by providing him with a "tiny island of freedom" and "a moment of spiritual transcendence" (Todorov, 1996, p. 93). Moreover, some inmates were able to sustain aspects of their humanity and continue to struggle to survive by virtue of moral convictions that were not lodged in religious or political transcending ideologies, such as devotion to a wife or child they hoped to see again, or "bearing witness" for the sake of future generations.

15 This is of course a debatable claim, as many psychologists view psychoanalysis as lodged in a so-called "scientific" worldview, one with strong positivistic and materialistic elements. The current wave of interest in neuroscience and psychoanalysis, "neuropsychoanalysis" as Mark Solms calls it, also suggests that psychoanalysis sees itself, or strives to be, a scientific account of human experience. Likewise, it is hard to read various relational psychoanalytic authors and not feel that a particular worldview, a rather fixed one, is in play. That is, psychoanalysis, in whatever version one is focusing on, can be regarded as a symbolic universe, which is reasonably and roughly a worldview, "a set of beliefs and assumptions that describe reality" (Koltko-Rivera, 2004, p. 3) that is created to legitimize the created institutional structure (Berger & Luckman, 1966). As Koltko-Rivera defines worldview, it is hard not to agree with my assertion that psychoanalysis has a worldview:

> a way of describing the universe and life within it, both in terms of what is and what ought to be. A given worldview is a set of beliefs that includes limiting statements and assumptions regarding what exists and what does not (either in actuality, or in principle), what objects or experiences are good or bad, and what objectives, behaviors, and relationships are desirable or undesirable. A worldview defines what can be known or done in the world, and how it can be known or done. In addition to defining what goals can be sought in life, a worldview defines what goals should be pursued. Worldviews include assumptions that may be unproven, and even improvable, but these assumptions are super ordinate, in that they provide the epistemic and ontological foundations for other beliefs within a belief system.
>
> (2004, p. 4)

The aforementioned is in sync with Ogden's (2016) claim, that "the current era of psychoanalysis might be thought of as the era of thinking about thinking," that is, "*the* way a person thinks, as opposed to *what* he thinks" (p. 17). For Buber and Marcel, such inordinate self-reflexion tends to be reductionistic, that is, it reduces God, others and the world into objects of one's own desires (Kramer & Gawlick, 2003, p. 165).

16 While Freud considered religious faith "a delusional remolding of reality" in *Civilization and Its Discontents*, psychoanalysis has, to some extent, progressed in its respect for the psychologically helpful function of religious faith for the individual and group (see my Chapter 4). Moreover, the positive role of personal illusion in cultural experience, such as in religious phenomena, aesthetic creation, play and the like, has been widely accepted by most analysts, thanks to Winnicott and others.

17 As Eigen notes, "The analyst works with the felt impact of the patient, and affective-ideological transformations of this impact" (1988, p. 66).

18 As Todorov points out, group membership, while almost always a helpful resource, was a morally ambiguous issue. For example, it could mean that a group member automatically helps all of the members of his group and does not concern himself with the needs of those who do not belong. The Communists, for example, fashioned insular groups "from which all those who did not share their convictions were excluded." Moreover, unlike religious believers, an enemy of the Communists, say a kapo or Nazi informer, would in some instances be killed by a group member. The Jehovah's Witnesses were the most tightly knit, their love for Jehovah being so passionate that they refused all accommodation and compromise with the Nazis.

However, according to Todorov, none of their fellow prisoners benefited from that love. He quotes Ravensbruck survivor Margarete Buber-Neumann, "If they took any risks at all, it was only in the service of Jehovah—and never of their fellow prisoners" (1996, 57–58, 83).

19 A selfobject refers to the person's experience of someone else as part of the self or as essential to satisfy a need of the self, such as for affirmation and idealization.

20 While relational versions of psychoanalysis have tried to correct this Freudian-based deficit, they nonetheless focus mostly on the interpersonal and intersubjective context in which the analyst and analysand are lodged, at a particular moment during the to and fro of treatment. They do not adequately consider the role of external reality, including external interpersonal reality outside the office setting, such as obedience to authority and group pressure, in human behavior. As in Freudian and other versions of psychoanalysis, relational psychoanalysis lacks a comprehensive and dynamic psychology of "everyday" situational behavior, how specific situational forces animate, if not determine, behavior regarding important personal and ethical matters (Marcus, 2020).

21 Buber has been questionably accused by Emil Fackenheim in his book *To Mend the World* as having "had a lifelong difficulty with the recognition of evil," perhaps rooted in his existential orientation of "inclusion," that is, "making present," imaging the emotional and intellectual experience of the other without losing oneself in the process (Lawritson, 1996, p. 297). Buber also seemed to have difficulty fathoming the existence of altruistic behavior in an extreme situation: "A man in hell cannot think, cannot imagine helping another. How could he?" (Anderson & Cissna, 1997, p. 59).

22 According to Gallagher, Marcel believed that "the Freudians only scratched the surface of symbol life," in that the "great symbols" point to what is eternal (Gallagher, 1962, 127). Jung and Fromm for example, opined on this theme in considerable detail.

23 Marcel believed that the faithful Christian is commanded to take the risk of the moral life. He writes, "Whence something like a breach which seems indeed to open in the middle of what one could call the field of human experience. Everything takes place in reality as on an earth shaken by a seismic shock. Since the coming of Christ we live in a split world" (Hernandez, 2011, p. 140).

24 Of course, from a psychoanalytic point of view, their extraordinary moral behavior was congruent with their "core" transcendent-pointing beliefs and values (roughly their ego-ideal) and thus enhanced their integrity and self-respect, and therefore avoided the toxic feeling that they did not live up to their moral ideals, a conclusion that probably would have made living with themselves intolerable. These are secondary considerations compared to their main motivation, which was to be for the other before themselves.

References

Akhtar, S. (2009). *Comprehensive dictionary of psychoanalysis*. London: Karnac.

Alexander, F. (1961). Mass-man in death camp and society. *New York Times Book Review*, October 8, p. 42.

Améry, J. (1980). (Trans. A. Rosenfeld & S. P. Rosenfeld). *At the mind's limits: Contemplations by a survivor on Auschwitz and its realities*. Bloomington: Indiana University Press.

Anderson, R., & Cissna, K. N. (1997). *The Martin Buber–Carl Rogers dialogue. A new transcript with commentary.* Albany: State University of New York Press.
Anderson, T. C. (2006). *A commentary on Gabriel Marcel's* The mystery of being. Milwaukee, WI: Marquette University Press.
Appelfeld, A. (1994). (Trans. J. M. Green). *Beyond despair: Three lectures and a conversation with Philip Roth.* New York: International Publishing.
Bauman, Z. (2008). *The art of life.* Cambridge: Polity.
Bass, A. (1998). Sigmund Freud: The question of a Weltanschauung and a defense. In P. Marcus & A. Rosenberg (Eds.), *Psychoanalytic versions of the human condition: Philosophies of life and their impact on practice* (pp. 412–446). New York: New York University Press.
Berger, P. (1967). *The sacred canopy.* Garden City, NY: Doubleday.
Berger, P., & Berger, B. (1972). *Sociology: A biographical approach.* New York: Basic Books.
Berger, P., & Luckman, T. (1966). *The social construction of reality: A treatise in the sociology of knowledge.* New York: Anchor.
Berkovitz, E. (1979). *With God in hell.* New York: Sanhedrin Press.
Bettelheim, B. (1960). *The informed heart.* Glencoe, IL: Free Press.
Bettelheim, B. (1979). *Surviving and other essays.* New York: Knopf.
Bettelheim, B. (1990). *Freud's Vienna and other essays.* New York: Knopf.
Bion. W. R. (1961). *Experiences in groups.* London: Tavistock.
Bouretz, P. (2007). Messianism and modern Jewish philosophy. In M. L. Morgan & P. E. Gordon (Eds.), *Modern Jewish philosophy* (pp. 179–191). Cambridge: Cambridge University Press.
Braiterman, Z. (1998). *(God) after Auschwitz: Tradition and change in post-Holocaust Jewish thought.* Princeton, NJ: Princeton University Press.
Breuer, J., & Freud, S. (1955). Studies on hysteria. In J. Strachey (Ed. & Trans.), *The standard edition of the complete psychological works of Sigmund Freud* (Vol. II, pp. 1–312). London: Hogarth Press. (Original work published 1893).
Buber, M. (1949). *The prophetic faith.* New York: Harper & Row.
Buber, M. (1957). (Trans. M. Friedman). *Pointing the Way. Collected Essays.* Atlantic Highlands, NJ: Humanities Press International.
Buber, M. (1960). (Trans. M. Friedman). *The origin and meaning of Hasidism.* New York: Horizon Press.
Buber, M. (1963). (Trans. O. Marx et al.). *Israel and the world: Essays in a time of crisis* (2nd ed.). New York: Schocken Books.
Buber, M. (1998). (Trans. M. Friedman & R. G. Smith). *The knowledge of Man: A philosophy of the interhuman.* New York: Prometheus Books.
Buber, M. (1988). *Eclipse of God: Studies in the relation between religion and philosophy.* (Introduction by R. M. Selzer. Translation of *Gottesfinsternis.*). Atlantic Highlands, NJ: Humanities Press.
Burt, D. X. (1999). Health, Sickness. In A. D. Fitzgerald (Ed.), *Augustine through the ages: An encyclopedia* (pp. 416–419). Grand Rapids, MI: Eerdmans.
Chopra, D. (2004). *The book of secrets: Unlocking the hidden dimensions of your life.* New York: Three Rivers.
Cooper, M. (2015). *Existential psychotherapy and counseling: Contributions to a pluralistic practice.* Los Angeles: Sage.
Douthat, R. (2020). The pandemic and the will of God. *New York Times, Sunday Review,* April 12, p. 9.
Eigen, M. (2014). *Faith.* London: Karnac.

Eigen, M. (1998). *The psychoanalytic mystic.* Binghamton, NY : ESF Publishers.

Eliach, Y. (1980). Jewish tradition in the life of the concentration camp inmate. In *The Nazi concentration camps: Proceedings of the Fourth Yad Vashem International Historical Conference* (pp. 195–206). Jerusalem, Israel: Yad Vashem.

Federn, E. (1980). *Witnessing psychoanalysis.* London: Karnac.

Fisher, D. J. (1991). *Cultural theory and psychoanalytic tradition.* New Brunswick, NJ: Transaction Publishers.

Friedman, M. S. (1986). *Martin Buber and the Eternal.* New York: Human Sciences Press.

Friedman, M. S. (2002). *Martin Buber: The life of dialogue* (4th ed.). London: Routledge.

Gallagher, K. (1962). *The philosophy of Gabriel Marcel.* New York: Fordham University Press.

Geertz, C. (1973). *The interpretation of cultures.* New York: Basic Books.

Fromm, E. (1973). *The anatomy of human destructiveness*, Greenwich: Fawcett Crest.

Goffman, E. (1961). *Asylums.* New York: Anchor Books.

Govrin, A. (2016). *Conservative and radical perspectives on psychoanalytic knowledge: The fascinated and the disenchanted.* London: Routledge.

Greenberg, T. M. (2016). *Psychodynamic perspectives on aging and illness* (2nd ed.). Heidelberg: Springer.

Greenberg, J. R., & Mitchell, S. A. (1983). *Object relations in psychoanalytic theory.* Cambridge, MA: Harvard University Press.

Hadot, P. (1995). (Ed. A. I. Davidson. Trans. M. Chase.). *Philosophy as a way of life.* Oxford: Blackwell.

Hale, N. G. (Ed.). (1971). (Trans. J. B. Heller). *James Jackson Putnam and psychoanalysis.* Cambridge: Cambridge University Press.

Halpern, C. (2002). *Suffering, politics, power: A genealogy in modern political theory.* Albany: State University of New York Press.

Hanly, C. (1993). Ideology and psychoanalysis. *Canadian Journal of Psychoanalysis.* *1*(2), 1–17.

Hernandez, J.G. (2011). *Gabriel Marcel's Ethics of Hope. Evil, God and Virtue.* London: Bloomsbury.

Hoare, C. H. (2002). *Erikson on development in adulthood: New insights from the unpublished papers.* Oxford: Oxford University Press.

Hordes, A. (1971). *Martin Buber: An intimate portrait.* New York: Viking.

Huberband, S., Gurock, J. S., & Hirt, R. S. (1987). *Kiddush Hashem: Jewish religious and cultural life in Poland during the Holocaust.* Hoboken, NJ: KTAV Publishing.

Johnson, A. G. (1995) *The Blackwell dictionary of sociology: A user's guide to sociological language.* Oxford, UK: Blackwell.

Kabatznick, R., & Marcus, P. (1986). Psychoanalysis and social psychology. *Journal of the American Academy of Psychoanalytic Dynamic Psychiatry, 14*(1), 115–123.

Kaufman, W. E. (1985). *Contemporary Jewish philosophies.* Detroit: Wayne State University Press.

Keekes, J. (2002). *The art of life.* Ithaca, NY: Cornell University Press.

Kogan, E. (1958). *The theory and practice of hell.* New York: Berkley.

Koltko-Rivera, M. E. (2004). The psychology of worldviews. *Review of General Psychology, 8*(1), 3–58.

Kramer, K. P., & Gawlick, M. (2003). *Martin Buber's I and Thou: Practicing living dialogue.* New York : Paulist Press.

Landes, D. (1983). Spiritual responses in the camps. In A. Grobman & D. Landes (Eds.), *Genocide: Critical issues of the Holocaust* (pp. 261–278). Chappaqua, NY: Russell Books.
Langer, L. L. (1987). *Holocaust testimonies: The ruins of memory.* New Haven, CT: Yale University Press.
Lawritson, J. D. (1996). Martin Buber and the Shoah. In M. Friedman (Ed.), *Martin Buber and the human sciences* (pp. 295–309). Albany: State University of New York Press.
Levi, P. (1986). *The drowned and the saved.* New York: Summit Books.
Levinas, E. (1969). (Trans. A. Lingis), *Totality and infinity: An essay on exteriority.* Pittsburgh, PA: Duquesne University Press.
Lingis, A. (2015). The babies in trees. In D. Ennis & A. Calcagno (Eds.), *Thinking about love: Essays in contemporary continental philosophy* (pp. 235–245). University Park: Pennsylvania State University Press.
Loewald, H. (1979). The waning of the Oedipus Complex. *Journal of the American Psychoanalytic Association, 37*, 751–775.
Marcel, G. (1965a). (Trans. K. Farrer). *Being and having: An existentialist diary.* New York: Harper & Row.
Marcel, G. (1965b). (Trans. E. Crauford). *Homo viator: Introduction to a metaphysic of hope.* New York: Harper and Row.
Marcel, G. (1973). *Tragic wisdom and beyond.* Evanston, IL: Northwestern University Press.
Marcel, G. (1984). Replies to Otto Friedrich Bollnow and Charles Hartshorne. In P. A. Schilpp & L. E. Hahan (Eds.), *The philosophy of Gabriel Marcel* (The Library of Living Philosophers, vol. 17; pp. 200–203; 367–370). La Salle, IL: Open Court.
Marcel, G. (1995). *The philosophy of existentialism.* New York: Carol Publishing.
Marcel, G. (2001a [1950] *Mystery of being. Volume I. Reflection and mystery.* South Bend, IN: St. Augustine's Press.
Marcel, G. (2001b [1951]). *Mystery of being. Volume II. Faith and reality.* South Bend, IN: St. Augustine's Press.
Marcus, P. (1999). *Autonomy in the extreme situation: Bruno Bettelheim, the Nazi concentration camps and the mass society.* Westport, CT: Praeger.
Marcus, P. (2013). *How to laugh your way through life.* London: Karnac.
Marcus, P. (2019). *The psychoanalysis of overcoming suffering: Flourishing despite pain.* London: Routledge.
Marcus, P. (2020). *Psychoanalysis, classic social psychology, and moral living: Let the conversation begin.* London: Routledge.
Marcus, P., & Rosenberg, A. (Eds.). (1998). *Psychoanalytic versions of the human condition: Philosophies of life and their impact on practice.* New York: New York University Press.
Mitchell, S. A. (2002). *Can love last. The fate of romance over time.* New York: W. W. Norton
Moore, D. J. (1996). *Martin Buber: Prophet of religious secularism.* New York: Fordham University Press.
Neve, M. (1992). Clare Winnicott talks to Michael Neve. *Free Associations, 3*, 167–184.
Ogden, T. H. (2016). *Reclaiming and unlived life. Experiences in psychoanalysis.* London: Routledge.
Ornstein, A. (1985). Survival and recovery. *Psychoanalytic Inquiry, 5*(1), 99–130.
Ornstein, A. (2001). Survival and recovery: Psychological reflections. *Harvard Review of Psychiatry, 9*(1), 13–22.

Palmer, G. (2006). Some thoughts on surrender: Martin Buber and the Book of Job. In M. Zank (Ed.), *New perspectives on Martin Buber* (pp. 185–202). Tubingen: Mohr Siebeck.

Pollack, R. (1996). *The creation of Dr. B.* New York: Simon & Schuster.

Rabinowicz, R. A. (Ed.). (1982). *Passover haggadah: The feast of freedom*, (2nd ed.). New York: Rabbinical Assembly.

Raines, T. (2002). *Rising to the light: A portrait of Bruno Bettelheim.* New York: Knopf.

Rose, N. (1996). *Inventing our selves.* Cambridge: Cambridge University Press.

Sartre, J. P. (1965). (Trans. B. Frechtman). *What is literature?* New York: Philosophical Library.

Schafer, R. (1976). *A new language for psychoanalysis.* New Haven, CT: Yale University Press.

Sutton, N. (1996). *Bettelheim: A life and a legacy.* New York: Basic Books.

Sweetman, B. (2008). *The vision of Gabriel Marcel: Epistemology, human person, the transcendent.* Amsterdam: Rodopi.

Todorov, T. (1996). *Facing the extreme: Moral life in the concentration camps.* New York: Henry Holt.

Treanor, B. (2006). *Aspects of alterity. Levinas, Marcel, and the contemporary debate.* New York: Fordham University Press.

Wiesel, E. (1974). Talking, and writing and keeping silent. In F. H. Littell & H. G. Locke (Eds.), *The German church struggle and the Holocaust* (pp. 269–277). Bloomington, IN: Wayne State University Press.

Wolf, A. J. (2004). Heschel's "Torah from Heaven." *Judaism, 53*(3–4), 303–304.

Chapter 6

Towards a spiritualized psychoanalysis

In this last chapter, I will integrate and expand the aforementioned material into a preliminary version of psychoanalysis conceived as a spiritual discipline. I should state from the onset that I do not propose an alternative to the multiplicity of psychoanalytic theories and practices. Rather, I am suggesting that psychoanalysis can be deepened and enlarged, and therefore, become more pertinent to our analysands, analysts, and those mental health professionals who are considering doing formal psychoanalytic training. Perhaps even more important for the future of our discipline—which is "under siege" and in decline (certainly in America and Europe), especially in terms of being perceived as the "go to" therapy for the average psychologically suffering person—is that by integrating a spiritual sensibility, such as using a Buberian/Marcelian angle of vision, we may make psychoanalysis a more summoning therapy to those individuals who want to sort out their serious personal problems in living.

To recap, for both Buber and Marcel, it was a new realm of morality they were pointing towards, one that was not focused on constraint and prohibition but rather on "a morality of aspiration to spiritual experience" (Anshen, 1967, p. 20). "Spirit" is a plane of relationship, "a response of man to his *Thou*," the realm of the between (Buber, 1958, p. 39). For Buber and Marcel, *Thou* does not specifically refer to you, he, she, or God, but rather points to the presence of wholeness and uniqueness emanating from sincere listening and responsible responding. Thou involves mutual stand-taking and mutual self-donation (Kramer & Gawlick, 2003, p. 19; Marcel, 1965a, pp. 106–107).[1] Both Buber and Marcel provide less of a detailed description and more of a "testimony" (Wood, 1999 p. 93) of transcendence and the transcendent: that through the I-Thou relationship, as a function of will (i.e., Marcelian availability or openness) and grace (the other's unprecedented, if not divinely inspired responsivity with the fullness of his whole being), the eternal/Absolute Thou is glimpsed/made present ("the grace of eternity incomprehensible to the human mind," said Buber (1964, p. 74)). In other words, the specific I-Thou relationship points in the direction of an all-embracing transcendence, which completes, consummates, and existentially grounds these specific relations (Kaufman,

1992, p. 68). As a result, the transformed participants engage the mystery of being with an upsurge of spiritual energy, always in relation to a human, non-human, or divine Thou.

Following Buber and Marcel, who as I have said were not systematic in their philosophies, I offer some initial comments that point in a direction I think would be helpful to making psychoanalysis a spiritual discipline. I will do this by organizing my comments based on three questions that every version of psychoanalysis explicitly or implicitly attempts to answer.

(1) What is the Buberian/Marcelian version of the world, their spiritual conception of the human condition? What are the central problematics that the individual struggles with within a larger social context?
(2) In light of this conception of the human condition, how is individual psychopathology (or problems in living) understood?
(3) How does this conception of the human condition inform this type of clinical psychoanalysis as it attempts to alleviate individual psychopathology?

Buber and Marcel on the human condition

While Buber and Marcel differ in aspects of their accounts on a number of points, especially in the mind of the specialist, there is astonishing similarity in terms of the main thrust of their thought: Buber and Marcel "together have walked a remarkably similar path," largely because they were both profoundly religious scholars (Wood, 1999, pp. 83, 94). In fact, Wood reports that Marcel told Paul Ricoeur that his entire oeuvre was a "generalization of his Christian faith," that his views on Christian existence and human existence were not plausibly separated as they reflected his perspective on artful living. Buber famously drew from Hassidic intraworldly mysticism, hallowing the everyday, as one of the touchstones of his general philosophy (ibid., p. 83). In fact, Buber noted that what was Jewish and most profoundly human were the same: "The most deep-seated humanity of our soul and its most deep-seated Judaism mean and desire the same thing" (1967a, p. 55). While my intention is not to convert the reader into a Judeo-Christian outlook and way of being-in-the-world, I do want to characterize the philosophical anthropology of these two dialogical personalist philosophers, for they have a version of the human condition, or at least a sensibility, that strikes me as not only summoning to the believer and non-believer, but possibly useful to psychoanalysis conceived as a spiritual discipline. While there have been some laudable attempts to mainly correlate (and compare and contrast) Jewish philosophy and Christian narrative into contemporary relational psychoanalysis (Hoffman, 2011; Oppenheim, 2017), my effort is focused more on how to integrate into mainstream psychoanalysis some of the insights of Buber and Marcel, one a Jewish and the other a Christian believing humanist (Ricoeur called Marcel's outlook "biblical" (Sweetman, 2011, p. 155)), such that a spiritual dimension of psychoanalysis can be nurtured and put into sharper focus. It is up to the reader to decide if any of these insights are theoretically and clinically useful.

A philosophical anthropology has been defined by a Buberian scholar as "the study of man's essential nature" (Wheelwright, 1967, p. 70) and by a Marcelian scholar as "what being human means" (O'Malley, 1984, p. 275). Both of these near-identical definitions assume that "wholeness and uniqueness" as they are manifested in participation in the immediacy of experience are central to understanding what being human means, that is, when later reflected upon once one has some critical distance (Friedman, 1996, p. 16). In fact, both Buber and Marcel recognize that we can only know the human and divine other through encounter, the immediacy of the present, though we are also geared to critically interpret the experience after (e.g., Marcel's primary and secondary reflection, problem solving and engaged encounter respectively). "Wholeness and uniqueness" for Buber is viewed in terms of the I-Thou relation as the gateway to the Eternal Thou, while for Marcel it is linked to the mystery of being, in contrast to the idea of problem (Wood, 1999, p. 83). Of course, while the claim that there is an "essential nature" of "what being human means" is a debatable one—given Foucault and other postmodern arguments that what constitutes "essential" and "human" has varied over time depending on who is making the judgment, that is, it depends on the *episteme* one is lodged in, the socio-intellectual reality,[2]—the fact is that Buber and Marcel do put forth in a highly sophisticated manner a narrative of the human condition that they believe is phenomenologically compelling and provides insights into what many believe "really matters" as one attempts to fashion a flourishing life in our "broken world," as Marcel called it (2008)[3]—that is, our world, where one's autonomy, integration, and humanity are blunted if not subverted by a society that is characterized by technomania, atomization, collectivization, pervasive anonymous bureaucracy, overreliance on so-called experts, a totalitarian potential, and the nuclear self-destructive possibility. Buber too decried the hierarchic and instrumental character of contemporary economic and political systems. For example, capitalist individualism potentiated egoism and narcissism and diminished collective solidarity, while bureaucratic state socialism diminished individual freedom and autonomy in favor of state power. In both instances, Buber saw the personification of I-It relationships, such that citizens were taken advantage of as a way to enhance individual and governmental wealth and power. Moreover, neither system cultivated the spiritual yearnings of individuals to hallow their everyday encounters with the Thou's who composed their communities (Baron, 1996, pp. 249, 250).

For Buber and Marcel, man is not conceptualized as a material entity or substance, but always in relation (i.e., a self-in-relation), and what characterizes this relation is an issue that both have tried to describe from a variety of points of view. Moreover, while both Buber and Marcel valued the rational faculty, they did not make this feature what defines the main thrust of human existence, for both philosophers were interested in man as he resides in the specific totality of circumstances, "the wholeness of man" (Buber, 1965, p. 123) and "being-in-a-situation" (Marcel, 2001, p. 139), as Buber and Marcel respectively described it. Clarifying some of these dynamic interactions was what mattered most to them, for it pointed to something "more," "higher," and "better" that could facilitate the best of human moral/ethical potential. It should also be mentioned that both Buber and Marcel's philosophical anthropology can be bracketed from their philosophy of religion, at least technically speaking (Friedman, 1986, p. 52). However, they both were believers (especially in their believing openness), and the eternal and Absolute Thou are embedded in their accounts of what it means to be a "whole, real man" and "homo viator" (itinerant being), as Buber (1965, p. 123) and Marcel (1965b) respectively characterized it. I will also treat this so-called religious/spiritual dimension as crucial to grasping their version of the human condition, and what it may usefully suggest to psychoanalysis.

Buber's philosophical anthropology hinges on his supposition of there being a "twofold principle of human life" (1998, p. 54), two movements between people, distance/detachment and relation/encounter. "The primal setting at a distance" (ibid., p. 50), as Buber calls it, refers to the individualized human capacity to view the other from afar as an independent, separate entity (unlike instinct-driven animals): "Distance provides the human situation" (ibid., p. 54). The second movement is "entering into relation" (ibid., p. 50): "Relation provides man's becoming in that situation" (ibid., 54). The I-It relation emanates from distance: it is one that is never spoken with the whole being, it is the relation of experiencing/using/knowing, it is situated in space/time, it is singular/one-sided (monological), it is controlling and affirms the subject-object duality. The I-Thou relation emanates from the relation: It is spoken solely with the whole being, it is an event/happening, it is spaceless/timeless, it is mutual/two-sided (dialogical), yielding and affirms interhuman betweenness (Kramer & Gawlick, 2003, p. 18). Buber also believed in "human nature" as characterized by "goodness" and "badness," conceived as directions not substances, what he called "polar reality" (Anderson & Cissna, 1997, p. 82). Such a polarity is characterized by "direction-aimlessness, yes-no, acceptance-refusal," the therapeutic goal being to strengthen the goodness and diminish the badness: "Man as man can be redeemed," said Buber (ibid.), for evil is a function of estrangement from the realm of I-Thou as a not-yet actualized possibility ("not-yet-being into being" (Buber, 1964, p. 85)).

For Buber, what constitutes the best of being human (what analysts might think of as requiring, for example, robust autonomy, integration, and humanity) is actualizing the innate capacity (the "inborn Thou," the drive for relation) to confirm a fellow person. Remember that for Buber only a "person" can enter into an I-Thou relation (whole, unique, and unified subject-to-subject), while an "individual" resides in an I-It relation (subject to object).[4] Confirmation means assuming a particular kind of existential orientation when face-to-face with another person, affirming, accepting, and supporting his wholeness and uniqueness, including challenging him when required. As Buber noted, "Man wishes to be confirmed in his being by man, and wishes to have a presence in the being of the other. The human person needs confirmation because man as man needs it" (Agassi, 1999, p. 16). "Making present" is Buber's evocative phrase for such mutual confirmation. It has been defined as concretely imagining what another person is wishing, feeling, perceiving, and thinking. In this form of engagement, each person perceives the other as an independent self, one who was once distant "from me" but cannot be dissociated from my distance "from him," and whose specific experience I am now willing and able to actualize, that is, make present. Such an event is only ontologically culminated when both persons intuit their inmost development of the self, a kind of self-becoming that has been potentiated through I-Thou dialogue (Friedman, 1986, p. 55).

As Buber and Marcel have noted, when such a meeting between two persons happens, they reside in a common existential realm that also is beyond their personal realm, what they call the "between," the interhuman (Buber) or intersubjective (Marcel). For Buber and Marcel, the between denotes the realm where real meeting occurs, primary togetherness, vital reciprocity, unforgettable common potentiation, and mutual bonding (Kramer & Gawlick, 2003, p. 24).[5] While it is tempting to reduce such meeting to mere psychological categories, both Buber and Marcel emphasize that the psychological or subjective experience does not constitute the I-Thou dialogue (whether spoken in words or silence), rather, it is correlated with it, or attends it. Buber calls this genuine dialogue "experiencing the other side" and "imagining the real" (different than psychoanalytic empathy, as I pointed out elsewhere), to emphasize that it is "making the other present" that is its ontological culmination. It is characterized by implementing "inclusion," imagining and embracing what the other person is feeling, thinking, and experiencing without relinquishing one's felt reality regarding what one is doing, actualizing the other's wholeness and uniqueness and regarding the other person as completely meaningful on his own terms (ibid., pp. 194–195).

Such a way of being-in-the-world demands responsibility and conscience. Friedman defines Buberian responsibility as "the response of the whole person to what addresses her in the lived concrete. The 'ought' must be bought back to lived life … from where it swings in the empty air" (i.e., no moral code can be judged credible prior to specific circumstances (1992, p. 47)). Like Levinas (and Marcel), for Buber egoism and altruism are comparable acts of the ego, self, or soul that arise "posterior to responsibility and the call of the other or the Thou-saying to the other"[6]; that is, the ethical relation is not simply a question of being selfcentric or selfless, rather it arises "in the presence of the other" (Lipari, 2004, p. 130). In fact, Buber describes a responsible person as "one who addresses me primarily, that is, from a realm independent of myself, and to whom I am answerable" (1965, p. 45).[7]

An evolved conscience "is the voice which calls one to fulfill the personal intention of being for which he was created" (Friedman, 1986, p. 57), that is, what he judges to be the "core" or "essential" beliefs and values of what he is as a whole, unique, and ethically inspired person. As Buber notes:

> The finger I speak of is just that of the "conscience," but not of the routine conscience, which is to be used, is being used and worn out, the play-on-the-surface conscience [the super-ego?], with whose discrediting they thought to have abolished the actuality of man's positive answer.

Rather, says Buber, "I point to the unknown conscience in the ground of being, which needs to be discovered ever anew, the conscience of the 'spark,' for the genuine spark is effective also in the single composure of each genuine decision" (1965, p. 69). Such a view of conscience means that the person has to choose "to be true to himself," in his wholeness, uniqueness, and ethicality, or he is susceptible to guilt, or even worse, a sense of humiliation that he is not the person he thought he was. Moreover, this process occurs not so much in oneself but through the other, in a manner that points to God. This is the moment when Buber's philosophical anthropology and philosophical theology (his philosophy of religion) are "mutually implicative" (Wheelwright, 1967, p. 86). As Friedman notes, "Ethical decision, for Buber, is thus both the current decision about the immediate situation that confronts one and, through this, the decision with one's whole being for God" (1986, p. 57). Exactly how one knows what one's destiny is, how one will authentically[8] fulfill the goal of creation in the direction of God, is not known by reference to an abstract, universal ethical system—and there, of course, lies the rub. For a person can engage in what some may judge as evil actions and still judge himself to be "true to himself," whole and unique and God-animated (e.g., Islamic terrorists). Thus, Buber (and Marcel) suggests that any concretely workable philosophical anthropology has to reference descriptive and positive normative considerations about what man is and "ought" to become. Both Buber and Marcel were not relativists (or skeptics) as usually understood. Marcel, for example, showed that secondary reflection (engaged participation in thought) permitted a modicum of rational, objective accessibility to the domain of personal experience, and he asserted that these deep experiences like faith, fidelity, hope, and love are objective in the sense they were the same for all human beings, and therefore he (like Buber) rejected relativism and subjectivism regarding experience (Sweetman, 2008). As I have said, both Buber and Marcel are allied with a believing humanism ("the humanism of the life of dialogue" (Friedman, 1967, p. 23)) lodged in a Judeo-Christian outlook and ethics, the latter being similar (despite obvious differences) to the morally and ethically "best" of all of the major religions and spiritualities associated with the Axial Age (a broadly described virtue ethics that emphasizes moral character) (Marcus, 2019).

Marcel's version of the human condition, "man as he really is" (O'Malley, 1984 p. 276), is encapsulated in his notion of man as homo viator. A homo viator, a spiritual wanderer, is someone who is mindfully open to the mysterious in himself and in others—ready, receptive, responsive, and responsible— to participate in the variety of enigmatic, transgressive, and transfiguring sacred presences in the world. At the center of the human condition is an "ontological exigence," a yearning for transcendence, which is manifest in all authentic living. This is "the exigence to penetrate to a level saturated with meaning and value," such as through faith, fidelity, hope, joy, and love (when phenomenologically grasped from *within* the present), that points to an "eternal fulfilling Presence," the empirical and Absolute Thou (Keen, 1967b, p. 155). As Marcel says, "We do not belong to ourselves: this is certainly the sum and substance, if not wisdom, of any spirituality worthy of the name" (1962, p. xiv). In other words, for Marcel, the soul or spirit of a person searches for those sacred presences that animate the world, but only if he is open to them with the fullness of his whole being: "All spiritual life is essentially dialogue," where the self and other meet in intimacy and involvement (1952, p. 137) That is, "The relationship that can be said to be spiritual is that of being with being ... What really matters is spiritual commerce between beings, and that involves not respect but love" (ibid., p. 211). What Marcel seems to be implying is that he is less a philosopher of the person or the personality as conventionally understood than of the personal; that is, the person is always in a shared situation, one of freedom to engage (i.e., "availability," Buber's relation) or disengage (i.e., "unavailability," Buber's distance) (O'Malley, 1984, p. 279).

Marcel's version of the human condition includes, for example, the key concepts of being and having, mystery and problem, primary and secondary reflection, and his phenomenological investigation of the concrete experiences that access being, that of faith, fidelity, hope, and love. While I have detailed these concepts in previous chapters, I do want to briefly remind the reader how these notions are interrelated, interdependent, and interactive, and point to what characterizes the homo viator, the human condition as Marcel describes it.

Being and having are philosophical clarifications that have bearing on a range of everyday human experiences, such as incarnation or human embodiment, intersubjectivity (Buber's interhuman), and what constitutes the person as uniquely human.[9] Marcel claimed that a person's connection to his own body is not one of common "possession," as if he owns his body the way he owns, for example, an inanimate object. Rather than say "I have a body," it is more correct or at least plausible to say, "I am my body." Freud famously said that "the ego is first and foremost a bodily ego" (1923, p. 26), that the ego originally emanates from bodily sensations, including, as others have pointed out, nursing and the avoidance of hunger, leading Freud to assume that bodily tension was the central motivational principle (although relational analysts have reinterpreted the aforementioned in terms of object-related fantasies). Marcel's point about the original, admittedly ambiguous connection to the body is that one cannot view one's body as a mere object, as if it were a problem to be solved, since the logical and emotional detachment that is necessary to do so cannot be easily accomplished (think of the difference between the way a surgeon relates to your extreme abdominal pain and you do). Indeed, the instant I judge my body as an object, it ceases being experienced as "my body," because the character of conceptual thought necessitates detachment from the object under investigation. That is, at the moment my body becomes "a body," it is viewed instrumentally and functionally. A body can be viewed both ways: as "my body" and as "a body." For example, although a leg may have been amputated, I am still "me," but "my body" qua object is different. Moreover, when my body is related to as "a body," I am unable to judge my bodily experiences as the totality of circumstances of my life (something personal, "me," is missing).

It is within this context that Marcel distinguishes having and being, two modes of relating to things and people (similar to Buber's I-It and I-Thou). "Having" occurs when we possess objects, it demands analysis and detachment from the self (e.g., Freud's "blank screen" so-called objective/neutral listening orientation), and aims for conceptual, abstract, and intellectual mastery and universal solutions (similar to Buber's I-It attitude). "Having" typically pertains to utterly external matters, and it suggests that one can dispose of things and assimilate otherness into its preexistent, familiar categories (we are "unavailable" in Marcel's language). Marcel is aware that such an attitude has its constructive role in how one relates to human beings, at least in certain instrumental contexts (e.g., the aforementioned surgeon operating on a patient), but it is, in general, fundamentally a degradation of the character of the aspiring self, and to the extent that one relates to humans as possessions, one faces catastrophic ramifications (e.g., "I have a wife whom I inadvertently treat like an object" versus "I cherish my wife whom I love"). In contrast, the realm of being is one in which experience is unified/integrated prior to conceptual analysis, in which the person engages reality in terms of presence and participation and has access to experiences that are subsequently diminished, if not misrepresented in terms of abstract thought. As we have seen in the last chapter, a simple example of the difference between having something and being something concerns an issue of great significance when it comes to say effectively responding to suffering; that is, one does not "have" hope or a redemptive belief amidst captivity, one "is" hope or such a belief. The mode of self-relation distinguishing these two attitudes prompts one to act less versus more active in terms of motivation and praxis.

In an attempt to further elaborate having and being, Marcel provides another seminal distinction, that of problem (the having mode, calling to mind I-It) and mystery (the being mode, calling to mind I-Thou), which are accessed through two kinds of critical reflection, primary and secondary. Primary reflection is problem-solving cognition, using "abstraction, objectification and verification," whereas secondary reflection seeks a broader, deeper, and altogether richer comprehension of the meaning and value of human existence "by a return to the unity of experience" (Keen, 1967a, pp. 18, 22). As Marcel points out, secondary reflection is not focused on things but on presences, and its contemplation does not start "with curiosity or doubt" as does primary reflection, but rather with "wonder and astonishment"; therefore, "it is humble in its willingness to be conformed to categories crafted that on which it is focused. It remains open to its object as a lover does to his beloved—not as a specimen of a class but as a unique being" (Keen, 2006, p. 701).

In other words, secondary reflection is the best way to illuminate the inner depths of personal experience, to access the self when it is approached as mystery. A mystery, says Marcel, "is something in which I am myself involved, and it can therefore only be thought of as a sphere where the distinction between what is in me and what is before me loses its meaning and its initial validity" (Marcel, 1965a, p. 117). Marcel's claim, which I still think is extremely relevant, is that most of the time we are lodged in primary reflection (e.g., Buber's I-It) and miss out on the existential benefits of secondary reflection (Buber's I-Thou), which refers to what is best about being uniquely human, such as faith, fidelity, hope, and love. For example, what philosophers of religion call the problem of evil, reconciling the omnipotent God with the existence of evil, relies on primary reflection and is thus geared to providing a universal objective solution; the question of how people make their personal suffering sufferable (how it deeply "cuts" into them and they still press forward) requires secondary reflection. Put succinctly, for Marcel and other existential thinkers, experience is both temporally and ontologically prior to reflection, though it is secondary reflection that follows primary reflection, such as in making suffering sufferable and the problem of evil. This being said, what Marcel was aiming for was an objective (or quasi-objective) rendering of the structures of human existence by describing common existentially compelling personal experiences accessed through secondary reflection.

As Marcel states, his "concrete" philosophy was aimed at "restoring the ontological weight to human experience" (1965a, p. 103), to encourage people to engage their personal existence as they relate to being at large, a form of life that honors both the visible and invisible presences in the world. For example, "availability," when manifested as fidelity, is a total commitment to the best interests of the other, implying a downward modification of one's narcissism (e.g., a self without an ego). In relationship to God, it transforms into faith; and availability in the face of suffering can become hope. For Marcel, one becomes most fully an authentic "I," most compassionately human (serving/sacrificing) through one's loving relationship with a Thou. Thus, intersubjectivity personifies Marcel's outlook on the human condition, it is the "realm of existence to which the preposition *with* properly applies," a relation that "really does bind" and brings "us together to the ontological level, that is *qua* beings" (2001a, pp. 178, 180–181). Marcel thus mainly understands and describes being in terms of intersubjectivity, the opposite of self-centeredness, such as faith, fidelity, hope, and love, the capacity for "openness to others," and "to welcome them without being effaced by them" (Marcel, 1973, p. 39). In his view, intersubjectivity is the prerequisite of human awareness, while communion, that mode of engagement that facilitates a sense of deep emotional and spiritual closeness, that is also profoundly creative (as it demands emotional/intellectual engagement) and transforms and enhances both people, is the form that an authentic life takes (Keen, 1967a, pp. 28–29).

Finally, like Buber, Marcel had significant religious aspect to his philosophical anthropology that affirmed the experience of the Absolute Thou (again for Marcel, experience, secondary reflection trumps primary reflection, intellectualizing, in matters of faith). Whether it is faith, fidelity, hope, or love, these ways of accessing being are best grasped by referencing a transcendent reality, an infinite being. The Absolute Thou (of which God is the symbol, as is Buber's eternal Thou) is the transcendent reality that the spiritual aspirant makes an unconditional promise to, an existential commitment that apprehends and intuits that while it includes his own personal efforts, it ultimately emanates from and is affirmed through the Absolute Thou. In this context, life is regarded as a "gift" of divine grace (a "blessing," as the believer might say), one that one is dutybound to uphold through striving for holiness, especially in being other-directed, other-regarding, and other-serving in the deepest and most expansive manner possible. This is opposite, says Marcel, to viewing life through the lens of the broken world, where pessimism, cynicism, and nihilism make it feel like a "dirty joke" (Sweetman, 2011, p. 119).

To summarize, both Buber and Marcel, qua dialogical personalist philosophers, appear to be emphasizing some of the following features of the human condition as they conceive it.

1. Both philosophers believe that the human cast of the mind is fundamentally spiritual. That is, it aspires to "something more," "something higher," and "something better," what can be called transcendence, which references a transcendent realm and/or infinite being, the intuitively felt presence of the eternal or Absolute Thou. The essential aspect of the eternal/Absolute Thou (and of others and the world) cannot be known, it is inexpressible, and what matters most is He can be addressed in dialogue. In this process, human subjectivity, or at least a particular form of subjectivity, is transcended.
2. Both philosophers focus on "the wholeness of one's being and the wholeness of what is," that is, it is the "lived sense of the whole itself" as opposed to the abstract, fragmentary conceptual conundrums of conventional philosophy (and, in some instances, psychoanalysis) that matters most (Wood, 1999, p. 83). Their focus was more on praxis or practical wisdom for life and less on a philosophical superstructure to buttress it.
3. Both philosophers emphasize the centrality of dialogue with the Thou, whether formulated in terms of Buber's I-Thou or Marcel's mystery of being, which occurs in relation to a Thou. I-It relations are analogous to Marcel's problem, while I-Thou is analogous to his mystery (though Marcel used I-It, that is "I and a he," and I-Thou terms (Keen, 1967a, p. 29)); they represent two ways of relating to others and the world and imply a

non-self-centric mode of self-relation. The overarching goal of the Thou relation is the transformation of one's entire outlook and behavior, one's way of being-in-the-world. It requires will, that is, openness and intention, and grace, the uncoerced openness of the other. This is an improvised openness that can be described as mysteriously divinely inspired (Buber) and availability (Marcel), for "Thou-ism" to become dispositional. Feelings always attend to or accompany every Thou but do not define or constitute the meeting. Feelings are ways of participating with and in the other. They accompany faith, fidelity, hope, and love, as well as uplifting responses to the beauty and power of nature that Buber and Marcel appreciated and described in their writings on "Thou-ism." "Love," says Buber, is "responsibility of an I for a Thou" (1958, pp. 14–15); it always occurs between an I and a Thou and is not something that one simply feels in one's mind. For Marcel, "To say that one loves a being ... means ... Thou, at least, thou shalt not die," and "I love less for my own sake, than for what I can hope to obtain from another, and more for the sake of the other" (Marcel, 2001a, pp. 98, 61).

4. Both philosophers were worried that the "It" mode has become the dominating way of relation, in part, potentiated by the hyper-scientific/technological world we reside in, that while having its helpful and necessary role in everyday existence, has brought on extreme alienation, dis-ease, and contributed to the general sense of being "under siege." As Buber noted, "Without It man cannot live. But he who lives with It alone is not a man" (1958, p. 34).
5. Both philosophers emphasize the intuitively felt presence of mystery. Any Thou, including the eternal and Absolute Thou, is a sensed Presence in the here-and-now and not content or substance, analogous to listening to music or, metaphorically, perceiving a light that becomes more intense and radiant. For the homo viator, transcendence pursues hope and rebirth as it intuits mystery, something eternal, some infinite dimension, below the surface of everyday reality, that becomes the existential basis for justifying his way of being-in-the-world (i.e., a life devoted to holiness, as Buber and Marcel would describe it).
6. Both philosophers are deeply committed to a set of valuative attachments as manifesting what they regard as the "best" of being human. Put differently, they believe there is a perpetual and everlasting structure of value intrinsic in the universe, which has an objective presence if accessed using secondary reflection, as Marcel called it. Buber and Marcel emphasize the acknowledgment of radical alterity, or otherness, as a prerequisite of any Thou-ism. What sounds obvious to most thoughtful people today, that notwithstanding differences in individual outlook, beliefs and values, and historical situatedness, Buber and Marcel (and of course Levinas) affirm the significance of the existential reality that the other, qua other, is not me. In other words, for Buber and Marcel, any dialogue between two people, or

with an inanimate object, animal, and with God, must recognize in what manner the otherness of the other is manifested. The goal is simply to appreciate the unique otherness of the other without assigning our own meaning/understanding onto and into them and never to strive in other ways to assimilate or appropriate the other into ourselves (Lipari, 2004, p. 128). A lot easier said than done![10]

7. As the aforementioned quotations from Buber and Marcel on love indicate, the emphasis in their outlooks is on recognizing and affirming the other's otherness, and thus they both imply that a downward modification of individual narcissism and egocentricity is a prerequisite for autonomous, integrated, and humane existence (ibid., p. 129). In fact, Buber and Marcel suggest that the I become a whole, unique, and unified self only in relation to the other. "All real living is meeting," Buber says (1958, p. 11), while Marcel declares, "All spiritual life is essentially dialogue" (1952, p. 137).
8. As the aforementioned quotations on love as responsibility suggest, Buber and Marcel put an emphasis on ethical obligation to the other (Lipari, 2004, p. 129). As Wood noted, for Buber (but also for Marcel), ethics was situational, though both thinkers make references to an "absolute principle": "The principle is the integrity, i.e., the undividedness, both the self and the Other, which must be established and preserved in every situation" (and this means being attuned to manifestations of the Thou) (Wood, 1969, p. 103). Buber claimed that the "task of human life is not to become 'good' but to become 'holy,' i.e., really related to the transcendent Thou," which implies living the good (ibid., p. 104). Marcel concurs; he believed that man was created in the image of God (hence, our duty is to imitate God), and this means he has an essential dignity, that is, the sacred is "the mysterious principle at the heart of human dignity" (1963, p. 128). Indeed, "integrity and dignity are terms which, though not identical, are indissolubly linked" (ibid., p. 162). Both Buber and Marcel were devoted in their own unique ways to strongly felt, flexibly and creatively applied, transcendent-pointing moral beliefs and values that are primarily other-directed, other-regarding, and other-serving, as the "royal road" to holiness. Such an outlook and behavior is not only a conscious valuative commitment, but it always emerges within the intersubjective realm, a situation that demands context-dependent, setting-specific, attuned responsivity to the other's otherness. Probably before Levinas, Marcel declared that the other's death matters more than his own: "[T]he consideration of one's own death is surpassed by the consideration of the death of a loved one … the only thing worth preoccupying either one of us was the death of someone we loved" (1973, p. 131).
9. Both Buber and Marcel describe language not so much in instrumental, pragmatic, communicative terms, but, says Buber, "The mystery of the coming-to-be of language and that of the coming-to-be of man are one" (Agassi, 1999, p. 154). In other words, communication via language

> is responsible responding, Marcelian availability to presence, a world-construction with the other (the "between"), one that tends to be affect-integrating, meaning-giving, and action-guiding. The act of speaking, of opening oneself to the other's otherness (to address God/man, which is presence-animated), is different than the instrumental, pragmatic substance of speech (to express, which is content-animated). Thus, self-becoming and world-construction occur to the extent that one is ready, reactive, responsive, and responsible with the fullness of one's whole being to the other's otherness (Lipari, 2004, p. 131).

Put succinctly, for Buber and Marcel, their roughly similar concept of the person is that he is a homo viator, a spiritual wanderer or itinerant being who longs for the immanent, unique, unprecedented, and singular Thou. He engages in a groping, ambiguous search towards the light. Moreover, every particular I-Thou encounter points to an all-embracing transcendence (a transsubjective reality that is discovered/encountered, not created), an ineffable, inexhaustible, glimpsed Presence (the eternal/Absolute Thou) apprehended and intuited with our being, not our mind's eye (a "blinded intuition" says Marcel), which completes, consummates, and existentially grounds the specific I-Thou encounter (Kaufman, 1992, p. 68). Thus, for Buber and Marcel, the most impressive instantiation of "Thou-ism" as dispositional, as a way of being-in-the-world, is holiness (the restoration of the sacred in everyday life in harmony with the lived Presence, in affinity with eternity). That is, an orientation towards life that is infused with a form of ethicality, an outlook and behavior that are centrally animated by other-directed, other-regarding, and other-serving considerations as well as praiseworthy virtue ethics.[11] As Marcel noted, "Philosophically, the road to the other leads through the depths within myself" (O'Malley, 1984, p. 281), and amidst this self-exploration and lived existence much can go painfully astray, our next topic.

Buber and Marcel on individual psychopathology (or problems in living)

While Buber and Marcel, or at least my rendering of their ideas about a spiritualized human condition, often use religious language, I deliberately did not systematically "translate" these ideas into somewhat similar secular, psychoanalytic concepts, for I believe, as does Oppenheim, that there are "vibrant possibilities of religious language for revealing unanticipated dimensions of our intersubjective lives" (2017, p. 71). Of course, the very different language games of religion/philosophy and psychoanalysis can be amalgamated only tentatively and provisionally, with "fear and trembling," for they are different forms of discourse that can be deceptive and misinforming, especially when translated. Thus, cautious optimism seems to make the most sense. Likewise, while Buber, Marcel, and psychoanalysts often use rather high-falutin theoretical language/

formulations in their discussions of dialogue and the like, clinicians should never forget that they must engage the suffering analysand on his own terms (especially emotionally), person-to-person, in the immediacy of the present, "man as being in a situation," as Marcel called it (Sweetman, 2011, p. 114). In short, Buber and Marcel would agree with the popular expression, "keep it real."

In this section, I try to present what Buber and Marcel view as psychopathology (henceforth, problems in living), mainly their general causes that have bearing on some psychoanalytic notions for helping analysands with their pained lives, as this is the bailiwick of psychoanalysis. In the next section I take up the issue of how Buberian/Marcelian dialogue can help bring about greater self-awareness, self-understanding, self-overcoming, and self-transformation, especially through embracing their aforementioned spiritual sensibility.

While Buber wrote a few pieces and gave some lectures on psychological topics, like the Freudian unconscious (which he challenged),[12] and participated in dialogue with Carl Rogers (Agassi, 1999), for the most part, he dealt with general themes of existential guilt, trust, mutuality, and reciprocity, and what constituted the ideal attitude of the therapist to the patient, client, or analysand. Much of what Buber described has been loosely appropriated into psychoanalysis, in particular, in contemporary relational approaches, at least to some degree (Aron, 1996), sometimes not giving him credit for foreshadowing many of the key ideas (Aron, Grand, & Slochower, 2018; Charles, 2018). As Aron pointed out, "among all twentieth-century philosophers, Martin Buber elaborated a philosophy of dialogue that most closely resonates with the relational psychoanalytic approach and its emphasis on mutuality" (Aron, 1996, p. 154).[13] Indeed, researchers have found that the analyst must be willing and able to exude what researchers say are the five essential elements of psychotherapeutic support—presence, holding, caring, challenging, and confirming (Heery & Bugental, 2005, p. 257). The analyst, as I conceive him, must be ever mindful of the key finding of psychotherapy effectiveness research, that it is not the particular theory or technique that is used by the psychotherapist that matters most.[14] As Bion quipped, "I would [rely on theory only] … if I were tired and had no idea what was going on … the analyst you become is you and you alone—that is what you use" (Ogden, 2016, pp. 109, 111). Rather, as Buber and Marcel would no doubt not be surprised to learn, effectiveness is best predicted, that is, achieved, by the therapist-patient "alliance," or the degree to which the patient feels bonded, trusting, and part of a collaborative partnership (Ardito & Rabellino, 2011). Sounding like Buber (on confirmation) and Marcel (on availability), Thomas H. Ogden, a prominent analyst, notes that "what is mutative, I believe [in psychoanalysis] is the experience of oneself in the context of being with another person who recognizes you to be the person you are and the person you are in the process of becoming" (2016, p. 179).

Marcel also wrote about themes that are pertinent to the question of individual problems in living, such as maintaining personal dignity in the face of the mass society, fidelity, and betrayal in relationships, the body/mind relationship, and generating hope in the face of despair (Marcus, 2013). For the most part, Buber and Marcel were mainly concerned with what they viewed as the dehumanizing tendencies in our world, those that undermined autonomy, integration, and humanity, and alienated people from "Thou-ism" and other forms of spiritually animated, transcendence-pointing, affect-integrating, meaning-giving, and action-guiding ways of being-in-the-world. Both philosophers were especially troubled by the lack of willingness and ability to restore the sacred into everyday life, rooted in a faith in an immanent/transcendent God, whether it was hallowing the everyday as Buber called it (addressing the eternal Thou) or accessing being through faith, fidelity, hope, and love, as Marcel described it (the Absolute Thou).

Like any form of psychoanalysis, what constitutes problems in living or psychopathology will depend on the underlying version of the human condition, the philosophical anthropology of the thinker that is in play. For both Buber and Marcel, it is a specific kind of relatedness that matters most, what reaches towards the Thou. This is the opposite of inordinate narcissism, egocentricity, and other forms of selfcentricism, which Buber and Marcel, and for that matter, all of the great personages of the Axial period and those contemporary thinkers influenced by them, put forth as the "highest" ethical/moral ideal. Indeed, all of the great religious and spiritual traditions lodged in the Axial period advocate the spiritual aspirant's willingness and ability to love deeply and widely, including putting the anonymous other before oneself, such as taking care of the orphan, widow, and poor and welcoming the stranger. In other words, like Buber and Marcel, these Axial traditions asserted that transcendence is achieved through the inter-human encounter and expanded and deepened sociality, especially through embracing an existential comportment that is mainly other-directed, other-regarding, and other-serving. As the other great dialogical philosopher Levinas put it, "Through the relations with the Other, I am in touch with God" (1989, p. 17).

For Buber (and to a large extent Marcel), it is the wounding "disconfirmation that causes 'mental illness'" (Friedman, 1985, p. xii). Disconfirmation, as I have said, is the opposite of confirmation of otherness: fully engaging the unique presence of the other, affirming, accepting, and supporting him and, when indicated, gently but firmly opposing him (Kramer & Gawlick, 2003, p. 202).[15] Confirmation helps promote "healing through meeting," as Buber called it (Agassi, 1999, p. 17), while disconfirmation tends to undermine one's autonomy, integration, and humanity, this being a fertile breeding ground for the development of later neurotic, psychotic, and other serious problems in living. Most importantly and obviously, when disconfirmation occurs within the context of the vulnerability and exposure of "the earliest stages of life," it "must be a major factor in psychopathology" (Friedman, 1985, p. 123). It is common knowledge that parental caregiving that is nurturing and stable, that is characterized by accurate empathy, attunement, sensible structure, limits, and boundaries, and the like tends to fashion children who are reasonably "healthy" adults, capable of deep and wide love and creative and productive work. The opposite kind of parenting, that tends to be neglectful and abusive, usually leads to profound problems in living for the child when he becomes an adult. In a word, for Buber "the roots of neurosis lie both in the patient's closing himself off from the world," Marcel's unavailability, "and in the pattern of society itself and its rejection and non-confirmation of the patient," Marcel's "broken world" (Farber, Howe & Friedman, 1956, p. 53). As Buber said, "Egoism is not self-love but a lack of love" (1964, p. 92), while Marcel noted that "True love is humble" (2001a, p. 83).

In *I and Thou*, Buber takes up one of the causes of problems in living, in a section called "What is self-contradiction," which suggests what the origins of severe psychological problems, even psychosis, may be:

> If a man does not represent the *a priori* of relation in his living with the world, if he does not work out and realize the inborn *Thou* [the human tendency toward relationship evoked by the parental caregiver who responds to the child's effort to relate] on what meets it, then it strikes inwards. It develops on the unnatural impossible object of the *I*, that is, it develops where there is no place at all for it to develop. Thus, confrontation of what is over against him takes place within himself, and this cannot be relation, or presence or streaming interaction, but only self-contradiction.

Moreover, says Buber,

> The man may seek to explain it as a relation, perhaps as a religious relation, in order to wrench himself from the horror of the inner double-ganger [roughly, a ghostly double of a living person, particularly one that haunts its fleshy compliment]; but he is bound to discover again and again the deception in the explanation. Here is the verge of life, flight of an unfulfilled life to the senseless semblance of fulfilment, and its groping in a maze and losing itself even more profoundly.
>
> (1958, pp. 69–70)

What Buber is suggesting is that what tends to bring about severe psychological problems in living, even psychotic or psychotic-like conditions, is the suffering person's near-total estrangement of the I to the Thou. This is instantiated when the suffering person is totally (or near-totally) unavailable, as Marcel would call it; he is cut off from any efforts to be compassionately encountered, to give and, especially, to receive love. Instead, he resides largely in the phantasmagoric imaginings of his unhinged mind, projecting his "craziness" outwardly to a world that inevitably feels menacing or worse, perhaps in conversation with an imaginary Thou. Such people are like a "windowless monad," a selfcentric way of being-in-the-world, that while at certain times functions like a protective cocoon, more often than not is experienced as a personal "concentration camp"

(Appelfeld, 1994, p. 17). For example, I am currently treating three chronically, severely depressed analysands, all highly medicated and very intelligent, though grossly underfunctioning in work and love. The aforementioned description was woven into interpretations I gave them about their impoverished and self-referential way of being-in-the-world (depression is intensely narcissistic), and they all concurred that I was accurate. However, as they all told me, and I agreed, their problem is how to get liberated from their self-made, self-encapsulating "concentration camp," not having the will, let alone the ability, to do so. All of these analysands feel hopeless, helpless, and hapless, and I often feel likewise in my treatment of them.

Implicit in the previously cited Buber quotations is his claim that maintaining a modicum of wholeness and unity is what keeps a person from falling victim to serious problems in living. Drawing from the essay "Spirit and Body of the Hasidic Movement," Buber notes, "The more dissociated [fragmented] the soul, the more it is at the mercy of its sickness and attacks, the more concentrated it is, the more it is able to master them. It is not as if it conquered the body; rather through its unity it ever again saves and protects the unity of the body" (ibid.). Buber's point here is that the relation of a person, a "soul" to the totality of circumstances of his life, its "organic life," to a large extent relies on the extent the person/soul is whole and unified (ibid.). In other words, for Buber, to the extent that one feels, thinks, and acts in a way that reflects a robust degree of wholeness and unity (that is instantiated by, for example, autonomy, integration, and humanity), one is less prone to problems in meaning, purpose, and direction, as well as specific conventionally described psychological conditions (that have their own idiosyncratic trajectory).

As I said earlier, the terms *wholeness* and *unity* are hard to define, let alone in a manner that is agreed upon, and they are to some extent not "politically correct" psychological terms compared to other postmodern tropes, like multiplicity or plurality of selves and the like. Postmodernism has put forth a fragmented and decentered self that has no essence, only images, and while I have some sympathy with this perspective, wholeness and unity as Buber, Marcel, and others describe them ("the core of the person" (Buber, 1964, p. 40) a "personal center" (Buber, 1958, p. 133)) strike me as necessary aspects of a credible self-conception, let alone one that leads to artfully fashioning a spiritually animated flourishing life. By wholeness, Buber (and Marcel) does not mean an unchanging, conclusive condition in which the person engages in this or that action according to a specific definition/criterion (it is not a fixed content or belief). While Buber uses the term to describe a body-mind-spirit integration such that no single component has greater weight (roughly a kind of unity), this too is not the main thrust of his notion of wholeness. Rather, wholeness is best understood as a constituent aspect of self-in-relation, and its actualization is a direction of movement that ebbs and flows and is context-dependent and setting-specific (Kramer & Gawlick, 2004, p. 100). Wholeness is instantiated only through relation, through availability as Marcel calls it, that is, meeting the other in their whole, unique presence, willing and able to respond with the fullness of their whole being in dialogical encounter. Drawing from Marcel, Treanor calls this the "porous unity of the self" (2006, p. 66). Says Buber:

> "With the whole being" can be described most simply thus: I enter into the act or event which is in question with all the available forces of my soul without conflict, without even latent much less perceptible conflict.
>
> (1964, p. 52)

It is at this point that Buber's religious/spiritual perspective is in sharpest focus. As Ventimiglia (2008) aptly put it, for Buber "people are sick because they have gone away from what makes them whole. They have lost God, because without genuine dialogue [which requires wholeness, unity], God cannot be known" as a lived reality (p. 616). In other words, to the extent that one cannot engage in I-Thou encounters (which ebbs and flows with I-It), whether with humans (e.g., persons), nature (e.g., a tree), spirit becoming forms (e.g., art), or directly with the eternal Thou (e.g., prayer), one is not able to glimpse the power and source of what is Beautiful, True, and most importantly Good in life, the eternal Thou (which can never become an It). And without glimpsing the fringe of the eternal Thou (or perhaps its secular equivalent if religious language is objectionable, for as Buber and Marcel suggested, all names of God are holy because they not only speak *of* God but *to* him (Gordon, 2011, p. 213)),[16] one is less willing and able to effectively take a stand, make a decision, and bear witness on matters of ultimate concern (Kramer & Gawlick, 2003, p. 65). These limitations too are a fertile breeding ground for later serious problems in living. Most importantly, without glimpsing the eternal Thou, one is not willing and able to effectively become a partner with God, the source and presence of genuine relationship, which in effect forms the living bond among all separated beings.[17] Such estrangement from God implies estrangement from man, and thus the person begins a downward spiraling that usually leads to a hyper-selfcentric mode of being-in-the-world. As Ventimiglia noted, for Buber "psychopathology is found in the breakdown of interpersonal relationships" (2006, p. 616), the unwillingness and inability to at least episodically jettison the It world for the Thou one: "A soul is never sick alone," says Buber, "but is always a between-ness also, a situation between it and another existing being" (1967b, p. 142). In short, psychopathology is that which works against being with and for the other as Thou, that is, that impedes, obstructs, truncates, or blunts a transcendence-pointing, existential comportment that is other-directed, other-regarding, and other-serving, that is the "bedrock" of artfully fashioning a holy life as Buber and Marcel call it. Levinas put this point just right, "The concern for the other breaches concern for the self. This is what I call holiness. Our humanity consists in being able to recognize the priority of the other"; "The priority of the other person begins in this self-effacing gesture in ceding our place. This is the road that can lead to holiness" (2001, pp. 234, 191).

For Marcel, problems in living are related to what he calls the "the spirit of abstraction," the root cause of the estrangement, nihilism, and potential violence of modern man, including the violence that is turned inwards and warps one's outlook and degrades one's behavior, that is, one's autonomy, integration, and humanity. The spirit of abstraction, which is exemplified in primary reflection, is defined as follows: "As soon as we accord any category, isolated from all other categories, an arbitrary primacy, we are the victims of abstraction" (2008, p. 116)—for example, function and functionality (which assumes that practical and utilitarian concerns should trump moral and esthetic ones), and the idealization of technology (technomania as opposed to the sensible use of technology). Marcel does understand and appreciate the usefulness of abstraction (as does Buber with the It world), just as he appreciates and understands the usefulness of technology, but what he is against are the deleterious, dangerous effects of the spirit of excessive abstraction, especially as they play out in everyday relations with others (e.g., our utter dependence on "gadgets" that gives us a smooth material life at the expense of our "inner reality," including enacting "spiritual activity directed towards higher ends" (Sweetman, 2011, pp. 118, 122). Abstraction is a consequence of forgetting, disregarding, and not honoring concrete reality from which the abstraction is derived—for example, disavowing that the enemy a soldier is ordered to kill is a thinking, feeling person, perhaps with a wife and children; forgetting that a patient diagnosed as psychotic is a unique individual with a painful family history that drove him into his psychosis and is not reducible to his medical ascription; that a thing of nature, like a daffodil, is more than, and different from, its scientifically described structure and characteristics (Keen, 1967a, p. 13–14).

And finally, perhaps worst of all, there is the danger that our personal way of self-defining and self-fashioning may become mainly animated by the alienating spirit of abstraction. According to Marcel, "it is pretty certain ... that we are tending to become bureaucrats, and not only in our outward behavior, but in our relations with ourselves. This is as much as to say that between ourselves and existence we are interposing thicker and thicker screens" (2001a, p. 191). Such unavailability is a specific style of life, a specific kind of deficit, a passive inertness, an emptiness, and the egoism and narcissism it generates, such as arrogance and pride, are derivative aspects of this inadequacy (Bollnow, 1984, p. 182). For Marcel, it is this spirit of abstraction that is at the root of so much dehumanization and violence that characterizes our "broken world" at its worst, as in totalitarianism where the human person is reduced to a destroyable object, evidenced in Nazi and other forms of industrialized and mass killings. The broken world signals that we are losing the domain of being and availability, the basis of genuine human relationships and the spirit of transcendence (Sweetman, 2011, p. 7). Moreover, according to Marcel, such a life attitude, mindlessly governed by the spirit of abstraction, is the basis for the less extreme, but still very toxic, everyday loss of appreciation for, and affirmation of, the dignity and sacredness of all human beings and the physical environment. This is especially exemplified in our truncated, if not dehumanized and dehumanizing, everyday relations with others, as manifested in common discourtesy and unkindness, and our disrespectful attitude towards our physical environment. Keen summarizes the matter just right:

> The results of such a [functional] way of thinking are disastrous for human dignity. As the capacity to love, to admire, and to hope dries up, the functional man loses the ability, and even the desire, to transcend his situation of alienation and captivity. His world loses its mysterious character, it becomes "purely natural," and all things are explained by reference to the categories of cause and effect. With the eclipse of mystery goes the atrophy of the sense of wonder.
>
> (Keen, 1967a, p. 10)

For Marcel, qua believer, without viewing oneself and the world with a sense of sacred attunement, that we are God's highly fallible human creatures, humble, grateful, serving (not servile!), devoted to using our "gifts" in a joyful and meaning-saturated, communal and responsible for and to the other manner, we are doomed to a life of hopelessness and the belief that life is pointless and human values are worthless. Needless to say, by knowingly or unknowingly being ensconced in the spirit of abstraction in our self and other relations, we are "sitting ducks" to develop a wide range of forms of conventionally described psychological distress. Indeed, even analysts can relate to their analysands in a manner that reflects the spirit of abstraction (as can psychotherapists with their patients and clients), such as when they get "stuck" in primary reflection without moving into the synthesizing, recollecting activity of secondary reflection. That is, analysts can lose sight of the fact that the person they are conversing with is a concrete, embodied, situated existence and not simply a fee-paying "case" (like other such cases with a function, roles, and characteristics) that he views as abstracted elements of existence as if they were an independent system (a He, She, or It), rather than as a Thou (Treanor, 2006, pp. 67, 74).

If availability, conceived as a dispositional form of relation to others that points to the transcendent (what Marcel also calls the intersubjective, Buber's interhuman), reflects the willingness and ability to give to the other, to offer up one's emotional, intellectual, spiritual, and material assets for the other's well-being, then unavailability is its opposite. There is a correlation between how one treats others and oneself: the more one is unavailable, sealed-off from dialogical communication/participation and communion/presence, the less one is willing and able to give generously and hospitably, with bounty and plenitude, as one is self-enclosed, self-occupied, and selfcentric. Unavailability then is exemplified for example in pride—that presentation of the self that indicates excessive self-value, an unreasonable sense of superiority as to one's talents, beauty, wealth, or rank—in technomania and technolatry, and in an over-valuing of function and functionality, where other considerations should be operative, if not given precedence. As Marcel notes, all forms of unavailability reflect alienation, from others and from oneself: the more I treat the other as an it or a thing, the more I see myself that way. Likewise, the more I can relate to the other as a Thou, the more I can view myself similarly. And finally, the more the other relates to me in a manner that reflects unavailability, the more I feel like an it or an object, while the more availability from the other, the more I feel like a presence (Treanor, 2006, pp. 73, 75). Treanor quotes Marcel on this point, a fitting quote to conclude this section:

> It will perhaps be made clearer if I say the person who is at my disposal [available] is the one who is capable of being with me with the whole of himself [like Buber's "wholeness and uniqueness"] when I am in need; while the one who is not at my disposal [unavailable] seems merely to offer me a temporary loan raised on his resources. For the one I am a presence; for the other I am an object [i.e., if we consider others as means for self-serving ends, rather than as singular individuals, dialogue cannot occur].
>
> (Marcel, 1995, p. 40)

For Marcel then, serious problems in living are related to unavailability, not only from ill-conceived, ill-advised, and ill-fated activities and contexts that one is inordinately engaged or ensconced in, such as the aforementioned technomania, atomization, collectivization, pervasive anonymous bureaucracy, over-reliance on so-called experts, a totalitarian potential, and the nuclear self-destructive possibility. Just as important is the unavailability that reflects inner lifelessness, that is, the unavailable person has engaged in a process of self-objectification, he is self-enclosed and selfcentric, and while he engages in a variety of activities, he ends up feeling "encumbered," as Marcel calls it, "used up" (e.g., productive in a wasteland) by the many things he has superficially grafted onto his feeble, unskillfully cobbled-together self-identity (Hernandez, 2011, p. 22). These so-called pseudo- or pseudo-like acquisitions reflect a person who has lost, or not found, his own authentic voice (becoming who one is as Nietzsche called it)[18] and is therefore not willing and able to be present. Indeed, to put it colloquially and religiously, to be existentially "MIA" or "AWOL" is analogous to a "crippling moral evil," an offense that Marcel equates with sin (even "original sin"), in which function rather than value are what animates relationships (ibid.). While original sin may be a hard concept for analysts to embrace, what Marcel means sounds exactly right to me: that all people "are born with limited capacities to pursue the good, and left to our own devices all of us will betray ourselves and our fellow man" (Pattison, 1988, p. 89). In other words, like Saint Augustine and Freud, Marcel believed that we are fundamentally flawed creatures, frequently selfish, impatient, dishonest, envious, mean-spirited, and flawed in our capacity to love and in our relations with others—the main interest of Marcel, Buber, and, of course, psychoanalysis. As Marcel, Buber, and Freud noted, unless checked by moral force, by conscience, and by moral action, we are all prone to the everyday "inhumanity" (or worse) towards others, especially to those dear to us, which is often the basis for our own subversion in terms of guilt and other forms of unhappiness. The aforementioned calls to mind Freud's death instinct and Klein's claim that aggression was a projection of the individual's inherent self-destructive drive.

For Buber and Marcel, the analysand's problems in living are perhaps best understood in terms of their being "ethically disabled." As Jacobs describes it, their mode of being-in-the-world, "their characters are such that sound ethical considerations," that is, strongly felt, flexibly and creatively applied, transcendent-pointing moral beliefs and values, that are primarily other-directed, other-regarding, and other-serving (the "royal road" to holiness), are "inaccessible to them" (2001, p. 1). Moreover, such analysands have a seriously limited and restricted capacity for moral self-transformation, "for ethical self-correction" (ibid., p. 74). In Buberian/Marcelian language, an ethically disabled analysand is more-or-less consistently and significantly estranged from the Beautiful, True, and most importantly, the Good. Such an analysand can be said to lack ethical integrity and "good" character, the "irreproachable" "character" that Freud believed was a prerequisite to being a competent treating analyst (Freud, 1905, p. 267).

Stated differently, in general, to the extent that the seemingly natural inclinations of the selfishness/infantile narcissism of the self, the ego, and the soul dominate one's life conduction (roughly, the It-world), especially in one's interhuman relations, one is more likely to suffer in terms of guilt, anxiety, depression, and alienation. As Freud noted, "Narcissism is the universal and original state of things, from which object-love is only later developed, without the narcissism necessarily disappearing on that account" (Freud, 1917, p. 416). If this infantile narcissism is not transformed into "healthy" narcissism (e.g., realistic self-esteem without being closed-off to the needs/desires of others), the person's willingness and ability to effectively love and work are significantly impaired, if not forever arrested. This is a basic, widely accepted spiritual/moral insight of all major ancient religious/spiritual wisdom traditions associated with the Axial period (Marcus, 2019). Like Freud and his followers, Buber and Marcel recognize that overcoming, even significantly modulating, our inherent selfishness, infantile narcissism, and tendency toward egocentricity is no easy task. The *tzadikkim* (righteous people) and saints (like Father Kolbe, Janusz Korczak, and Miep Giese mentioned in Chapter 5) who live lives of holiness, radical selflessness, and kindness (a life-long process of self-becoming) characterize the ideal way of being-in-the-world that Buber and Marcel had in mind.[19]

Thus, many problems in living, and in their extreme, severe psychopathology as analysts would describe it, emanate in part from the selfish self-undermining, if not taking over, of the ethical/moral self. The needs and aspirations of the selfish self, the ego, and the soul have fairly consistent priority over the life-affirming needs of the other (the It world dominates one's existence with little or no Thou). When the ego is tied to the self in this manner, the fundamental isolation and loneliness of the subject that Marcel and Buber claim is endemic in our "broken world" remains continuous and steady.

Psychoanalysis, with its interest in narcissistic pathologies, has provided much insight into the development and tragic course of such a way of being. For Buber and Marcel, to the extent that one avoids, ignores, or is ignorant of one's responsibility for the other, including what we do carelessly, inadvertently, and unconsciously, one can be said to be ethically disabled, lacking in autonomy, integration, and most importantly, humanity.

In this view, to the extent that one can embrace and live strongly felt, flexibly and creatively applied transcendent-pointing moral beliefs and values, that are primarily other-directed, other-regarding, and other-serving, can one be described as an "evolved" person (who can live Thou) or a "healthy" ex-analysand, patient, or client, as analysts and psychotherapists would call it. Pathology, so to speak, can be conceptualized as those habits of mind, heart, and behavior that impede the movement of transcendence towards responsible subjectivity, towards living a life characterized by love, justice, peace, and what have been broadly described as virtue ethics. Indeed, from a Buberian/Marcelian point of view, a person's capacity for critical, ethical self-reflection, acknowledging when moral requirements and obligations to the other have not been properly met and responded to (Buber/Marcel's Thou and Marcel's availability), is a good prognostic indicator for a successful analysis, especially when psychoanalysis is conceptualized as a spiritual discipline.

In mainstream psychoanalytic terms, the above refers to the transmutation of narcissism from infantile to more "mature" or "healthy" forms and the development of wide-ranging, free, flowing, and unrestrained (i.e., non-neurotic) emotional capacities, especially to give but also to receive love. Psychoanalysis has been masterful in its ability to describe, understand, and ameliorate the many developmental, conflictual, and other impediments that blunt, impair, and block individuals' capacity to live a life guided by deep and expansive love and creative and productive work.

As I have tried to suggest throughout this book, there are conceptual and practical advantages to the psychoanalyst's embracing a Buberian/Marcelian perspective on the subject matter that is at the heart of psychoanalysis, namely, reducing the suffering of analysands (hence, psychoanalysis as a spiritual discipline). In particular, I have suggested that pain, sorrow, conflict, and other forms of suffering are fruitfully viewed in terms of helping the analysand give meaning to his suffering by developing an ethical response to it, one that enacts strongly felt, flexibly and creatively applied, transcendent-pointing moral beliefs and values that are primarily other-directed, other-regarding, and other-serving. Whether it is my own or the other's suffering, the way to make such suffering "sufferable," at least in general terms, is to perceive it as an ethical/moral problem requiring such a self-transcending way of thinking, feeling, and acting. Such a Buberian/Marcelian-inspired angle of vision provides fresh, thought-provoking ways of understanding previously inadequately illuminated aspects of love, work, faith, and suffering, as well as such clinically pertinent issues as responsibility, trust, guilt, anxiety, mortality saliency, spirituality/religiosity, and so forth.

In this context, for Buber and Marcel, personality or character is best understood as ethical/moral subjectivity—ready, reactive, responsive, and responsible—with the fullness of one's whole being to the other's otherness, his emotional, intellectual, spiritual, and material needs and reasonable desires (Levinas has greatly opined on this theme). This ethical/moral subjectivity is where a kind of "resource for moral recognition," "ethically sound practical reasoning," and ultimately, moral "recovery" or repossession of ourselves is concentrated (Jacobs, 2001, p. 43). In other words, personality or character can be viewed as the affect-integrating, meaning-giving, and action-guiding nexus for enacting our strongly felt, flexibly and creatively applied, transcendent-pointing moral beliefs and values that are primarily other-directed, other-regarding, and other-serving. In this view, a personality or character disorder, at least most generally, can be defined as the habitual conscious and unconscious ways that a person is inadequately responsive, misguided, and/or deaf to ethical/moral considerations, that is, to the summoning call of the other as one's normative horizon of feeling, thought, and action. All such personality disorders are trapped in the It world and are unavailable in the extreme.

For example, in narcissistic personality disorder, the person's habitual way of perceiving, relating to, and thinking about the other is marked by grandiosity, envy, and an inordinate need for admiration. Such unavailability is an outlook, a way of being, that cuts him off from properly empathizing with and responding to the reasonable needs and desires of the other. Instead, the other is exploited to advance his own ends, that is, to have his excessive need for self-aggrandizement, self-importance, and specialness affirmed again and again. The borderline personality individual, who has marked lability in his sense of self, emotions, and impulse control, has volatile, unstable, and explosive interpersonal relationships that make it near impossible to consider the other's needs and wishes in any sustained and reasonable manner. His fear of abandonment, his inordinate need for idealization and quick sense of devaluation, and his boundless rage all diminish, if not arrest, his ability to give and receive love. He too is radically unavailable. Likewise, the paranoid person whose inner life is typified by all-encompassing distrust and suspiciousness of others, such that their intentions are viewed as malicious, makes him largely incapable of giving to and serving the other. Frequently questioning the devotion, honesty, and reliability of friends and acquaintances, giving humiliating or menacing interpretations to inoffensive comments or benign events, being prone to holding grudges and disinclined to forgive insults and hurts, and imagining infidelity in his partner make him unable to reach out and say Thou, to care properly for the other in any genuinely other-regarding manner. The dependent personality, characterized by an inordinate infantile need to be nurtured and taken care of, often leading to submissiveness, demanding and clinging relatedness, and fears of separation and abandonment, is severely limited in his ability to love, let alone experience "mature" love that respects the separateness and autonomy of the other. Such a person is steeped in the misery of the It world; he is as, Marcel would say, unable to participate in being or being-with, a "closed-in-ness" and "holding back'" (Marcus, 2013, p. 204).

Likewise, the mode of being in the world of schizoid, avoidant, antisocial, and obsessive-compulsive personalities can also be fruitfully analyzed in terms of their ethical/moral meaning and significance, as evidenced in their diminished capacity to respond empathetically (or Buber's imagining the real, saying Thou) to the other's needs for love and justice—the schizoid's aloofness and indifference to social relationships and his emotional restrictedness, coldness, and prickliness; the avoidant's detachment from the social world, social anxiety, and low self-esteem; the antisocial's harmful, disruptive, inconsiderate interpersonal approach, always at the expense of the other's rights and needs; the obsessive-compulsive's tendency to control others, his perfectionism, cheapness, fussy orderliness, and lack of positive emotional expressiveness. In all of these and other personality disorders, the individual is ethically/morally corrupted, unable to respond with the fullness of his whole being to the reasonable needs and desires of the other in a genuinely other-regarding, other-serving manner. As a result of their truncated ties to empathy (and imagining the real), those analysands with personality or character disorders, whether they acknowledge it or not, are suffering greatly, for they reside in a loveless hell.

Buber and Marcel on treatment considerations

Many of Buber's notions connected to his philosophy of dialogue have been briefly discussed or referenced in a few publications reflecting mainstream psychoanalytic clinical practice (and more so in existential and Gestalt psychotherapy). The emphasis has been largely on how Buberian notions correlate, if not foreshadow, seminal ideas circulating in contemporary relational psychoanalysis. For example, Buber is briefly referenced/discussed about mutuality and reciprocity (Aron, 1996), dialogue (Ehrenberg, 1992), the interhuman, the between (Aron & Starr, 2013), and the imagined real (Cooper, 2000).[20] And Buber's notion of what the "end of therapy" is resonates with relational theorists: "The specific 'healing' relation would come to an end the moment the patient thought of, and succeeded in, practicing 'inclusion' and experiencing the event from the doctor's pole as well" (1958, p. 133).[21] For the most part, however, as the psychoanalyst/philosopher Donna Orange (who wrote a short, appreciative chapter on Buber) puts it: "the philosopher of dialogue [versus monologue], inclusion [aka imagining the real versus psychoanalytic empathy], and confirmation [the interhuman], has gone largely unnoticed in the psychoanalytic world," and Buber's clinical understandings ought to "embrace us and inspire us in our work with those who have rarely if ever been really met with the interhuman" (2010, pp. 15, 33). Indeed, as I have noted throughout this book, for example, Buber's aforementioned notions, especially "healing through meeting" all speak to what any version of psychoanalysis must effectively enact over and over again to help the analysand fashion a flourishing life. For as Friedman has correctly pointed out, Buber's assertion in *I and Thou* that "All real living is meeting" stresses the key "element of human existence in which we relate to others in their uniqueness and otherness and not just as a content of our experience" (Friedman, 1992, p. 55). That is, the psychological, the intrapsychic, is only a correlate or accompaniment of the dialogical, which is the most important touchstone of what Buber (and Marcel) view as reality (ibid.).[22] Dialogue thus suggests a "new kind of mind," as David Bohm aptly put it,[23] it moves through the analysand and analyst and is not lodged "in any or even in all of the individual participants"; instead, it resides "in a whole that is incommensurable with the sum of the finite parts." This is the soul-altering shift from identity logic to the openness of genuine dialogue (Metcalfe & Game, 2008, p. 345).

What Orange said about Buber being "largely unnoticed in the psychoanalytic world" is even more true when considering Marcel. For example, Hoffman (2011), who discusses relational psychoanalysis and the Christian narrative (i.e., the redemptive notions of incarnation, crucifixion, and resurrection), including liberally drawing from Marcel's admiring student Paul Ricoeur, never once mentions Marcel's work. Though Marcel did not engage in any specific psychological/psychotherapy studies as far as I know, as I have tried to show in a previous publication, his work on the intersubjective has a grossly underappreciated positive significance for psychoanalysis, especially when conceived as a spiritual discipline (Marcus, 2013). This being said, rather than mainly correlate Buber/Marcel's understandings of various psychoanalytic concepts as they relate to clinical practice (Oppenheim, 2017; Hoffman, 2011; Jewish and Christian narratives, respectively),[24] I want to focus on how their specifically spiritual insights (as defined above and throughout this book) can be helpfully integrated into mainstream clinical practice, such that they become part of the answer to the question, how does psychoanalysis, specifically a Buberian/Marcelian-inspired philosophy of dialogue, help an analysand artfully fashion a flourishing life? This is a life that Buber and Marcel would regard as consummated, culminated, and existentially grounded in the eternal/Absolute Thou and instantiated in a skillfully and wisely lived holy life (that implies autonomy, integration, and humanity).

For both Buber and Marcel, the key mechanism of change is to actualize transcendence in the healing dialogue between the analyst and analysand and, more importantly, enacting this transcendence-pointing outlook and behavior into one's everyday life. Transcendence, at least in its most elemental sense, means reaching out towards the other and his unique otherness. Such a centrifugal movement also implies a centripetal movement, one that is away from selfcentric ways of being-in-the-world. This is the difference between an existential orientation that is mainly being for the other versus being for oneself. Like all Axial-inspired thinkers, Buber and Marcel assume there is a "transcendent dimension in the core their [human] being," of which love, justice, peace, and other celebrated ethical/moral virtues were its instantiation (Armstrong, 2006, p. xvii). For Buber and Marcel, both believing humanists, transcendence was lodged in the intuitively sensed source and power of the eternal and Absolute Thou, respectively, the word God being its symbol, not the other way around. For example, in *I and Thou* Buber says that God "is the Being that is directly, most nearly, and lastingly, over against us, that may properly only be addressed and not expressed"; he is the "Absolute Person" who is encountered every time we meet our fellow human being or the world as "Thou" (Friedman, 1986, p. 15). Marcel was committed to what he called the "authentic, vertical transcendent, that is the transcendence, holiness, and sanctity of Christ and the martyrs"; he too believed that a life of holiness was the overarching goal of a well-lived life (Heffernan, 2017, pp. 17, 20). Says Marcel,

> When I myself speak here of a recourse to the transcendent, I mean, as concretely as possible, that our only chance in the sort of horrible situation I have imagined [the materialism and degradation associated with the broken world] is to appeal, I should perhaps *not* say to a power, but rather to a level of being, an order of the spirit, which is also the level and order of grace, of mercy, of charity..
>
> (Sweetman, 2011, p. 115)

Moreover, transcendence means "the absolute, impassable gulf which opens between the soul and Being whenever Being refuses us a hold" (e.g., giving oneself up to God as in the joined hands of the believer, who is amidst an unchangeable ordeal of suffering, or the non-believer, like the artist, who experiences the transcendent in "the most authentic and profound way") (ibid., p. 72, 116).

As I have said, for Buber and Marcel, transcendence, the reaching out to the other as a Thou, always implicates the absolute/Eternal Thou, in fact, they are mutually implicative ("meetings stand," said Buber, "under freedom and under grace" (1964, p. 20)). It is this aspect of their thought that is often underplayed, if even stated (or rejected) by most of the aforementioned contemporary relational psychoanalysts.[25]

Overall, I have tried to suggest that human existence, including problems in living and psychopathology, is best illuminated in terms of Buber and Marcel's spiritually animated dialogical philosophy and believing humanism (Buber's self-description). In this context, psychoanalytic treatment becomes a way of helping analysands move from ethical disablement or impairment towards a fuller, deeper, wider, and freer expression of their transcendence-pointing striving for holiness (a word/placeholder that one should not be afraid of using in analytic circles). In such a view, the individual is, at least in some sense, consciously or unconsciously always moving towards the transcendent, towards something more, higher, and better, conceived in ethical/moral terms as the Good, which implicates the eternal/Absolute Thou, as Buber and Marcel have suggested. For Buber and Marcel, while experiencing the transcendent is in some sense doable, this in no way means that it is conceptually understandable or can be accurately and completely described, for by definition it is beyond our human ways of thinking and speaking (it is only intimated). Marcel puts the matter just right:

> There is an order where the subject finds himself in the presence of something entirely beyond his grasp. I would add that if the word "transcendent" has any meaning it is here—it designates the absolute, unbridgeable chasm yawning between subject and being, insofar as being evades every attempt to pin it down.
>
> (1973, p. 193)

In this context, the self's responsibility for and to the other is central, and while its purest expression is possibly in martyrdom, it can take on many different forms, including the mutuality and reciprocity that both Buber and Marcel have described. What matters for Buber and Marcel is that the movement is toward the Thou, with its eternal and infinite echoes. That is, it is through the encounter with the eternal/Absolute Thou, through revelation that mainly takes place in the interhuman realm, that the homo viator finds/creates his unique destiny. This destiny is potentiated and instantiated by the love, justice, and peace he shows towards others in his earthly existence.[26]

Thus, one way to see the role of the analyst is to expand the analysand's awareness and understanding of what conscious and unconscious personal factors (e.g., thoughts, feelings, wishes, and fantasies) —and especially his strongly felt beliefs and values—impede, diminish, or take the place of his transcendent striving for something more, higher, and better (I have liberally drawn on Jacobs (2001) for the following comments). Drawing from Ogden, Aron, himself a Jewish believer who has "ideas about God with which I grew up and that continue to speak to me spiritually," has implied a similar overarching goal of psychoanalysis when he noted that "the ultimate value of psychoanalysis is for the analysand to choose life, to choose vitality, meaning, and authenticity" (2004, pp. 445, 449). This includes, for example: (1) deconstructing the many ways that analysands defend, insulate, and deceive themselves from feeling appropriate guilt, shame, remorse, and self-reproach for their misdeeds towards others (e.g., Buber's existential guilt versus neurotic guilt);[27] (2) understanding why the analysand is unmoved to reflect on, and critically reevaluate his selfish and immoral acts (not honoring the other), or even perceive that he has acted selfishly or hurtfully towards others. This involves analyzing the analysand's beliefs and values, especially within the context of his personal background and moral history, including the vulnerability, anxiety, pain, confusion, and conflict (i.e., the traumatic) that almost always sustains such ill-conceived and ill-fated beliefs and values and self-serving behavior;[28] and (3) understanding why the analysand is often unmoved by constructive criticisms of his immoral actions and associated feelings and thoughts, why they do not self-correct. The analyst needs to help the analysand work through his conscious reasons and unconscious motivations for willingly causing suffering to others, for being unjust (e.g., unfair) in his relationships. This means encouraging the analysand to see how his various moral lapses, often rooted in interference by his selfishness and inordinate desire for self-affirmation and gratification, make his own and his loved one's lives miserable. As Buber noted, "Where there is faith and love, a solution may be found even to what appears to be a tragic contradiction" (1957, p. 144).

Thus, we can say, that in such a Buberian/Marcelian-inspired form of psychoanalysis, we are always doing "character analysis." "Great character," says Buber, is "one who by his actions and attitudes satisfied the claim of situations out of deep readiness to respond with his whole life, and in such a way that the sum of his actions and attitudes expresses at the same time the unity of his being in its willingness to accept responsibility" (1965, p. 114). Responsibility is the response of the whole person to what addresses him in the immediacy of the lived concrete situation. The aim is to help the analysand recognize and deeply appreciate, in the widest sense, ethical/moral considerations (without moralizing) that negatively impact the other and oneself. Most importantly, this means being motivated by strongly felt, flexibly and creatively applied, transcendent-pointing moral beliefs and values that are primarily other-directed, other-regarding, and other-serving, which according to Buber and Marcel is the "royal road" to holiness. In a Buberian/Marcelian-glossed psychoanalytic language, this means helping the analysand become a morally autonomous and integrated individual, one who has the effective cognitive, emotional, and motivational capacity to be stably devoted and attached to the Beautiful, True, and most importantly, the Good. From the analyst's point of view, this means learning how to genuinely listen, a subject of great interest in analytic theory but beyond the scope of this chapter. For Buber and Marcel, genuine listening means motivating and encouraging in the analysand the will and ability to skillfully, artfully, and wisely create his own meanings (including beliefs, values, and truths) in the immediacy of the present, which quite likely will be very different than the analysts (Gordon, 2011, p. 207).[29] Says Buber,

> Genuine conversation, and therefore every actual fulfilment and relation between men, means acceptance of otherness. When two men inform one another of their basically different views about an object, each aim to convince the other of the rightness of his own way of looking at the matter, everything depends so far as human life is concerned, on whether each thinks of the other as the one he is, whether each, that is, with all his desire

> to influence the other, nevertheless unreservedly accepts and confirms him in his being this man and in his being made in this particular way.
>
> (1998, p. 59)

What kind of inner attitude does the analysand need to fashion the aforementioned way of being in the world? First, it requires that the analysand ask different and tough questions of himself. While the typical analysand asks, "Why do I exist rather than not," the Buberian/Marcelian–inspired analysand also asks, "Have I the right to be, am I worthy of being?" The typical analysand asks, "What do I hope for, what do I desire to be happy?" The Buberian/Marcelian–inspired analysand also asks, "What must I do?" In other words, the psychoanalyst prompts the analysand to ask additional existential questions, ethical/moral questions that cut deeper and are altogether more disruptive. The Buberian/Marcelian–inspired analysand's words do not follow Descartes—I think or I want or even I feel—but rather, as Levinas says, are like Abraham's response to the summoning call of God to serve Him, "Here I am." In this context, the meaning, truth, and value of the analysand's life are to a large extent approached in terms of his response to the other's call; the analysand lives less in terms of his self-serving desire, as for power or acquisitions, and more in terms of the Beautiful, True, and especially the Good—a life devoted less to questing after fame and fortune and more to service to others. For Buber and Marcel (and Levinas), responsibility for others thus becomes the fundamental meaning of his self-identity. Put differently, it is a question of giving themselves/availability or withholding themselves/unavailability. To do otherwise is what Buber called *"vegegnung,"* a made-up word for "'mismeeting' or 'miscounter' to designate the failure of real meeting [sometimes traumatically so] between men" (1973, p. 18).

Psychoanalysis as a spiritual discipline can be thus viewed in terms of helping the analysand, conceived as a homo viator, to artfully fashion a flourishing life. That is, the analysand is a spiritual itinerant on a "journey" that leads from "appearance to reality, bondage to liberation, confusion to insight, darkness to light" (Erikson, 2006, p. 5). As Buber noted, the goal is in part the "regeneration of an atrophied personal centre" (1958, p. 133).[30] That is, "inner transformation simply means surpassing one's present factual constitution; it means that the person one is intended to be penetrates what has appeared up until now, that the customary soul enlarges and transfigures itself into the surprise soul" (Buber, 1957, p. 206). He begins with critical questions: How do I view myself? How do I find myself situated in the world? Answering these questions involves the analysand looking at himself as an object of study, based largely, though not entirely, on the frame and filter of his childhood experiences. In other words, these questions assume that what one takes oneself to be, shapes who we are and how we live our life (Kelly, 2013). Second, the analysand critically asks, how can I develop the will and ability to go about transforming myself into something I regard as better? This involves viewing one's God-given freedom (as Buber and Marcel might say) as a Foucauldian-animated self-transformative practice. Such a practice of freedom is both retrospective (how do I get free of myself, such as from my inordinate narcissism and egocentricity?) and prospective (how do I self-transform as an ethical commitment to becoming better, such as being for the other), based on what resources one has in the present (Koopman, 2013). For Buber and Marcel, these are mainly dialogical resources that implicate the eternal/Absolute Thou, and include freely embracing a way of life that is primarily other-directed, other-regarding, and other-serving, a holy life, that in many ways is instantiated in the "best" of the Judeo-Christian moral outlook, as with the ethicality we associate with the Hebrew prophets and with Jesus.[31] Exactly how this is done, what practices and processes are enacted, is of course up to the analysand and analyst to work out between them, though it typically depends on the "language game," the version of psychoanalysis the analyst is allied with. The point, however, is that these practices of freedom become enmeshed in one's way of being-in-the-world and represent a particular form of life reflecting the aforementioned self-transformative processes and ethical/moral commitments. For Buber and Marcel, such a spiritual outlook is grounded in the free, flowing, and unrestrained dialogical relation of I-Thou: "This fragile life between birth and death can nevertheless be a fulfillment—if it is a dialogue" (Buber, 1966, p. 19). From a dialogical point of view then, this so-called maturity, or what I would more aptly call practical wisdom, "is neither knowingness nor independence [though these qualities are not to be underappreciated], but an ability to live well in time and space, so that life is graced by a capacity for wholeness and wonder"—in other words, a spiritually animated form of dialogical mindfulness in which the aforementioned process "leads back to the holiness of the whole" (Metcalfe & Game, 2008, pp. 355, 356).

Final word

The idea of psychoanalysis conceived as a spiritual discipline, particularly one that is lodged in the dialogical personalism of Buber and Marcel, may seem like a version that is so top-heavy with "god-talk" and religious/spiritual categories and language that it is beyond the way mainstream psychoanalysis (including its postmodern tendencies) views itself, let alone operates in the clinical context (i.e., accusing me of bringing God, or even worse, moralism, in through the back door). However, as Orange noted, "Dialogic philosophy [e.g., she highlights Buber, though not Marcel] is a better resource than 'postmodernism' for our clinical practice" (2010, p. 12). Moreover, as Oppenheim noted, in contemporary psychoanalysis, such as in the works of "Mitchell, Benjamin, and Hoffman, there are moments of breakthrough, but also a persistent underlying, literalist suspicion concerning religious concepts and values" (2017, p. 153). As I pointed out in my introductory chapter, while there has been some appropriation of Eastern religion/spirituality (Vaidyanathan & Kripal, 2002, Hinduism) into psychoanalysis, mainly Buddhist ideas (Molino, 2013), the fact is not much has been done by analysts, qua believers (of some hybrid variety) who are lodged in Judeo-Christian outlook and morality. It is up to the reader to decide whether the aforementioned resonates with their personal experience. For the believer, I am sure a lot of it does, but there is no security or guarantee, as Buber and Marcel repeatedly stated. This lack of security and guarantee, even plausibility, is that much truer for those non-believers who don't feel addressed by Buber and Marcel, who don't have the analogous faith experiences they describe, and who point to a lack of objective (or quasi-objective) criteria or methods for understanding the relation to the eternal/Absolute Thou. I urge such readers, which is by far most analysts and other mental health professional, to approach this book (and other such books) without preconceived opinions and judgments (Buber, 1964, p. 96). Marcelian availability—ready, reactive, responsive, and responsible—is the only port of entry into the mystery of being, including of the eternal and infinite Being.

This being said, my position is not as anachronistic as one might think. For example, as early as 1953, Hans Loewald, a Freudian with revisionist tendencies, opined that the "mature individual" is "able to reach back into his deep origins and roots of being [his 'soul' as Buber/Marcel might say] find[ing] in himself the oneness from where he stems [the ultimate 'ground' of his being] and understand[ing] this in his freedom as his bond of love with God," with the noncorporeal "whole" cosmic consciousness, ethicality. Loewald's "god-talk" is his way of describing the cosmic vision and oceanic sentiment, its associated ethical outlook, and the analytical goal of helping analysands become "spiritual beings," as he called them, to achieve the "highest form of awareness … the freedom for faith and love" (1953, pp. 13, 14, 15). Loewald never backed off this point of view, as far as I know.

The late Lewis Aron, one of the major proponents of contemporary relational psychoanalysis, who appreciated Buber's (and other Jewish thinkers') philosophy of dialogue, wrote in 2004, "Indeed, psychoanalysis may be envisioned as a form of worship, in which contact is made with the Almighty through immersion in the richness and depth of the inner life and in communion with the Other" (2004, p. 450). Moreover, sounding like Buber and Marcel, Aron noted that "being deeply engaged with God, imitating God's ways, may paradoxically help keep us [analysts] from playing God" (ibid.). He approvingly referenced Michael Eigen's book on Judaism and psychoanalysis (1998) that "described psychoanalysis as a form of prayer" (ibid.) which aims to expand and deepen the person's sense of discovered/created identity.

Hoffman (2011), herself a believer who is lodged in non-fundamentalist, conservative, and evangelical Christian theology, provides a theoretical and clinical perspective on relational psychoanalysis and the Christian narrative. Her claim is that intersubjectivity as understood in Christian theology and intersubjectivity in relational psychoanalysis (i.e., Jessica Benjamin's theory of mutual recognition) are correlated in important ways, though also different.

She twins three phases of psychoanalytic treatment—identification, surrender, and gratitude—with the Christian notions of incarnation, crucifixion, and resurrection. Hoffman is clearly inspired by her faith in a transcendent God that is in play in the clinical context; for example, she declares: "A loving force for life, Hegel's *Geist* [Spirit], God's grace, is operative in the evolution of culture and the transformation of individual lives in the consultation room" (p. 219). She also refers to the divinely inspired "gift[s]" of faith, love, and hope (pp. 166–167), and plausibly shows via a detailed clinical study that there is a creative way of not only correlating, but integrating some spiritual and psychoanalytic dynamics within the clinical context.

Eigen (2012, 2014), another hybrid believer, strongly influenced by Bion in his psychoanalytic outlook, also draws from the Judeo-Christian outlook and morality (and Eastern as well as other sources) in his understanding of the role of religion/spirituality in clinical psychoanalysis. One of the key notions animating Eigen's book on mysticism (1998) is the experiencing of God, not inevitably as a Being external to the self or a personal God (though it could be), but mainly in our personal and group lives, in the delights and anguish of the life and death of the self. Calling to mind Marcel's homo viator, psychoanalysis is conceived as "a psychospiritual journey" (ibid., p. 160). For example, he noted,

> I feel that what you call that other dimension [the spiritual/divine] is here, always here. Whatever you call God or spiritual reality is right here, in our lives. We are creating it and it is creating us through the way we are with each other, how we make each other feel. Do our interactions make a more kindly world or a less kindly world? It reminds me of what Judaism says—that my words are creating angels and devils."
>
> (Eigen, 2014, pp. 98–99)[32]

His book *Faith* is replete with such terms as "holy," "sacred," "I believe in miracles," and "goodness," all words that resonate with Buber and Marcel's dialogical personalism (ibid., 99, 100).[33] Finally, Eigen powerfully affirms an existential attitude that has animated my study:

> There is no reason to place artificial limits on where or how far therapy should go. Throughout my career I have heard that therapy is not a religion, and must stop short of the religious dimension. Perhaps this is true for many practitioners but it has never been so for me. Therapy is a holy business for me and was so from my first session, as patient and as therapist.
>
> (1998, pp. 41–42)

I can cite other psychoanalytically lodged authors who affirm aspects of the aforementioned Judeo-Christian faith/God/religion/spirituality nexus, but I think the point has been made that it is time for mainstream psychoanalysis to seriously engage with the dialogical personalist philosophies of Buber and

Marcel, and other likeminded religious/spiritual thinkers. For their insights can profoundly enhance our discipline and directly "speak" to our current (and potential) analysands, patients, and clients who are trying to make their suffering sufferable, including from interhuman/intersubjective "hunger," if not "starvation," neglect, and abuse, as Buber and Marcel have detailed it. Moreover, our critics who view psychoanalysis as a "has been" discipline may come to realize in following Mark Twain's famous attributed quip, "The reports of my death are greatly exaggerated."

Notes

1 Wholeness and uniqueness also imply *unity*; in fact, Buber and Marcel use this word in their descriptions of I-Thou relations and in many contexts. For example, Buber speaks about "wholeness, unity, and uniqueness" in *Between Man and Man* (Friedman, 1986, p. 56), while Marcel refers to recollecting oneself as a "unity" via secondary reflection and "suprapersonal unity" in *The Mystery of Being* (2001b, p. 182). There is little doubt that a sense of unity is an important aspect of one's self-conception, though too much unity can be detrimental (e.g., over-coherence). Exactly what unity of self means, and how it is instantiated in "real life," is a hugely complex issue, with no consensus among scholars (the same is true for wholeness and uniqueness). For example, philosopher Stephen L. White (1991) claims that the unity of the self is manifested in personal identity and moral responsibility and is probably best conceptualized in terms of normative considerations. Buber and Marcel might well have been sympathetic with this formulation. To make matters even more complex, Buber said, "No man can know his own unity" (Buber, 1967b, p. 171), yet he also wrote "Genuine life is unification" (1957, p. 34).

2 See Sweetman (2008) for a thoughtful response to aspects of the postmodern critique as it pertains to Marcel. See also Treanor's (2006) impressive defense of Marcel from Levinas's criticisms, a thinker he claims significantly overlapped with Marcel on many substantial points. Likewise, see Atterton and colleagues (2004) on dialogue and the difference between Buber and Levinas; again, there is considerable theoretical and practical overlap between these dialogical thinkers despite the pilpul of the specialists. In fact, Lipari (2004) makes a strong case for the Buber–Levinas encounter as one characterized by "failed" encounters for communication ethics (miscommunication and misrecognition), in that they did not listen to the other and embrace their otherness. Says Lipari, Buber and Levinas agreed with each other a lot more than they disagreed on substantial points, notwithstanding their apparent unconscious need to distinguish themselves qua original thinkers for self-serving reasons. As I have said, while these giants (Buber, Levinas, Marcel) had their idiosyncratic trajectories, and certainly do differ on specific philosophical/theological points, in many ways they arrived at the same or a very similar endpoint in terms of everyday praxis, including as it pertains to fashioning a flourishing life. Love, said Marcel, is the "essential ontological datum," and Buber and Levinas would agree with the gist of this claim (1965a, p. 167).

3 It is worth mentioning that Thomas Ogden, one of the original independent thinkers in psychoanalysis, noted, "Most fundamentally the analytic relationship exists for the purpose of helping the analysand make psychological changes ["psychological

growth"] that will enable him to live his life in a more fully human way" (2004, pp. 109, 3). Exactly what is meant by a "more fully human way" is not detailed, nor are any criteria provided for its instantiation; rather, it appears to be assumed that most readers know what this means.

4 Marcel also distinguishes between the individual and the person. The former is "the *one* in the fragmented state," like a "statistical factor"; but for the "absolute person, the already-fragile distinction between the relatively passive act of confronting and the active one of assuming is completely abolished; the absolute person tends to posit itself as wholly responsible for history" (Sweetman, 2011, p. 78).

5 It should be noted that somewhat similar to Buber and Marcel, Foucault believed that non-reciprocity and dissymmetry in relationships can indicate domination, such as the social superiority and contempt for the other in ancient Greece (Gros, 1994, p. 532).

6 Levinas claims that there is a "primordial responsibility for the other," however, he does not demonstrate or "prove" that this so-called responsibility is an assumed universal, inherent structure of being, rather than, for example a socially constructed meaning and valuative attachment that he and every good man embraces (Levinas, 2001, p. 182).

7 Loewald notes that a for "mature" person responsibility means "to own up to our own history, to be responsible for our unconscious," which implies that it is one's responsibility to be the author of one's existence, including behaving towards others in an other-directed, other-regarding and other-serving manner (1978, p. 21).

8 Authenticity is one of those evocative philosophical/psychological terms that is hard to define and instantiate, in fact, there is no consensus on exactly what it means and refers to. For example, Charles Rycroft (1995, p. 10) points out, while psychoanalysis frequently makes distinctions between actions and behavior "which are done in good and bad faith, which are true and false to the self," it has no rigorous way "of making the distinction, nor the similar one between 'sincere' and 'insincere,'" although clinical work often relies on the analyst being able to make such fine distinctions. Authenticity might be serviceably defined for my purposes as each person for the most part, is the author and creator of his way of being-in-the-world (his modality of existence).

9 In clarifying these basic Marcelian concepts, I have liberally drawn from Sweetman's books (2008, 2011) and his other writings on Marcel as they are eminently clear and accessible to the non-specialist and specialist alike. Likewise, Treanor (2006) and his other writings on Marcel were very useful.

10 I should remind the reader that what is "me" and the "other," let alone uniquely me and the other, is hardly an easy distinction to make. For what constitutes these similarities and differences, and what criterion to use to discern them, is a hugely complex matter which philosophers have been opining about for a very long time, with no majority agreement. Someone should write a Foucauldian-inspired genealogical study of these terms.

11 Virtue ethics means different things to different people, though Nietzsche/Foucault scholar Ansell-Patterson (2013, p. 425) noted, "We can describe both Nietzsche and Foucault [non-believers] as modern-day virtue ethicists," for they strive to free the potential of individual self-choice and personal self-fashioning from oppressive homogenization and normalization. Buber and Marcel would probably not agree with the gist of this formulation. As Sweetman (2008; 2011) notes, virtue ethics

refers to the theory that emanates from Aristotle; it would not generally be used to describe the perspectives of Nietzsche and Foucault, who opposed the notion of human nature. Buber and Marcel would favor traditional virtue ethics to some degree since they support an objective account of human nature. They would not support developing the self through self-fashioning, since this suggests relativism, which they did not adhere to.

12 According to Friedman, Freud and other versions of psychoanalysis "places the unconscious within the person alone, reality is seen as psychic rather than interhuman" (Agassi, 1999, p. 230). I am not sure that Friedman's point still applies with the force it had in 1999, given contemporary developments in psychoanalysis. Buber also criticized Freud and Jung for their "psychologism," not dealing with the ontic dimension of human existence (cosmic phenomena are understood as psychic), among other issues, in his correspondence and elsewhere (1964, p. 81). As Buber noted, in "psychologizing of the world," the "non-psychic reality is obliterated, that this fundamental relation of I to a world [e.g., Being] ceases to be able to be a relation I to Thou" (Buber, 1967b, p. 144).

13 The notion of mutuality is a significant one in contemporary relational psychoanalysis, beginning with Sandor Ferenczi's "mutual analysis." Such analysts as Ehrenberg (1974), Mitchell (1993), Ogden (1994), and Aron (1996) have extensively treated this subject, asserting that the analytic process is co-produced or "co-constructed" by the analysand and analyst, and a degree of self-disclosure by the analyst is necessary and useful to the analysand. For Buber, in contrast to Carl Rogers, "equality" does not exist between the analyst and analysand, mainly because of their objectively different social roles. The analyst is the "expert" provider of a therapeutic service and the analysand is the suffering consumer. This means, according to Buber, that the power dynamics are asymmetrical from the get-go in favor of the analyst who sees with less neurotic or other distortion what is going on (he has a somewhat detached presence, says Buber), and the analysand is not typically geared to know and understand the analyst in a similar manner (though in the transference, this certainly occurs). Thus, Buber equates equality to similar role-dependent attitudes, within the totality of circumstances of the analytic dyad, that make the analyst and analyst unequal. For Rogers, equality cannot be judged this way. That is, equality is accomplished "in moments of mutual recognition of basic personness, even if the participants have dissimilar role limitations" (Anderson & Cissna, 1997, p. 38). Likewise, for Rogers, and many relational analysts, analysts and analysands can engage in "mutual listening on equal *experiential* footing, even if not on fully equal *role* footing" (ibid., p. 41). In other words, when the relationship is critically evaluated externally and analytically, it looks unequal, yet experientially, at least in good analysis, there is a sense by both participants that there is an "equal validity as persons" (ibid., p. 45). Whether there can ever be an absolutely equal relationship is debatable, especially since it is hard to generate a credible and verifiable way of making such a judgment. Buber made clear that "'asymmetry' is only one of the possibilities of the I-Thou relation"; similarly, "'mutuality' has many 'gradations' and cannot not be regarded as the rule." There also are "various stages of the I-It state," depending on one's estrangement from the Thou relation (1964, p. 28, 57).

14 Indeed, there is an abundance of psychotherapy outcome studies in "the contemporary American psychoanalytic literature" that indicates the relevance of a warm, genuine, and open rapport and a "positive alliance" that matters most, and tellingly,

"not necessarily the analysis of it [the alliance, including the transference], or the preoccupation with discussing it" (Curtis, 2009, p. 113).

15 Confirmation includes acceptance, which means not making heavy-handed ethical/moral judgments and embracing the patient on his own terms. Confirmation, which includes a trust aspect, says Buber to Carl Rogers, is "accepting the whole potentiality of the other and making even a decisive difference in his potentiality. Of course, we can be mistaken again and again in this, but it's just a chance between human beings" (Agassi, 1999, p. 266). In other words, acceptance involves accepting the analysand in the immediacy of the present and acceptance of his potentiality, qua person. This can involve challenge if not confrontation always in the context of a trusting relationship, that is, truth spoken lovingly (Anderson & Cissna, 1997, pp. 92, 95).

16 It is worth mentioning that most people in Western society have a god-image of some kind, whether they are believers or non-believers. Moreover, the god the non-believer repudiates may be pertinent to understanding the analysand's self-conception, and most importantly, it may illuminate his valuative attachments and subsequent behavior, as it does in the case of the believer (Rizzuto, 1979).

17 As Buber said, the "most essential concern" in his work is "the central significance of the close association of the relationship to God with the relation to one's fellow-men" (1965, pp. 123–124).

18 This means becoming unique, singular, unrivaled, self-fashioning, and self-legislating (Ansell-Pearson, 2015).

19 Buber and Marcel recognize a duality of structure to human existence, that is, man is fundamentally selfcentric (Marcel's original sin); witness an infant where his utterly self-serving needs are the bedrock of his existence (an It existence). However, there is also a reaching towards the other; initially, this is the infant's need-satisfying reaching towards the object, the parental caregiver, but as the child evolves into a person, including deepening and expanding his capacity for ethical/moral transformation (emotional, cognitive, and behavioral), he can encounter the other, and he longs for interhuman/intersubjective relation, to say Thou. As Buber noted,

> Through the fact that he enters into essential reciprocity, man becomes revealed as man; indeed, that only with this and through this does he attain to that valid participation in being that is reserved for him; the saying ofThou by the I stands in the origin of all individual human becoming.
>
> (1965, p. 209)

20 I am indebted to Oppenheim, (2017), who itemized the four aforementioned psychoanalytic references.

21 Buber apparently got this idea from Carl Rogers during their dialogue in 1957, a year before *I and Thou* was published. Said Rogers: "If this client comes to the point where he can experience what he is expressing, but also can experience my understanding of it and reaction to it, and so on, that really therapy is just about over." Buber responded, "Yes. This is just what I mean" (Anderson & Cissna, 1997, p. 39).

22 Buber believed that it is not possible to have "dialogue with oneself," mainly because "it lacks the otherness and surprise [of mutuality] necessary for real dialogue" (Anderson & Cissna, 1997, p. 70). However, one can argue that the otherness of the unconscious as analysts usually formulate it, and the surprise associated with

realizing something new about oneself, all in the context of analytic conversation, constitutes a reasonable family resemblance to Buber's criterion. This being said, as Bion quipped, "Life is full of surprises. Most of them bad" (Eigen, 1998, p. 134). Buber's notion of the unconscious is "the ground of being of the person" (1964, p. 39).

23 Metcalfe & Game (2008) differentiate the mind in dialogue; it is ecological and not Euclidean, "it is not what one subject gives to another, but is the sense of differences within a network characterized by feedback" (p. 353).

24 This is not to say that there isn't a lot to learn from Oppenheim and Hoffman, who at times interestingly go beyond correlations and try to show how Jewish and Christian narratives can amplify relational psychoanalytic notions. And to be fair, both authors do from time to time attempt to synthesize the religious and psychological traditions as have other authors.

25 Oppenheim (2017) singles out Jessica Benjamin for particular criticism in this regard, claiming that "Buber's understanding of mature religiosity stands in dialectical opposition to Benjamin's [negative] portrayal," and he accuses her of not reckoning with his work on intersubjectivity (let alone Marcel's), calling it "the missing Buber" (pp. 67, 68). In contrast, is Jones (1991), an Episcopal priest and psychoanalytically glossed clinical psychologist who in the last chapter of his praiseworthy book *Toward Psychoanalysis of the Sacred* declares:

> If there is no escaping dependency on a selfobject milieu, there is nothing childish about acknowledging connection to a self-sustaining universal matrix. If selves necessarily stand in relation, it is not necessarily irrational to ask if this complex of selves in relation does not itself stand in relation.
>
> (1991, p. 135)

26 As Buber put it, "Creation is not a hurdle on the road to God, it is the road itself. We are created along with one another and directed to a life with one another" (1965, p. 52). Marcel believes similarly: "My deepest and most unshakeable conviction... is that... it is not God's will at all to be loved by us *against* the Creation, but rather glorified *through* the Creation and with the Creation as our starting point (1965a, p. 135). It should be emphasized, however, that for Buber and Marcel such a destiny is almost always preceded by and interspersed with forms of suffering that need to be metabolized and survived, and/or a Buddhist-like emptiness, a positive void that involves an "unselving" (Eigen, 1998, p. 154). Analyst Marion Milner calls this emptiness "expectant waiting" that is the psychological staging ground for transcendence (Raab, 2000, p. 188).

27 For Buber, there is "original guilt," which is equated with withholding oneself and remaining in oneself (Marcel's unavailability); "existential guilt," which is an ontic, interhuman domain the person resides in: "He has injured an order of the human world whose foundation he knows and recognizes as those of his own existence and of all common human existence"; and "neurotic guilt," which is "groundless," a subjective/psychological feeling inside a person (Buber, 1998, pp. 116, 117). Neurotic guilt is what psychoanalysis tends to focus on, though most guilty feelings are a hybrid phenomenon constituted by the aforementioned three forms of guilt. Marcel also discusses existential guilt, "guilt with which a person as such has burdened himself," and is not comprehended using such categories as repression, violating an unconscious taboo, and making conscious (Sweetman, 2011, p. 147).

28 Ogden (2016) describes something similar in his notion of trauma "that is left 'unlived'" (p. 3), that has not been emotionally metabolized mainly because the analysand is "bound, tied and gagged" (my words, e.g., dissociated, deadened) by his inability to freely and critically think/feel. The analytic context, a "sacred space" as a colleague called it (p. 7), permits such emotional processing of the truth of experience to occur.

29 Metcalfe and Game, both educators, offer a beautiful description of the reciprocal nature of speaking and listening, one that is in sync with my reading of Buberian/Marcelian dialogue as it applies to psychoanalysis as a spiritual discipline: "Dialogue is not an excess of giving, or even a sequence of giving and then receiving, but a receiving that gives and a giving that receives. It is the ability to listen that allows teachers [analysts] to know what is called for at any stage of the class" [the analysis] (2008, p. 352). Indeed, listening demands the analyst's will and ability to "attend imaginatively to another's language," and most importantly perhaps, "the analyst is able to hear only what he, potentially at least, is able to say" (Farber, 1956, p. 115). As Buber said, "The good teacher [analyst] educates by his speech and silence... he must be a really existing man and he must be really present to his pupils [analysands]; he educates through contact" (Buber, 1967b, p. 102).

30 Buber also uses the phrase "the atrophy of the spirit within" to designate what needs to change (1957, p. 118).

31 Buber says that that Goethe was a free person capable of genuine dialogue with nature; Socrates engaged in such dialogue with his fellow humans, while Jesus had an un-narcissistic personal relation with the Father.

32 In an interview, Eigen says that by God he mainly means "a biblical God, the God of Abraham, Isaac and Jacob"; however, he then humbly qualifies his testimonial and says, "Hey, well, what I mean by God could be anything, because I don't know" (1998, p. 193).

33 Sounding very similar to Buber and Marcel, Eigen notes, "If I do not draw from the Holy Spirit on a daily basis, I become a semi-collapsed version of myself. We are sustained directly by God, not only through others. We are sustained by others, not only by God" (1998, p. 163).

References

Agassi, J. B. (1999). (Ed.) *Martin Buber on psychology and psychotherapy: Essays, letters, and dialogues*. Syracuse, NY: Syracuse University Press.

Anderson, R., & Cissna, K. N. (1997). *The Martin Buber–Carl Rogers dialogue: A new transcript with commentary*. Albany: State University of New York Press.

Ansell-Pearson, K. (2015). Questions of the subject in Nietzsche and Foucault. In J. Constancio, M. J. M. Branco, & B. Ryan (Eds.), *Nietzsche and the problem of subjectivity* (pp. 411–435). Berlin: De Gruyter.

Anshen, R. N. (1967). Credo perspectives. Their meaning and function. In M. Buber (1967). (Trans. M. Friedman). *A believing humanism—My testament, 1902–1965* (pp. 11–19). New York: Simon & Schuster.

Appelfeld, A. (1994). (Trans. J. M. Green). *Beyond despair: Three lectures and a conversation with Philip Roth*. New York: International Publishing.

Ardito, R. B., & Rabellino, D. (2011). Therapeutic alliance and outcome of psychotherapy: Historical excursus, measurements, and prospects of research. *Frontiers of Psychology, 2,* 270. https://doi.org/10.3389/fpsyg.2011.00270

Aron, L. & Starr, K. (2013). *A psychotherapy for the people: Toward a progressive psychoanalysis.* New York: Routledge.

Armstrong, K. (2006). *The great transformation: The beginning of the religious traditions.* New York: Knopf.

Aron, L (1996). *A meeting of minds. Mutuality in psychoanalysis.* Hillsdale, NJ: Analytic Press.

Aron, L. (2004). God's influence on my psychoanalytic vision and values. *Psychoanalytic Psychology, 21*(3), 442–451.

Aron, L., Grand, S., & Slochower, J. (2018). (Eds.). *De-idealizing relational Theory: A critique from within.* London: Routledge.

Atterton, P., Calarco, M., & Friedman, M. (Eds.). (2004). *Levinas and Buber: Dialogue and difference.* Pittsburgh, PA: Duquesne University Press.

Baron, L. (1996). Introduction. In M. Friedman (Ed.), *Martin Buber and the human sciences* (pp. 249–251). Albany: State University of New York Press.

Bollnow, O. F. (1984). The concept of availability. In P. A. Schilpp & L. E. Hahn (Eds.), *The philosophy of Gabriel Marcel* (pp. 177–199). La Salle, IL: Open Court.

Buber, M. (1957). (Trans. M. Friedman). *Pointing the way: Collected essays.* Atlantic Highlands, NJ: Humanities Press.

Buber, M. (1958). (Trans. R. G. Smith). *I and Thou* (2nd ed.). New York: Charles Scribner's Sons.

Buber, M. (1964). (Eds. S. Rome and B. Rome) *Philosophical interrogations.* New York : Holt.

Buber, M. (1965). (Trans. R. G. Smith). *Between man and man.* New York: Macmillan.

Buber, M. (1966). *The way of response.* New York: Schocken.

Buber, M. (1967a). (Ed. N. N. Glatzer). *On Judaism.* New York: Schocken.

Buber, M. (1967b). (Trans. M. Friedman). *A believing humanism: My testament, 1902–1965.* New York: Simon & Schuster.

Buber, M. (1973). (Ed. M. Friedman). *Meetings.* LaSalle, IL: Open Court.

Buber, M. (1998). (Ed. M. Friedman; Trans. M. Friedman & R. G. Smith). *The knowledge of man: A philosophy of the interhuman.* New York: Harper & Row.

Charles, M. (Ed.). (2018). *Introduction to contemporary psychoanalysis.* London: Routledge.

Cooper, S. H. (2000). *Objects of hope: Exploring possibility and limit in psychoanalysis.* Hillsdale, NJ: Humanity Books.

Curtis, R. C. (2009). *Desire, self, mind, and the psychotherapies: Unifying psychological science and psychoanalysis.* Lanham, MD: Jason Aronson.

Ehrenberg, D. B. (1974). The intimate edge in therapeutic relatedness. *Contemporary Psychoanalysis, 10,* 423–437.

Ehrenberg, D. B. (1992). *The intimate edge. Extending the reach of psychoanalytic interaction.* New York: Norton.

Eigen, M. (1998). *The psychoanalytic mystic.* Binghamton, NY: ESF Publishers.

Eigen, M. (2012). *Kabbalah and psychoanalysis.* London: Routledge.

Eigen, M. (2014). *Faith.* London: Karnac.

Erikson, S. A. (2006). *Philosophy as a guide to living* (course guidebook). Chantilly, VA: The Teaching Company.

Farber, L. H. (1956). Martin Buber and psychiatry. *Psychiatry, 19*(2), 109–120.

Farber, L. H., Howe, R. L., & Friedman, M. S. (1956). Martin Buber and psychotherapy: What is effective in the therapeutic process. *Pastoral Psychology*, 7, 46–53.
Freud, S. (1905). On psychotherapy. In J. Strachey (Ed. & Trans.), *The standard edition of the complete psychological works of Sigmund Freud* (vol. 7, pp. 257–268). London: Hogarth.
Freud, S. (1917). Introductory lectures on psycho-analysis. In J. Strachey (Ed. & Trans.), *The standard edition of the complete psychological works of Sigmund Freud* (vol. 16, pp. 243–463). London: Hogarth.
Freud, S. (1923). The ego and the Id. In J. Strachey (Ed. & Trans.), *The standard edition of the complete psychological works of Sigmund Freud* (vol. 19, pp. 3–36). London: Hogarth.
Friedman, M. (1967). Martin Buber's credo. In M. Buber (1967). (Trans. M. Friedman), *A believing humanism—My testament, 1902–1965* (pp. 21–30). New York: Simon & Schuster.
Friedman, M. (1985). *The healing dialogue in psychotherapy*. Northvale, NJ: Jason Aronson.
Friedman, M. (1986). *Martin Buber and the Eternal*. New York: Human Sciences Press.
Friedman, M. (1992). *Religion and psychology: A dialogical approach*. New York: Paragon House.
Friedman, M. (1996). Martin Buber's "Narrow Ridge" and the human sciences. In M. Friedman (Ed.), *Martin Buber and the human sciences* (pp. 3–25). Albany: State University of New York Press.
Gordon, M. (2011). Listening as embracing the other: Martin Buber's philosophy of dialogue. *Educational Theory*, *61*(2), 207–219.
Gros, F. (1994). Course Context. In Gros, F. (Ed.), G. Burchell (Trans.) *Michel Foucault. The Hermeneutics of the Subject. Lectures at the College De France. 1981–1982.* (pp. 507–550). New York: Picador.
Heerry, M., & Bugental, J. F. T. (2005). Meaning and transformation. In E.V. Deurzen & C. Arnold-Baker (Eds.), *Existential perspective on human issues* (pp. 253–264). Basingstoke: Palgrave Macmillan.
Heffernan, G. (2017). The meaningless life is not worth living: Critical reflections on Marcel's critique of Camus. *Marcel Studies*, *2*, 1–22.
Hernandez, J. G. (2011). *Gabriel Marcel's ethics of hope. evil, God and virtue*. London: Bloomsbury.
Hoffman, M.T. (2011). *Toward mutual recognition. Relational psychoanalysis and the Christian narrative*. London: Routledge.
Jacobs, J. (2001). *Choosing character: Responsibility for virtue and vice*. Ithaca, NY: Cornell University Press.
Jones, J. W. (1991). *Contemporary psychoanalysis & religion: Transference and transcendence*. New Haven: Yale University Press.
Kaufman, W. E. (1992). *Contemporary Jewish philosophies*. Detroit: Wayne State University Press.
Keen, S. (1967a). *Gabriel Marcel*. Richmond, VA: John Knox Press.
Keen, S. M. (1967b). Gabriel Marcel. In P. Edwards (Ed.), *Encyclopedia of philosophy* (vol. 5, pp. 153–155). New York: Macmillan.
Keen, S. M. (2006) Gabriel Marcel. In D. M. Borchert (Ed.), *Encyclopedia of philosophy* (2nd ed., vol. 1, pp. 701–703). New York: Macmillan.
Kelly, M. G. E. (2013). Foucault, subjectivity, and technologies of the self. In C. Falzon, T. O'Leary, & J. Sawicki (Eds.), *A companion to Foucault* (pp. 510–525). Malden, MA: Wiley-Blackwell.

Koopman, C. (2013). The formation and self-transformation of the subject in Foucault's ethics. In C. Falzon, T. O'Leary, & J. Sawicki (Eds.), *A companion to Foucault* (pp. 526–543). Malden, MA: Wiley-Blackwell.

Kramer, K. P., & Gawlick, M. (2003). *Martin Buber's I and Thou: Practicing living dialogue.* New York: Paulist Press.

Levinas, E. (1989). (Ed. S. Hand). *Difficult freedom: Essays on Judaism.* Baltimore, MD: Johns Hopkins University Press.

Levinas, E. (2001). (Ed. J. Robbins). *Is it righteous to be? Interviews with Emanuel Levinas.* Stanford, CA: Stanford University Press.

Lipari, L. (2004). Listening to the Other: Ethical implications of the Buber-Levinas encounter. *Communication Theory, 14*(2), 122–141.

Loewald, H. (1953). Psychoanalysis and modern views on human existence and religious experience. *Journal of Pastoral Care,* 7(1), 1–15.

Loewald, H. (1978). *Psychoanalysis and the history of the individual: The Freud lectures at Yale.* New Haven, CT: Yale University Press.

Marcel, G. (1952). (Trans. B. Wall). *Metaphysical journal.* Chicago: Henry Regnery.

Marcel, G. (1962). Foreword. In K. T. Gallagher (Ed.), *The philosophy of Gabriel Marcel.* New York: Fordham University Press.

Marcel, G. (1963). *The existential background of human dignity.* Cambridge, MA: Harvard University Press.

Marcel, G. (1965a). (Trans. K. Farrer). *Being and having: An existentialist diary.* New York: Harper & Row.

Marcel, G. (1965b). (Trans. E. Crauford). *Homo viator: Introduction to a metaphysic of hope.* New York: Harper & Row.

Marcel, G. (1973). *Tragic wisdom and beyond.* Evanston, IL: Northwestern University Press.

Marcel, G. (1995). *The philosophy of existentialism.* New York: Carol Publishing.

Marcel, G. (2001a [1951]). *Mystery of being. Volume II. Faith and reality.* South Bend, IN: St. Augustine's Press.

Marcel, G. (2001b) *The mystery of being. Volume I: Reflection and mystery.* South Bend, IN: St. Augustine's Press.

Marcel, G. (2008). *Man against mass society.* South Bend, IN: St. Augustine's Press.

Marcus, P. (2019). *The psychoanalysis of overcoming suffering: Flourishing despite pain.* London: Routledge.

Marcus, P. (2013). *In search of the spiritual: Gabriel Marcel, psychoanalysis, and the sacred.* London: Karnac.

Metcalfe, A., & Game, A. (2008). Significance and dialogue in learning and teaching. *Educational Theory, 58*(3), 343–356.

Mitchell, S. (1993). *Hope and dread in psychoanalysis.* New York: Basic Books.

Molino, A. (Ed.) (2013). *Crossroads in psychoanalysis, Buddhism, and mindfulness: The word and the breath.* Lanham, MD: Jason Aronson.

Ogden, T. (1994). *Subjects of analysis.* Northvale, NJ: Jason Aronson.

Ogden, T. H. (2004). *Reverie and interpretation: Sensing something human.* Lanham, MD: Jason Aronson.

Ogden, T. H. (2016). *Reclaiming unlived life: Experiences in psychoanalysis.* London: Routledge.

O'Malley, J. B. (1984). Marcel's notion of the person. In P. A. Schilpp & L. E. Hahn (Eds.), *The philosophy of Gabriel Marcel* (pp. 275–294). La Salle, IL: Open Court.

Oppenheim, M. (2017). *Contemporary psychoanalysis and modern Jewish philosophy*. London: Routledge.
Orange, D. M. (2010). *Thinking for clinicians. Philosophical resources for contemporary psychoanalysis and the humanistic psychotherapies*. London: Routledge.
Pattison, E. M. (1988). The Holocaust as sin: Requirements in psychoanalytic theory for human evil and mature morality. In S. A. Luel & P. Marcus (Eds.), *Psychoanalytic reflections on the Holocaust: Selected essays* (pp. 71–94). New York: University of Denver Press and KTAV Publishers.
Raab, K. A. (2000). Creativity and Transcendence in the Work of Marion Milner. *American Imago*, 57(2), 185–214.
Rizzuto, A.-M. (1979). *The birth of the living God*. Chicago: University of Chicago Press.
Rome, S., & Rome, B. (Eds.). *Philosophical interrogations: Interrogations of Martin Buber, John Wild, Jean Wahl, Brand Blanshard, Paul Weiss, Charles Hartshorne, Paul Tillich*. New York: Holt, Rinehart and Winston.
Rycroft, C. (1995). *A critical dictionary of psychoanalysis*. Middlesex: Penguin Books.
Sweetman, B. (2008). *The vision of Gabriel Marcel: Epistemology, human person, the transcendent*. Amsterdam: Rodopi.
Sweetman, B. (Ed.). (2011). *A Gabriel Marcel reader*. South Bend, IN: St. Augustine's Press.
Treanor, B. (2006). *Aspects of alterity: Levinas, Marcel, and the contemporary debate*. New York: Fordham University Press.
Vaidyanathan, J. G., & Kripal, J. (Eds.). (2002). *Vishnu on Freud's desk: A reader in psychoanalysis and Hinduism*. Oxford: Oxford University Press.
Ventimiglia, D. (2008). Martin Buber, God, and psychoanalysis. *Psychoanalytic Inquiry, 28*, 612–621.
Wheelwright, P. (1967). Buber's philosophical anthropology. In P. A. Schilpp & M. Friedman (Eds.), *The philosophy of Martin Buber* (The Library of Living Philosophers, vol. 12, pp. 69–96). La Salle, IL: Open Court.
White. S. L. (1991) *The unity of self*. Cambridge, MA: MIT Press.
Wood, R. E. (1969). *Martin Buber's ontology*. Evanston, IL: Northwestern University Press.
Wood, R. E. (1999). The dialogical principle and the mystery of being: The enduring relevance of Martin Buber and Gabriel Marcel. *International Journal for Philosophy of Religion, 45*(2), 83–97.

Index

For Product Safety Concerns and Information please contact our EU
representative GPSR@taylorandfrancis.com
Taylor & Francis Verlag GmbH, Kaufingerstraße 24, 80331 München, Germany

www.ingramcontent.com/pod-product-compliance
Ingram Content Group UK Ltd.
Pitfield, Milton Keynes, MK11 3LW, UK
UKHW022031061126
477531UK00003B/160
* 9 7 8 0 3 6 7 7 5 4 0 1 3 *